Intensive Care: Nursing and Medicine

Intensive Care: Nursing and Medicine

Editor: Camilia Brooks

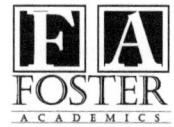

www.fosteracademics.com

www.fosteracademics.com

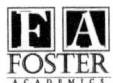

Cataloging-in-Publication Data

Intensive care : nursing and medicine / edited by Camilia Brooks.
    p. cm.
Includes bibliographical references and index.
ISBN 978-1-63242-871-4
1. Intensive care nursing. 2. Critical care medicine. 3. Emergency medicine.
4. Intensive care units. I. Brooks, Camilia.
RT120.I5 I58 2020
616.028--dc23

Foster Academics,
118-35 Queens Blvd., Suite 400,
Forest Hills, NY 11375, USA

ISBN 978-1-63242-871-4 (Hardback)

Contents

Preface

Every book is a source of knowledge and this one is no exception. The idea that led to the conceptualization of this book was the fact that the world is advancing rapidly; which makes it crucial to document the progress in every field. I am aware that a lot of data is already available, yet, there is a lot more to learn. Hence, I accepted the responsibility of editing this book and contributing my knowledge to the community.

Intensive care is a technologically-advanced and resource-intensive area of healthcare. It is concerned with the provision of care and support to patients with acute and life-threatening conditions. Patient management is crucial in intensive care medicine. Intensive care nursing operates with the objective of providing the utmost level of care to unstable patients. Individuals who require frequent nursing assessments and life sustaining drugs and technology are given such quality of care. Intensive care is provided to patients when they require cardiac, respiratory and renal support, and after surgery when patients are considered unstable. The ever growing need of advanced intensive care is the reason that has fueled the research in the field of intensive care medicine and nursing in recent times. From theories to research to practical applications, case studies related to all contemporary topics of relevance to this field have been included in this book. The extensive content of this book provides the readers with a thorough understanding of the subject.

While editing this book, I had multiple visions for it. Then I finally narrowed down to make every chapter a sole standing text explaining a particular topic, so that they can be used independently. However, the umbrella subject sinews them into a common theme. This makes the book a unique platform of knowledge.

I would like to give the major credit of this book to the experts from every corner of the world, who took the time to share their expertise with us. Also, I owe the completion of this book to the never-ending support of my family, who supported me throughout the project.

Editor

Protective effect of early low-dose hydrocortisone on ventilator-associated pneumonia in the cancer patients

David Lagier[1][*], Laura Platon[1], Jérome Lambert[2], Laurent Chow-Chine[1], Antoine Sannini[1], Magali Bisbal[1], Jean-Paul Brun[1], Karim Asehnoune[3], Marc Leone[4], Marion Faucher[1] and Djamel Mokart[1]

Abstract

Background: Ventilator-associated pneumonia (VAP) is a care-related event that could be promoted by immune suppression caused by critical diseases, malignancies and cancer treatments. Low dose of hydrocortisone was proposed for modulation of immune response in the critically ill population.

Methods: In this monocentric observational study, all cancer patients mechanically ventilated for more than 48 h were included. Effect of low-dose hydrocortisone administered during the first 48 h of mechanical ventilation was evaluated applying inverse probability weighting analysis after propensity score assessment. VAP impact on 1-year mortality, ICU length of stay and mechanical ventilation duration was secondarily determined.

Results: Within this cohort, 190 cancer patients were followed. VAP was confirmed in 22.1% of cases in the early hydrocortisone group and confirmed in 42.6% of cases in the no or late hydrocortisone group. Early hydrocortisone exhibited a protective effect on the risk of VAP (OR 0.23; 95% CI 0.12–0.44; $P < 0.0001$). VAP was associated with 1-year mortality (HR 1.60; 95% CI 1.10–2.34; $P = 0.017$) and increased ICU length of stay (mean extra length of stay: 4.2 days; 95% CI 0.6–7.8).

Conclusions: Immune modulation with low-dose hydrocortisone administered in the first days of mechanical ventilation could protect from VAP occurrence in cancer patients.

Keywords: Ventilator-associated pneumonia, Neoplasms, Immunomodulation, Hydrocortisone, Propensity score

Background

Recently introduced aggressive treatments have significantly decreased the overall mortality rate in cancer patients [1]. These new approaches come at the price of a steep rise in infections and treatment-related toxicities [2]. Immune suppression with or without neutropenia is a major concern in this setting. On the other side, critical conditions found during sepsis or acute respiratory failure induce a complex immune response making severely ill patients prone to secondary ICU-acquired infections, such as ventilator-associated pneumonia (VAP) [3]. During sepsis, hydrocortisone improves the phagocytic abilities of neutrophils, decreases the blood concentration of anti-inflammatory cytokines (interleukin-10) and increases the blood concentrations of the host defence against infection (interferon γ and interleukin-12) [4, 5]. By balancing the inflammatory response, hydrocortisone might also decrease the growth and virulence of bacteria [6, 7]. In septic shock, low-dose hydrocortisone improves shock reversal irrespective to adrenal response to corticotropin [8]. Moreover, it has been shown that low-dose hydrocortisone can reduce the incidence of hospital-acquired pneumonia in intubated patients with multiple

*Correspondence: david.lagier@ap-hm.fr
[1] Intensive Care Unit, Paoli-Calmettes Institute, 232 Boulevard de Sainte-Marguerite, 13009 Marseille, France
Full list of author information is available at the end of the article

trauma [9]. Survival of cancer patients with acute respiratory failure has improved over time to about 60% [10]. Nevertheless, invasive mechanical ventilation remains associated with a 28-day mortality rate of about 50% [11]. In non-selected populations, VAP is a common hospital-acquired pneumonia and occurs in up to 30% of patients receiving mechanical ventilation for more than 48 h. The main objective of our study was to evaluate the preventive role of early treatment with low-dose hydrocortisone regarding incidence of VAP in cancer patients. The prognostic impact of VAP on 1-year mortality, mechanical ventilation duration and ICU length of stay was secondarily assessed.

Methods

Study population

In this monocentric observational study, all consecutive cancer patients requiring invasive mechanical ventilation for more than 48 h that have been admitted to our ICU between January 1, 2009, and December 31, 2013, were prospectively followed. We excluded from the study patients that needed two or more invasive mechanical ventilation periods during their ICU stay. The Paoli-Calmettes Institute Institutional Review Board approved this observational study (No. IPC-2017-077). No consent was needed in this observational study.

Diagnosis of VAP

All ventilated patients were daily screened for new respiratory or septic events. VAP was suspected if a recent and persistent infiltrate on chest radiograph was associated with at least two of the following criteria: hyperthermia (> 38 °C) or hypothermia (< 36 °C), purulent tracheal secretions and worsening of gas exchange. Because of its high variability and poor specificity in the onco-haematological context, leucocyte count was not taken into account. Quantitative microbiological culture of 10^6 colony-forming unit (CFU)/mL of a typical pathogen from endotracheal aspirate or 10^4 CFU/mL from bronchoalveolar lavage fluid confirmed VAP [12, 13]. Early VAP was defined as a VAP diagnosed before the 5th day of invasive mechanical ventilation. An adjudication committee (two senior ICU physicians) systematically reviewed VAP diagnosis to determine whether it meets protocol-specified criteria. It was blinded to hydrocortisone status.

VAP bundles

In our ICU, VAP prevention strategy included 30° semi-sitting position, endotracheal cuff pressure control, chlorhexidine 0.2% daily oral care and a sedation protocol based on the Richmond Agitation Sedation Scale with daily sedation discontinuation. No selective digestive or oropharyngeal decontamination was used. Enteral

nutrition was gradually implemented as early as possible. Parenteral nutrition was used if contraindication or poor tolerance to enteral route was present. Anti-acid treatment was pursued during mechanical ventilation periods irrespective of the hydrocortisone status.

Low-dose hydrocortisone treatment

In this study, low-dose hydrocortisone was usually prescribed in case of refractory septic shock with persistent arterial hypotension despite high-dose vasopressor therapy ($\geq 0.8 \ \mu g \ kg^{-1} \ min^{-1}$ of norepinephrine) or as an alternative therapy in case of sepsis with previous curative corticosteroid therapy. In case of sepsis and ongoing curative corticosteroid therapy, the treatment was switched for hydrocortisone. Fifty milligrams was administered intravenously every 6 h according to our local protocol.

Data collection

All data were extracted and analysed by senior physicians using our ICU management software (MetaVision ICU, iMDsoft Inc.®, Dedham, MA, USA). As previously described [10], baseline data were recorded upon ICU admission: gender, age, cancer type, cancer stage classified in four categories (newly diagnosed, complete remission, partial remission and evolutive disease), main ICU admission purpose (septic shock, acute respiratory failure, coma and others), presence of neutropenia, history of haematopoietic stem cell transplantation (HSCT) and recent exposure to antibiotics or curative corticosteroids (during the 10 days before admission). SOFA score [14] was also reported at the time of endotracheal intubation. Several approaches implemented during the first 48 h after endotracheal intubation, including vasopressors, renal replacement therapy, substitutive steroids therapy for refractory shock, granulocyte colony-stimulating factors (G-CSF), enteral nutrition and antibiotherapy (adapted or empirical), were recorded. VAP microbiological evidences were also documented. ICU mortality was evaluated. ICU survivors were prospectively followed after ICU discharge until the end of the study and 1-year survival was determined.

Statistical analysis

Data are presented as median (interquartile range) for quantitative variables and count (percentages) for qualitative variables. Binary outcome (i.e. the occurrence of VAP) was analysed using a Chi-square test or the non-parametric Wilcoxon rank-sum test as appropriate. The multivariate analyses were performed using a logistic model. The primary outcome of the study was to evaluate the prevention of VAP using early low dose of hydrocortisone. VAP incidence was reported to the incidence per

1000 ventilator days. Effect of early low-dose hydrocortisone on incidence of VAP was studied using propensity score analysis to take into account the non-randomized design of this study. Early hydrocortisone group was defined by hydrocortisone treatment initiated during the first 48 h of invasive mechanical ventilation. Patients treated by hydrocortisone for more than 48 h before tracheal intubation were excluded from this analysis. Propensity score, which is the probability that a patient will receive low-dose hydrocortisone, was assessed using a logistic regression model with baseline covariates as explanatory variables and treatment with low-dose hydrocortisone as the outcome. An inverse probability weighting (IPW) analysis was then performed to assess the average treatment effect of low-dose hydrocortisone assessed by comparison of two pseudo-population, one where nobody would have received low-dose hydrocortisone and one where everybody would have received it. Cumulative incidence of VAP in ICU was estimated taking into accounts competing risk of discharge of ICU (either death or discharge alive).

Association between baseline variables, describing patient's condition at ICU admission or at intubation, and overall mortality was assessed by univariable analysis using Cox proportional hazard models. Multivariable analysis including variables significantly associated with death was performed using a Cox proportional hazard model with VAP as a time-dependent variable. Variable selection was based on Akaike information criteria (AIC). Since VAP is a time-dependent event, it cannot be treated as a baseline covariate. Hence, a Mantel–Byar analysis was performed to assess and graphically display the effect of VAP on 1-year mortality. To estimate extra length of stay (in ICU-discharged patients) and extra duration of intubation (in extubated patients) due to VAP, we used a multistate model that takes into account time to VAP.

Results

Between January 1, 2009, and December 31, 2013, 208 patients were included in the study. Among them, 18 have been excluded for multiple periods of invasive mechanical ventilation. Among the 190 patients included in the final analysis, 55 (28.9%) develop a confirmed VAP. Early VAP onset was found in 12 patients (21.8% of the total VAP). Microbiological data are outlined in Table 1. Substitutive corticotherapy with low-dose hydrocortisone was prescribed in 122 (64.2%) cases and was predominantly used in patients without VAP ($P = 0.003$; Table 2). The median mechanical ventilation duration was 11 (6–18) days. ICU and 1-year mortality rate were 56 and 77%, respectively (Table 3).

Table 1 Microbiological documentation depending on the timing of VAP

	Early VAP ($n = 12$)	Late VAP ($n = 43$)
P. aeruginosa	4	10
E. coli	2	6
K. pneumoniae	1	6
E. cloacae	1	3
Enterococcus sp	2	8
Staphylococcus sp	1	2
Stenotrophomonas sp	0	5
Other Gram-negative bacteria	1	3

Effect of early low-dose hydrocortisone

Nine patients received hydrocortisone for more than 48 h before tracheal intubation and were excluded from this analysis. Global VAP incidence in the 181 patients included in the analysis; incidence was 25.5/1000 ventilator days. Stratified according to cortisone, incidence was 20.3/1000 ventilator days in the group receiving early low-dose hydrocortisone and 32.7/1000 ventilator days in the group receiving no or late low-dose hydrocortisone. A prior multivariable analysis has identified early hydrocortisone treatment as the only independent variable significantly associated with the VAP occurrence (OR 0.41; 95% CI 0.2–0.8; $P < 0.01$). The propensity score was constructed using the following relevant variables: age, neutropenia and admission purpose at admission, as well as SOFA score, vasopressors, antibiotherapy (adapted, empirical, none) and enteral nutrition at the time of intubation. Standardized differences in the unweighted population and in the weighted population are shown in Fig. 1. VAP was confirmed in 22.1% of cases in the early hydrocortisone group (25 out of 113 patients) and confirmed in 42.6% of cases in the no or late hydrocortisone group (29 out of 68 patients). Using IPW analysis, early hydrocortisone exhibited a protective effect on the risk of VAP (OR 0.23; 95% CI 0.12–0.44; $P < 0.0001$, Fig. 2).

VAP prognostic impact

Considering VAP as a time-dependent covariate, univariate analysis (Table 2) revealed that VAP is not associated with 1-year mortality (HR 1.41; 95% CI 0.98–2.03; $P = 0.06$). After multivariate adjustment (Table 2), an independent and significant association is revealed between VAP and 1-year mortality (HR 1.60; 95% CI 1.10–2.34; $P = 0.017$, Fig. 3). Regarding initial vs late onset VAP, there indeed was a difference in prognosis, with late onset VAP being associated with a higher mortality [HR 1.74 (95% CI 1.17–2.58)], but early VAP being not significantly different from no VAP [HR 0.98

Table 2 Patient's characteristics

Variables	Patients without VAP (n = 135)	Patients with VAP (n = 55)	P
Male gender, n (%)	87 (64.4)	41 (74.5)	0.23
Age (year), median (IQR)	59.2 (52.2–65.8)	60.4 (50.2–67.1)	0.99
Cancer type			0.39
Haematological malignancy, n (%)	95 (70.4)	35 (63.6)	
Solid tumour, n (%)	40 (29.6)	20 (36.4)	
Cancer stage			0.91
Diagnosis, n (%)	36 (26.7)	15 (27.3)	
Complete remission, n (%)	29 (21.5)	13 (23.6)	
Partial remission, n (%)	31 (23)	14 (25.5)	
Evolutive, n (%)	39 (28.9)	13 (23.6)	
HSCT, n (%)	47 (24.7)	14 (25.4)	0.43
Admission purpose			0.32
Septic shock, n (%)	59 (43.7)	21 (38.2)	
Acute respiratory failure, n (%)	51 (37.8)	27 (49.1)	
Coma, n (%)	14 (10.4)	2 (3.6)	
Others, n (%)	11 (8.1)	5 (9.1)	
Clinical sepsis upon admission			0.042
Respiratory, n (%)	79 (58.5)	31 (56.4)	
Non-respiratory, n (%)	31 (23)	6 (10.9)	
None, n (%)	25 (18.5)	18 (32.7)	
Characteristics upon admission			
Neutropenia, n (%)	54 (40)	18 (32.7)	0.41
Antibiotherapy, n (%)	104 (77)	43 (78.2)	1
Corticosteroids (curative), n (%)	32 (23.7)	19 (34.5)	0.15
SOFA score (day of intubation), median (IQR)	11 (8–14)	11 (8–13)	0.28
Characteristics at the first 48 h of MV			
Vasopressors, n (%)	99 (73.3)	44 (80)	0.36
Renal replacement therapy, n (%)	28 (20.7)	9 (16.4)	0.55
Substitutive hydrocortisone, n (%)	96 (71.1)	26 (47.3)	0.003
G-CSF, n (%)	20 (14.8)	9 (16.4)	0.82
Enteral nutrition, n (%)	40 (29.6)	21 (38.2)	0.3
Antibiotherapy			0.09
Adapted, n (%)	41 (30.4)	11 (20)	
Empirical, n (%)	89 (65.9)	38 (69)	
None, n (%)	5 (3.7)	6 (10.7)	

HSCT haematopoietic stem cell transplantation, *G-CSF* granulocyte colony-stimulating factors, *MV* mechanical ventilation, *IQR* interquartile range

(0.39–2.46)]. VAP resulted in a significantly longer ICU stay for patients discharged [mean extra length of stay: 4.2 days (95% CI 0.6–7.8)] and a longer, although not significant, mechanical ventilation duration for patients extubated [mean extra duration: 1.7 days (95% CI − 1.5 to 5.0)].

Discussion

We report herein on 190 onco-haematology patients admitted to ICU and treated with mechanical ventilation over 4 years. We showed the protective effect of low-dose hydrocortisone administered in the first days of mechanical ventilation regarding VAP occurrence. An association was found between VAP occurrence and 1-year mortality. The deleterious impact of VAP on ICU length of stay was also demonstrated. To our knowledge, this is the first study reporting prognosis data with regard to VAP in the specific cancer population.

VAP is a controversial topic [15–17]. In the global ICU population, VAP incidence and attributable mortality are uncertain [18, 19]. In a systematic review of published randomized trials [20], VAP-cumulated incidence

Table 3 Predictors of 1-year mortality: univariate and multivariate analysis

Variables	Univariate			Multivariate		
	HR	95% CI	P	HR	95% CI	P
Male gender	0.89	0.64–1.24	0.49			
Age	0.99	0.98–1	0.13			
Cancer type						
Haematological malignancy	1	(Reference)	0.91			
Solid tumour	0.91	0.65–1.28				
Cancer stage						
Complete remission	1	(Reference)	0.02	1	(Reference)	0.03
Diagnosis	1.37	0.87–2.16		1.44	0.88–2.35	
Partial remission	0.82	0.50–1.33		0.98	0.57–1.68	
Evolutive	1.54	0.99–2.41		1.77	1.10–2.87	
HSCT	1.28	0.86–1.92	0.23			
Admission purpose						
Others	1	(Reference)	0.055			
Septic shock	0.96	0.54–1.71				
Acute respiratory failure	0.62	0.34–1.11				
Coma	0.66	0.31–1.43				
Clinical sepsis upon admission						
None	1	(Reference)	0.02	1	(Reference)	0.04
Respiratory	1.67	1.09–2.56		1.65	1.03–2.65	
Non-respiratory	1.91	1.16–3.15		1.78	1.01–3.15	
Characteristics upon admission						
Neutropenia	1.41	1.02–1.94	0.04			
Antibiotherapy	1.18	0.80–1.72	0.4			
Corticosteroids (curative)	1.03	0.73–1.45	0.89			
SOFA score (day of intubation)	1.10	1.06–1.15	0.0001	1.11	1.05–1.17	0.0002
Characteristics at the first 48 h of MV						
Vasopressors	1.34	0.93–1.94	0.11			
Renal replacement therapy	1.45	1.00–2.12	0.06			
Substitutive hydrocortisone	1.28	0.92–1.77	0.28			
G-CSF	1.85	1.23–2.78	0.005	1.65	1.03–2.65	0.042
Enteral nutrition	1.17	0.68–2.00	0.58			
Antibiotherapy						
Adapted, n (%)	1	(Reference)	0.83			
Empirical, n (%)	0.85	0.6–1.22				
None, n (%)	0.96	0.5–1.86				
VAP	1.41	0.98–2.03	0.06	1.60	1.10–2.34	0.017

HSCT haematopoietic stem cell transplantation, *G-CSF* granulocyte colony-stimulating factors, *MV* mechanical ventilation, *VAP* ventilator-associated pneumonia

varies from 9% to more than 40% depending on the study and the given population. This heterogeneity is mainly explained by the lack of consensual definition [17, 21] and by the variability in VAP bundles implementation rates [22, 23] in the different ICUs. In this study, we used an association of clinical and bacteriological criteria to diagnose VAP in reference to the 2005 ATS/IDSA guidelines [12]. This definition is slightly different from the definition of probable VAP according to the last CDC definition of ventilator-associated events [24], which emphasize on FiO2 and positive end-expiratory pressure adjustment in response to worsening oxygenation. However, the prognostic significance of that current CDC definition remains to be established [25]. The cumulative incidence of VAP in our cohort was 28.9%. Despite regular use of validated VAP bundles in our ICU, this remains relatively high. Cancer treatments and malignancy-related immunosuppression could explain the

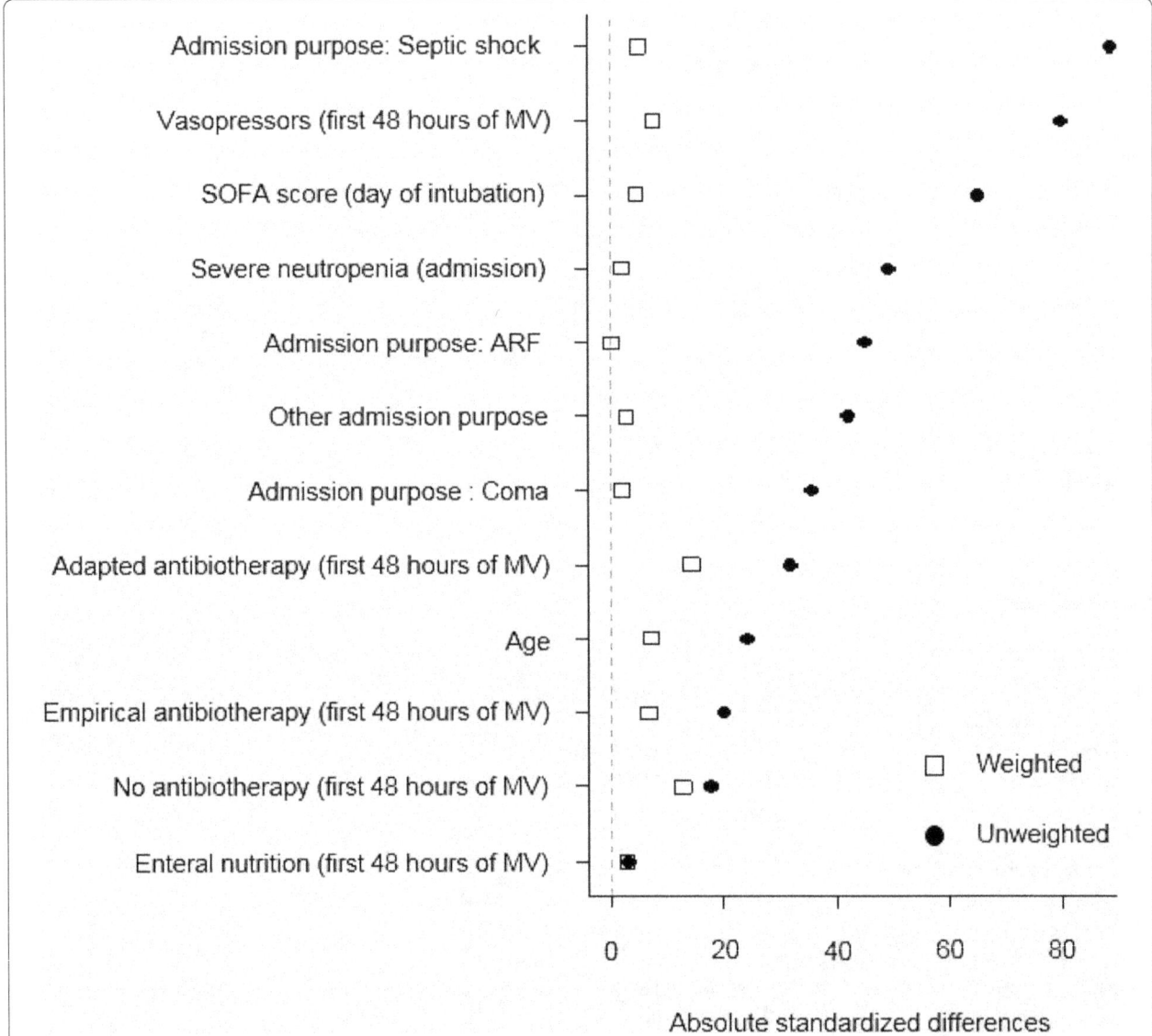

Fig. 1 Covariate imbalance (assessed by standardized mean differences) between the two groups of patients receiving and not receiving early HC in the unweighted (original) and weighted populations

higher susceptibility to develop nosocomial infections in the onco-haematological population.

Theoretically, VAP is a delayed event that happens after 48 h of mechanical ventilation. The pathophysiology of nosocomial infections combines the bacterial colonization induced by the invasiveness of general ICU cares (endotracheal intubation, catheter, etc.) and a state of susceptibility to infection [26]. It is well recognized that initial aggression induces a delayed state of profound immunodeficiency few days after the initial insult [3, 27]. More specifically, a biphasic evolution of immunological competence has been well described in sepsis [28] and trauma [29]. After an initial pro-inflammatory phase, a post-aggressive phase is characterized by a compensatory systemic anti-inflammatory state and an apoptotic depletion of immune cells [30, 31]. This delayed immunological status confers wider susceptibility to ICU-acquired infection [28] and viral reactivation. In the haematology population, ICU-induced immunodeficiency has also been described in neutropenic patients [32]. Monocyte and alveolar macrophage deactivation have been described after septic ARDS [33, 34] and could thus facilitate the occurrence of ICU-acquired infections. In order to counteract this phenomenon, low dose of hydrocortisone has been suggested to prevent post-aggressive immunosuppression. Indeed, hydrocortisone

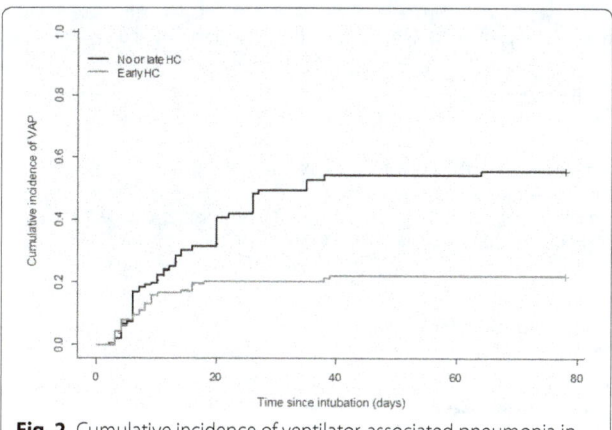

Fig. 2 Cumulative incidence of ventilator-associated pneumonia in the inverse probability of treatment weighting analysis

septic shock survival remains controversial [8, 35, 36]. Last study showed that it failed to prevent the development of septic shock in the severe sepsis population [37]. The HIPOLYTE study [9] has compared low-dose hydrocortisone to placebo in the first 28 days after a severe trauma. It showed a reduction in the incidence of hospital-acquired pneumonia with 4 more ventilation-free days. Despite hydrocortisone treatment, no significant reduction in norepinephrine treatment duration was found in this study. To be effective, hydrocortisone should be started earlier as possible in order to decrease the initial pro-inflammatory response and counteract the anti-inflammatory compensation. In immunosuppressed cancer patients, we focused on potential beneficial effects of the early initiation of substitutive hydrocortisone for VAP prevention. A reverse propensity score analysis was used to control bias and population heterogeneity inherent to non-randomized observational studies. After weighing on the most pertinent covariates, we found that early hydrocortisone prescribed around the intubation time was protective against the subsequent occurrence of VAP.

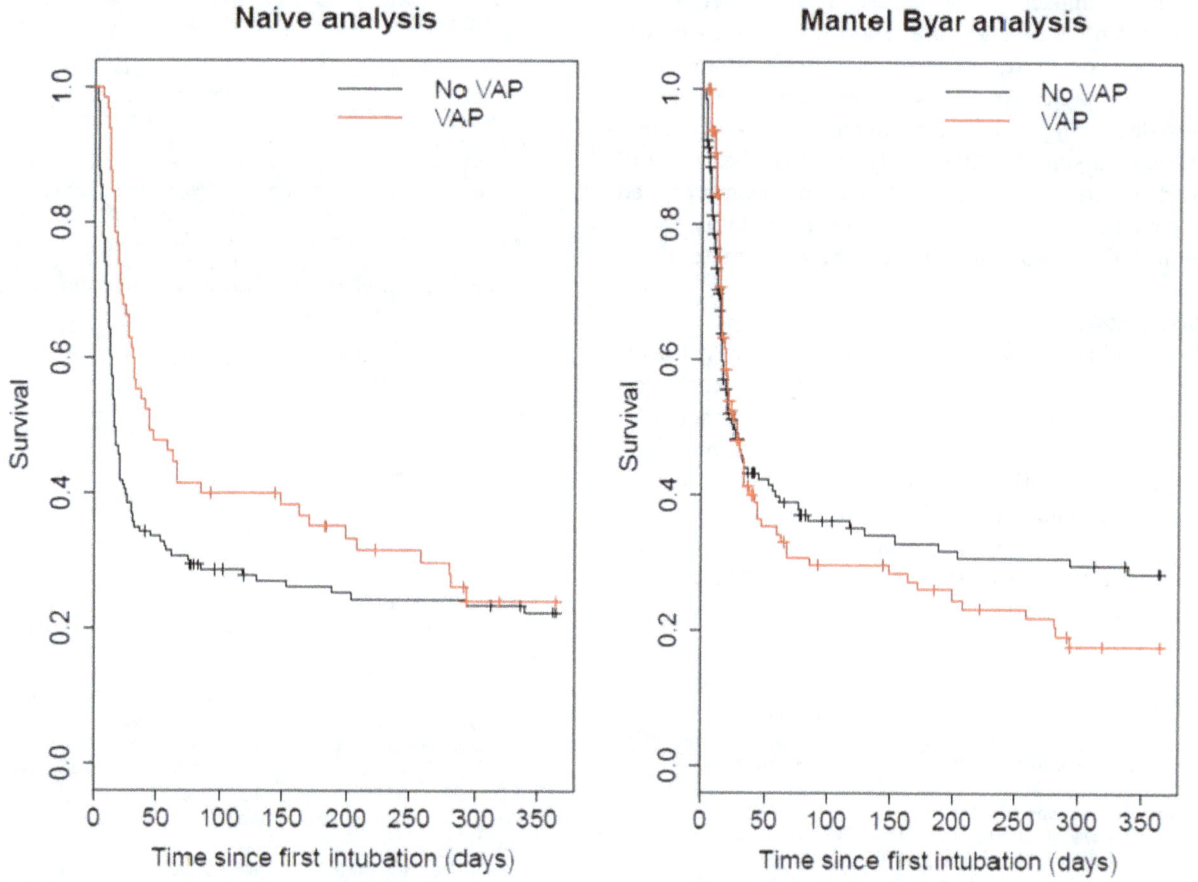

improves immune capacities, decreases blood concentrations of anti-inflammatory cytokines (interleukin-10) and increases host defence cytokines (interferon γ and interleukin-12) [4, 5]. However, despite positive hemodynamic effect, beneficial effect of substitutive corticotherapy on

Fig. 3 One-year survival according to ventilator-associated pneumonia status: naive analysis and time-dependent Mantel–Byar analysis

VAP impact on mortality remains debated [38, 39]. The overuse of traditional crude statistical test in past studies had led to conflicting results and overestimation of attributable mortality of VAP [21]. In our work, VAP was not associated with mortality in the naive-exposed–unexposed analysis. That result is surely related to the high mortality rates in the first days of ICU admission in the critically ill cancer patients. Indeed, a majority of patients did not have time to develop VAP before dying (competing risk). On the contrary, by considering VAP as a time-dependent variable and estimating survival from the time of VAP diagnosis, we showed that VAP was significantly associated with 1-year mortality.

Our study has limitations. First, despite the use of propensity score analysis, this study is observational and residual confounding factors and biases may exist. For example, exposure to chemotherapy with or without curative corticotherapy before ICU stay has not been taking into account. However, neutropenic status was included in the baseline covariates for the propensity score construction. Second, this is a monocentric study, so it is possible that our local protocol including VAP prevention bundle, diagnosis strategies and therapeutic management could influence the occurrence and the prognostic impact of the disease. Third, adherence to VAP prevention bundle is not reported in each treatment group and could induce a bias. Finally, systemic antibiotic treatment could play a preventive role on VAP occurrence depending on its spectrum and its duration. These data are missing, but it is likely that the liberal use of broad spectrum antibiotics in the immunocompromised patients, irrespective of the hydrocortisone status, would diminish the confounding effect of these parameters.

Conclusions

We found a positive effect of early low-dose hydrocortisone treatment in preventing VAP. Immunological aspects are crucial in the development of nosocomial infections, specifically in patients prone to immunological disorders. Critically ill cancer patients could benefit from the administration of low-dose hydrocortisone in the days surrounding mechanical ventilation initiation. This interesting result should be evaluated in a future large-scale randomized controlled trial.

Abbreviations
CFU: colony-forming unit; G-CSF: granulocyte colony-stimulating factors; HSCT: haematopoietic stem cell transplantation; ICU: intensive care unit; IPW: inverse probability weighting; VAP: ventilator-associated pneumonia.

Authors' contributions
DL, LP and DM were involved in design of the work, data collection, interpretation of the results and writing of the draft. JL was involved in design of the work, full statistical analyses, writing of the draft. LCC, AS, MB, JPB and MF were involved in design of the work, data collection and manuscript revision. ML and KA were involved in design of the work, interpretation of the results and manuscript revision. All authors read and approved the final manuscript.

Author details
[1] Intensive Care Unit, Paoli-Calmettes Institute, 232 Boulevard de Sainte-Marguerite, 13009 Marseille, France. [2] Biostatistics Department, Saint Louis Teaching Hospital, AP-HP, 1, Avenue Claude Vellefaux, 75010 Paris, France. [3] Department of Anesthesiology and Critical Care Medicine, Hotel Dieu, University Hospital of Nantes, 1 Place Alexis Ricordeau, 44903 Nantes, France. [4] Department of Anesthesiology and Critical Care Medicine, Hopital Nord, University Hospital of Marseille, Chemin des Bourrely, 13015 Marseille, France.

Acknowledgements
None.

Competing interests
The authors declare that they have no competing interests.

Funding
No financial support.

References
1. Mokart D, Pastores SM, Darmon M. Has survival increased in cancer patients admitted to the ICU? Yes. Intensive Care Med. 2014;40(10):1570–2.
2. Azoulay E, Pene F, Darmon M, Lengline E, Benoit D, Soares M, et al. Managing critically Ill hematology patients: time to think differently. Blood Rev. 2015;29(6):359–67.
3. van Vught LA, Klein Klouwenberg PM, Spitoni C, Scicluna BP, Wiewel MA, Horn J, et al. Incidence, risk factors, and attributable mortality of secondary infections in the intensive care unit after admission for sepsis. JAMA. 2016;315(14):1469–79.
4. Kaufmann I, Briegel J, Schliephake F, Hoelzl A, Chouker A, Hummel T, et al. Stress doses of hydrocortisone in septic shock: beneficial effects on opsonization-dependent neutrophil functions. Intensive Care Med. 2008;34(2):344–9.
5. Keh D, Boehnke T, Weber-Cartens S, Schulz C, Ahlers O, Bercker S, et al. Immunologic and hemodynamic effects of "low-dose" hydrocortisone in septic shock: a double-blind, randomized, placebo-controlled, crossover study. Am J Respir Crit Care Med. 2003;167(4):512–20.
6. Kanangat S, Meduri GU, Tolley EA, Patterson DR, Meduri CU, Pak C, et al. Effects of cytokines and endotoxin on the intracellular growth of bacteria. Infect Immun. 1999;67(6):2834–40.
7. Meduri GU, Kanangat S, Stefan J, Tolley E, Schaberg D. Cytokines IL-1beta, IL-6, and TNF-alpha enhance in vitro growth of bacteria. Am J Respir Crit Care Med. 1999;160(3):961–7.
8. Sprung CL, Annane D, Keh D, Moreno R, Singer M, Freivogel K, et al. Hydrocortisone therapy for patients with septic shock. N Engl J Med. 2008;358(2):111–24.
9. Roquilly A, Mahe PJ, Seguin P, Guitton C, Floch H, Tellier AC, et al. Hydrocortisone therapy for patients with multiple trauma: the randomized controlled HYPOLYTE study. JAMA. 2011;305(12):1201–9.
10. Azoulay E, Mokart D, Pene F, Lambert J, Kouatchet A, Mayaux J, et al. Outcomes of critically ill patients with hematologic malignancies: prospective multicenter data from France and Belgium—a groupe de recherche respiratoire en reanimation onco-hematologique study. J Clin Oncol. 2013;31(22):2810–8.
11. Lemiale V, Mokart D, Resche-Rigon M, Pene F, Mayaux J, Faucher E, et al. Effect of noninvasive ventilation vs oxygen therapy on mortality among immunocompromised patients with acute respiratory failure: a randomized clinical trial. JAMA. 2015;314(16):1711–9.
12. American Thoracic S. Infectious diseases society of A. Guidelines for the management of adults with hospital-acquired, ventilator-associated, and healthcare-associated pneumonia. Am J Respir Crit Care Med. 2005;171(4):388–416.
13. Kalanuria AA, Ziai W, Mirski M. Ventilator-associated pneumonia in the ICU. Crit Care. 2014;18(2):208.

14. Vincent JL, Moreno R, Takala J, Willatts S, De Mendonca A, Bruining H, et al. The SOFA (Sepsis-related Organ Failure Assessment) score to describe organ dysfunction/failure. On behalf of the Working Group on Sepsis-Related Problems of the European Society of Intensive Care Medicine. Intensive Care Med. 1996;22(7):707–10.

15. Borgatta B, Rello J. How to approach and treat VAP in ICU patients. BMC Infect Dis. 2014;14:211.

16. Klompas M, Platt R. Ventilator-associated pneumonia-the wrong quality measure for benchmarking. Ann Intern Med. 2007;147(11):803–5.

17. Nair GB, Niederman MS. Ventilator-associated pneumonia: present understanding and ongoing debates. Intensive Care Med. 2015;41(1):34–48.

18. Bekaert M, Timsit JF, Vansteelandt S, Depuydt P, Vesin A, Garrouste-Orgeas M, et al. Attributable mortality of ventilator-associated pneumonia: a reappraisal using causal analysis. Am J Respir Crit Care Med. 2011;184(10):1133–9.

19. Melsen WG, Rovers MM, Groenwold RH, Bergmans DC, Camus C, Bauer TT, et al. Attributable mortality of ventilator-associated pneumonia: a meta-analysis of individual patient data from randomised prevention studies. Lancet Infect Dis. 2013;13(8):665–71.

20. Safdar N, Dezfulian C, Collard HR, Saint S. Clinical and economic consequences of ventilator-associated pneumonia: a systematic review. Crit Care Med. 2005;33(10):2184–93.

21. Timsit JF, Zahar JR, Chevret S. Attributable mortality of ventilator-associated pneumonia. Curr Opin Crit Care. 2011;17(5):464–71.

22. Batra P, Mathur P, John NV, Nair SA, Aggarwal R, Soni KD, et al. Impact of multifaceted preventive measures on ventilator-associated pneumonia at a single surgical centre. Intensive Care Med. 2015;41(12):2231–2.

23. Pileggi C, Bianco A, Flotta D, Nobile CG, Pavia M. Prevention of ventilator-associated pneumonia, mortality and all intensive care unit acquired infections by topically applied antimicrobial or antiseptic agents: a meta-analysis of randomized controlled trials in intensive care units. Crit Care. 2011;15(3):R155.

24. Magill SS, Klompas M, Balk R, Burns SM, Deutschman CS, Diekema D, et al. Developing a new, national approach to surveillance for ventilator-associated events. Crit Care Med. 2013;41(11):2467–75.

25. Bouadma L, Sonneville R, Garrouste-Orgeas M, Darmon M, Souweine B, Voiriot G, et al. Ventilator-associated events: prevalence, outcome, and relationship with ventilator-associated pneumonia. Crit Care Med. 2015;43(9):1798–806.

26. Peleg AY, Hooper DC. Hospital-acquired infections due to gram-negative bacteria. N Engl J Med. 2010;362(19):1804–13.

27. Angus DC, Opal S. Immunosuppression and secondary infection in sepsis: part, not all, of the story. JAMA. 2016;315(14):1457–9.

28. Landelle C, Lepape A, Voirin N, Tognet E, Venet F, Bohe J, et al. Low monocyte human leukocyte antigen-DR is independently associated with nosocomial infections after septic shock. Intensive Care Med. 2010;36(11):1859–66.

29. Asehnoune K, Roquilly A, Abraham E. Innate immune dysfunction in trauma patients: from pathophysiology to treatment. Anesthesiology. 2012;117(2):411–6.

30. Grimaldi D, Louis S, Pene F, Sirgo G, Rousseau C, Claessens YE, et al. Profound and persistent decrease of circulating dendritic cells is associated with ICU-acquired infection in patients with septic shock. Intensive Care Med. 2011;37(9):1438–46.

31. Monneret G, Lepape A, Voirin N, Bohe J, Venet F, Debard AL, et al. Persisting low monocyte human leukocyte antigen-DR expression predicts mortality in septic shock. Intensive Care Med. 2006;32(8):1175–83.

32. Mokart D, Darmon M, Azoulay E. The alveolar macrophage and acute respiratory distress syndrome: A silent actor? Am J Respir Crit Care Med. 2014;189(4):499–500.

33. Mokart D, Kipnis E, Guerre-Berthelot P, Vey N, Capo C, Sannini A, et al. Monocyte deactivation in neutropenic acute respiratory distress syndrome patients treated with granulocyte colony-stimulating factor. Crit Care. 2008;12(1):R17.

34. Mokart D, Guery BP, Bouabdallah R, Martin C, Blache JL, Arnoulet C, et al. Deactivation of alveolar macrophages in septic neutropenic ARDS. Chest. 2003;124(2):644–52.

35. Annane D, Sebille V, Charpentier C, Bollaert PE, Francois B, Korach JM, et al. Effect of treatment with low doses of hydrocortisone and fludrocortisone on mortality in patients with septic shock. JAMA. 2002;288(7):862–71.

36. Kalil AC, Sun J. Low-dose steroids for septic shock and severe sepsis: the use of Bayesian statistics to resolve clinical trial controversies. Intensive Care Med. 2011;37(3):420–9.

37. Keh D, Trips E, Marx G, Wirtz SP, Abduljawwad E, Bercker S, et al. Effect of hydrocortisone on development of shock among patients with severe sepsis: the HYPRESS randomized clinical trial. JAMA. 2016;316(17):1775–85.

38. Nguile-Makao M, Zahar JR, Francais A, Tabah A, Garrouste-Orgeas M, Allaouchiche B, et al. Attributable mortality of ventilator-associated pneumonia: respective impact of main characteristics at ICU admission and VAP onset using conditional logistic regression and multi-state models. Intensive Care Med. 2010;36(5):781–9.

39. Melsen WG, Rovers MM, Koeman M, Bonten MJ. Estimating the attributable mortality of ventilator-associated pneumonia from randomized prevention studies. Crit Care Med. 2011;39(12):2736–42.

Mortality and detailed characteristics of pre-ICU qSOFA-negative patients with suspected sepsis

Izumi Nakayama[1], Junichi Izawa[2,3]*, Hideyuki Mouri[4], Tetsuhisa Kitamura[5] and Junji Shiotsuka[4]

Abstract

Background: Recent studies have suggested that quick Sequential Organ Failure Assessment (qSOFA) scores have limited utility in early prognostication in high-mortality populations. The purpose of this study was to investigate the association between pre-ICU qSOFA scores and in-hospital mortality among patients admitted to the ICU with suspected sepsis. This study also aimed to describe detailed clinical characteristics of qSOFA-negative (< 2) patients.

Methods: This single center, observational study, conducted in a Japanese tertiary care teaching hospital between May 2012 and June 2016, enrolled all consecutive adult patients admitted to the ICU with suspected sepsis. We assessed pre-ICU qSOFA scores with the most abnormal vital signs during the 24-h period before ICU admission. The primary outcome was in-hospital mortality censored at 90 days. We analyzed the association between pre-ICU qSOFA scores and in-hospital mortality.

Results: Among 185 ICU patients with suspected sepsis, 14.1% (26/185) of patients remained qSOFA-negative at the time of ICU admission and 29.2% (54/185) of patients died while in hospital. In-hospital mortality was similar between the groups (qSOFA-positive [≥ 2]: 30.2% [48/159] vs qSOFA-negative: 23.1% [6/26], $p = 0.642$). The Cox proportional hazard regression model revealed that being qSOFA-positive was not significantly associated with in-hospital mortality (adjusted hazard ratio 1.35, 95% confidence interval 0.56–3.22, $p = 0.506$). Bloodstream infection, immunosuppression, and hematologic malignancy were observed more frequently in qSOFA-negative patients.

Conclusions: Among ICU patients with suspected sepsis, we could not find a strong association between pre-ICU qSOFA scores and in-hospital mortality. Our study suggested high mortality and bacterial diversity in pre-ICU qSOFA-negative patients.

Keywords: Intensive care unit, Critical care, Bacteremia, Sepsis, quick Sequential Organ Failure Assessment (qSOFA) score, Infection, Mortality

Background

Early identification and interventions have been shown to improve sepsis outcomes [1, 2]. Recently, the quick Sequential Organ Failure Assessment (qSOFA) score was developed to promptly identify infected patients at risk of mortality. The original study showed that qSOFA-positive (≥ 2) patients had a 3- to 14-fold increase in in-hospital mortality compared to qSOFA-negative (< 2) patients [3]. With its simple and repeatedly measurable property, qSOFA has had a promising role in providing a more effective triage for infected patients [4].

However, recent studies have suggested that qSOFA has limited utility in early prognostication in high-mortality populations. One study showed that almost one-half of patients with infection remained qSOFA-negative even at the time of ICU admission [5]. In studies enrolling patients admitted to the ICU, the mortality of qSOFA-negative patients was greater than 10% [5–9]. Thus, the

*Correspondence: jizawa13@gmail.com
[2] Intensive Care Unit, Department of Anesthesiology, The Jikei University School of Medicine, 3-19-18 Nishi-Shinbashi, Minato-ku, Tokyo 105-8471, Japan

usefulness of qSOFA scores in high-risk populations has remained controversial.

We hypothesized that, for patients with suspected sepsis requiring ICU admission, the prognostic impact of qSOFA-positive was small. The purpose of this study was to investigate the association between pre-ICU qSOFA scores, assessed during the 24-h period before ICU admission, and in-hospital mortality among patients admitted to the ICU with suspected sepsis. Furthermore, we described detailed clinical characteristics of qSOFA-negative patients including clinical diagnosis, primary sites of infection, causative organisms, and comorbidities. Given this description, we aimed to disclose features of patients whose risk of mortality was difficult to estimate using qSOFA.

Methods

Study design, setting, and patients

This was an observational study conducted at the Okinawa Chubu Hospital, a tertiary care teaching hospital with 550 hospital beds and 14 ICU beds in Japan, between May 2012 and June 2016. The hospital institutional review board approved the study protocol (H28-14). Because of the retrospective approach of this study and de-identification of personal data, the board waived the need for informed consent.

We examined data of all adult (≥ 18 years) patients who were admitted to the ICU between May 2012 and June 2016. We identified consecutive patients with suspected sepsis through the following inclusion criteria: the documentation of the reason for ICU admission as 'bacteremia,' 'sepsis,' 'severe sepsis,' or 'septic shock' in the ICU register. Each documentation was based on the clinical judgment as having a severe infection requiring ICU admission. Two attending physicians reviewed the patient data and agreed on the clinical suspicion of infection. We excluded patients with cardiac arrest prior to ICU admission because we did not expect an additional predictive value of qSOFA in these patients.

Data collection

Data for analyses including age, sex, chronic health conditions, location prior to ICU admission, vital signs and qSOFA scores before ICU admission, the presence of rigor ('shaking chills'), primary site of infection, type of organisms, length of ICU stay, the prevalence of bacteremia and in-hospital mortality were collected from patient records. According to a previous report from our institution [10], we routinely classified the qualitative degree of rigor ('chills') as follows: 'mild chills,' feeling cold with the need for an outer jacket; 'moderate chills,' feeling very cold with the need for a thick blanket; and 'shaking chills,' a profound chill with generalized involuntary

bodily shaking, even under a thick blanket. Physicians were instructed to record the degree of chills when they suspected bacteremia in daily practice. We described the primary site of infection as bloodstream, respiratory, gastrointestinal, neurological, genitourinary, or musculoskeletal infection based on the clinical context. Bloodstream infection was defined as blood culture-positive infection including infective endocarditis, bacteremia from an unknown origin and catheter-related bacteremia. The primary infection site showed the following organism types, namely gram-negative bacterial infection, gram-positive bacterial infection, polymicrobial infection or fungal infection. Illness severity was assessed using the Acute Physiology and Chronic Health Evaluation (APACHE) II [11] and the Sequential Organ Failure Assessment (SOFA) scores [12] with the most abnormal measurements recorded during the first 24-h period after ICU admission (Additional file 1: Fig. S1). We used the worst SOFA scores and defined sepsis as a SOFA score of ≥ 2 according to the Sepsis-3 definition [4].

Measurement of the main exposure factors (Additional file 1: Fig. S1)

The qSOFA score had three criteria, assigning one point for alteration in mental status (Glasgow Coma Scale < 15), systolic blood pressure ≤ 100 mm, Hg or respiratory rate ≥ 22/min [4]. We evaluated pre-ICU qSOFA scores with the most abnormal vital signs at the time of clinical deterioration during the 24-h period before ICU admission. We set this time window to evaluate the performance value of pre-ICU admission qSOFA scores in prognosticating high-risk patients before ICU transfer. We also aimed to avoid the effect of therapeutic interventions during the ICU stay on qSOFA scores. According to a previous study, we defined qSOFA-positive or qSOFA-negative as a qSOFA score of ≥ 2 or < 2, respectively [3]. We also evaluated pre-ICU systemic inflammatory response syndrome (SIRS) with the most abnormal measurements during the 24-h period before ICU admission. SIRS-positive was defined as two or more of the following: temperature > 38 or < 36 °C, heart rate > 90 beats/min, respiratory rate > 20 breaths/min, or arterial carbon dioxide pressure < 32 mm Hg, white blood cell count > 12,000/μL or < 4000/μL [13]. In addition, we evaluated qSOFA scores and SIRS at the exact moment of ICU arrival using the first measurements of vital signs just after ICU admission.

Outcome measures

The primary outcome measure was in-hospital mortality, which was defined as any cause of death censored at 90 days after ICU admission. Other outcomes included the length of ICU stay, ICU stay ≥ 3 days, bacteremia and in-hospital mortality censored at 28 days after ICU admission. We defined bacteremia as 2 sets of blood culture with the same microorganism or 1 set of blood culture with bacteria, except for possible contaminated resources involving Coagulase-negative *Staphylococci*, *Corynebacterium* species, *Propionibacterium* species, *Bacillus* species, *Aerococcus* species, and *Micrococcus* species [14, 15].

Statistical analysis

Continuous data are presented as medians with interquartile range (IQR) and compared using the Mann–Whitney U test. Categorical data are presented as proportions and compared using a *Chi-squared* test or Fisher's exact test when appropriate. We used Kaplan–Meier plots to describe the survival between qSOFA-positive and qSOFA-negative patients and compared the survival curves with the log-rank test. As the primary analysis, the Cox proportional hazard regression model was used to assess the association between being qSOFA-positive before ICU admission and in-hospital mortality censored at 90 days after ICU admission. The hazard ratio (HR) and 95% confidence interval (CI) were calculated. The following variables were incorporated into the primary multivariable models: age, the presence of rigor ('shaking chills'), prior location to the ICU, and chronic health condition with immunosuppression. In the Kaplan–Meier description and the Cox regression analysis, if survival hospital discharge occurs within 90 days after ICU admission, we dealt with it as censoring. We also estimated the performance of pre-ICU qSOFA, pre-ICU SIRS, qSOFA at ICU arrival, and SIRS at ICU arrival in predicting sepsis by the Sepsis-3 and in-hospital mortality censored at 90 days. The crude risk ratios (RRs) with 95% CI and area under receiver operating characteristics (AUROC) were calculated. We used qSOFA scores and SIRS scores as continuous variables for the calculation of AUROCs. All statistical analyses were performed using R (The R Foundation for Statistical Computing, ver.3.2.4) and EZR (Saitama Medical Center, Jichi Medical University, ver.1.32), which is a graphical user interface for R [16]. All tests were two-tailed; p values of less than 0.05 were regarded as statistically significant.

Results

The patient flow diagram is presented in Fig. 1. We extracted 188 patients who were admitted to the ICU with suspected sepsis. After excluding 3 patients with prior cardiac arrest, we enrolled 185 patients for our analyses. At least 2 sets of blood cultures were obtained from all participants. The median age was 67 (IQR 57–79), and 61.1% (113/185) of patients were from the emergency room (ER) and 33.5% (62/185) of patients had at least

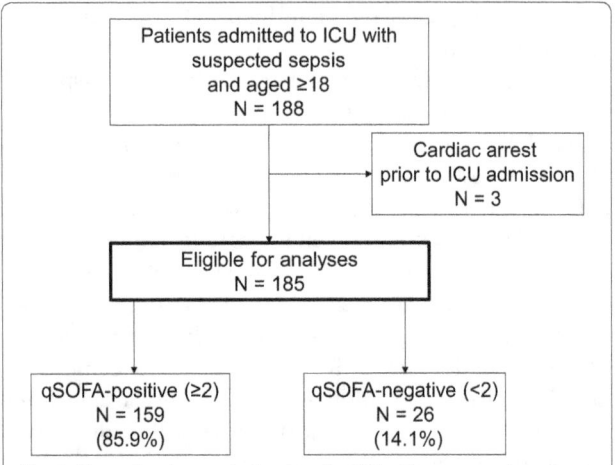

Fig. 1 Flow of patients admitted to the ICU with suspected sepsis from 2012 to 2016. *ICU* denotes intensive care unit, *qSOFA* quick Sequential Organ Failure Assessment

one chronic health condition. Among 185 patients, 85.9% (159/185) were qSOFA-positive and 89.7% (166/185) were SIRS-positive before ICU admission. The median APACHE II and SOFA scores were 21 (IQR 17–28) and 9 (IQR 5–11), respectively. In total, 91.9% (170/185) of patients fulfilled the Sepsis-3 definition, 53.0% (98/185) had positive blood culture, and 29.2% (54/185) died in hospital within 90 days after ICU admission.

Patient demographics, characteristics at the presentation of infection, and characteristics after ICU admission are presented in Table 1. While qSOFA-positive patients were presented with more deranged vital signs, qSOFA-negative patients were more frequently from the ward (qSOFA-positive: 35.8% [57/159] vs qSOFA-negative: 57.7% [15/26], $p = 0.050$) and more frequently had shaking chills (qSOFA-positive: 27.7% [44/159] vs qSOFA-negative: 53.8% [14/26], $p = 0.011$). Hematologic malignancy (qSOFA-positive: 5.7% [9/159] vs qSOFA-negative: 15.4% [4/26], $p = 0.090$) and immunosuppression (qSOFA-positive: 5.7% [9/159] vs qSOFA-negative: 15.4% [4/26], $p = 0.090$) were also observed more frequently in qSOFA-negative patients. The degree of organ dysfunction was similar between the groups in relation to respiration, coagulation, and liver and renal components of the SOFA scores.

The outcomes of qSOFA-negative patients were similar to those of qSOFA-positive patients (Fig. 2 and Table 2). The primary outcome, in-hospital mortality censored at 90 days after ICU admission, was not significantly different between the groups (qSOFA-positive: 30.2% [48/159] vs qSOFA-negative: 23.1% [6/26], $p = 0.642$). The other outcomes, ICU length of stay (qSOFA-positive: 3 [2–6] vs qSOFA-negative: 3 [2–5], $p = 0.787$),

Table 1 Characteristics before and after ICU admission in patients with suspected sepsis

	qSOFA-positive (≥ 2) (N = 159)	qSOFA-negative (< 2) (N = 26)	p value
Demographics			
Age (median [IQR])	67 [57–79]	68 [63–75]	0.791
Male (%)	95 (59.7%)	16 (61.5%)	1.000
Chronic health condition (%)			
Metastatic cancer	7 (4.4%)	1 (3.8%)	1.000
Chronic dialysis	22 (13.8%)	4 (15.4%)	0.767
Hepatic failure	15 (9.4%)	2 (7.7%)	1.000
Chronic respiratory failure	4 (2.5%)	1 (3.8%)	0.535
Hematologic malignancy	9 (5.7%)	4 (15.4%)	0.090
Immunosuppression	9 (5.7%)	4 (15.4%)	0.090
Characteristics at the presentation of infection			
Location prior to ICU admission (%)			0.050
Emergency room	102 (64.2%)	11 (42.3%)	
General ward	57 (35.8%)	15 (57.7%)	
Vital signs before ICU admission (median [IQR])			
Systolic blood pressure, mm Hg	82 [70–96]	105 [79–120]	0.004
Respiratory rate,/min	28 [24–30]	20 [20–24]	< 0.001
Glasgow coma scale	13 [9–15]	15 [15–15]	< 0.001
Heart rate,/min	116 [101–132]	110 [88–119]	0.047
Body temperature, Celsius	38.2 [37.2–39.1]	38.2 [37.1–39.2]	0.997
Shaking chills (%)	44 (27.7%)	14 (53.8%)	0.011
Characteristics after ICU admission			
APACHE II (median [IQR])	22 [17–29]	20 [15–24]	0.092
SOFA score (median [IQR])	9 [6–12]	6 [3–8]	0.001
SOFA respiration	2 [1–3]	1 [0–3]	0.112
SOFA coagulation	1 [0–2]	1 [0–2]	0.256
SOFA liver	0 [0–1]	0 [0–0]	0.296
SOFA central nervous system	1 [0–3]	0 [0–0]	< 0.001
SOFA renal	1 [0–3]	1 [0–2]	0.887
SOFA cardiovascular	3 [1–4]	1 [0–3]	< 0.001
Lactate, mmol/L (median [IQR])	2.5 [1.5–5.3]	1.5 [0.9–3.5]	0.075

qSOFA scores were assessed with the most abnormal vital signs during the 24-h period before the ICU admission. SOFA and APACHE II scores were calculated with the most abnormal measurements taken during the first 24-h period after the ICU admission

APACHE II Acute Physiology and Chronic Health Evaluation II, *ICU* intensive care unit, *IQR* interquartile range, *qSOFA* quick Sequential Organ Failure Assessment, *SOFA* Sequential Organ Failure Assessment

bacteremia (qSOFA-positive: 53.5% [85/159] vs qSOFA-negative: 50.0% [13/26], p = 0.833), and 28-day mortality (qSOFA-positive: 25.2% [40/159] vs qSOFA-negative: 19.2% [5/26], p = 0.627) were also similar between the groups. The Kaplan–Meier plots of survival showed no significant difference between the groups (p = 0.514). The Cox proportional hazard regression model revealed that pre-ICU qSOFA-positive was not significantly associated with in-hospital mortality (adjusted HR 1.35, 95% CI 0.56–3.22, p = 0.506).

Detailed microbiological results are presented in Table 3. Among primary sites of infection, bloodstream infection was more frequent in qSOFA-negative patients (qSOFA-positive: 18.2% [29/159] vs qSOFA-negative: 30.8% [8/26], p = 0.094). Among identified organisms, *Staphylococcus aureus* infection was more frequent in qSOFA-negative patients (qSOFA-positive: 8.8% [14/159] vs qSOFA-negative: 15.4% [4/26], p = 0.290). Of 26 qSOFA-negative patients, the most common site of infection was bloodstream infection (30.8% [8/26]), followed by genitourinary infection (23.1% [6/26]). Among qSOFA-negative patients who died in the hospital, all the patients had at least one chronic health condition.

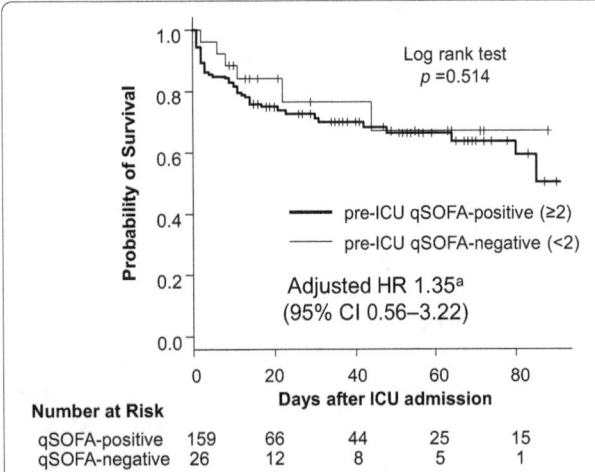

Fig. 2 Kaplan–Meier curves of in-hospital mortality censored at 90 days stratified as pre-ICU qSOFA-positive or qSOFA-negative. [a]Adjusted for age, the presence of rigor ('shaking chills'), prior location to the ICU and chronic health condition with immunosuppression. CI confidence interval, HR hazard ratio, ICU intensive care unit, qSOFA quick Sequential Organ Failure Assessment. The vertical tick marks on the curves denote censoring due to survival discharge

The performance of qSOFA and SIRS in predicting sepsis and mortality is shown in Table 4. The association between pre-ICU qSOFA or pre-ICU SIRS and in-hospital mortality censored at 90 days was not significant (qSOFA crude RR 1.38, 95% CI 0.62–2.74, AUROC 0.511; SIRS crude RR 0.92, 95% CI 0.45–1.85, AUROC 0.521). On the other hand, qSOFA at ICU arrival was significantly associated with in-hospital mortality censored at 90 days (crude RR 1.78, 95% CI 1.09–2.89, AUROC 0.586).

Discussion

Our study suggested that the prognostic impact of pre-ICU qSOFA, assessed during the 24-h period before ICU admission, was small among patients with suspected sepsis (HR 1.35, 95% CI 0.56–3.22). In this study, comprised of high-mortality (29.2%) patients, 14% (26/185) of patients remained qSOFA-negative even at the time of ICU admission. Moreover, the difference in in-hospital mortality was small (qSOFA-positive: 30.2% vs qSOFA-negative: 23.1%, $p=0.642$). Importantly, our study suggested that the risk of mortality in patients with bloodstream infection, immunosuppression or hematologic malignancy would be difficult to estimate using qSOFA scores. The results of our study may provide important implications for clinicians in early prognostication of patients with suspected sepsis and for developers of sepsis screening systems.

Among patients with suspected infection outside the ICU, qSOFA scores had greater prognostic accuracy than SIRS [3]. Since 1992, SIRS has gained widespread acceptance as the clinical definition of sepsis [13]. However, the specificity of SIRS ≥ 2 was too low and 70–90% of ICU patients, including non-infected patients, attained SIRS ≥ 2 during their ICU stay [17]. Along with the development of a new definition for sepsis, the qSOFA score has been generated to guide bedside clinicians in identifying infected patients at risk of in-hospital mortality or longer ICU stay [3]. The original study showed that qSOFA-positive patients had a 3- to 14-fold increase in in-hospital mortality compared to qSOFA-negative patients when qSOFA scores were assessed during the 72-h period around the onset of infection. Further external validation studies have shown that qSOFA scores had greater prognostic accuracy than SIRS among patients presenting to the ER [18–20].

However, recent studies have suggested that qSOFA has limited utility in early prognostication in high-mortality populations. In a retrospective analysis of a large adult ICU patient database, qSOFA assessed during the first 24-h following ICU admission had little additional predictive value for mortality over SIRS [6]. In recent studies consisting of patients admitted to the ICU or patients

Table 2 ICU stay and in-hospital mortality in ICU patients with suspected sepsis

	qSOFA-positive (≥ 2) (N=159)	qSOFA-negative (<2) (N=26)	p value
ICU length of stay (median [IQR])	3 [2–6]	3 [2–5]	0.787
ICU stay ≥ 3 days (%)	94 (59.1%)	15 (57.7%)	1.000
Bacteremia (%)	85 (53.5%)	13 (50.0%)	0.833
In-hospital mortality (%)			
28-day mortality	40 (25.2%)	5 (19.2%)	0.627
90-day mortality	48 (30.2%)	6 (23.1%)	0.642

qSOFA scores were assessed with the most abnormal vital signs taken during the 24-h period before the ICU admission

In-hospital mortality was defined as any cause of death censored at 28 days or at 90 days after the ICU admission

ICU intensive care unit, IQR interquartile range, qSOFA quick Sequential Organ Failure Assessment

Table 3 Microbiological results in ICU patients with suspected sepsis

	qSOFA-positive (≥ 2) (N = 159)	qSOFA-negative (< 2) (N = 26)	p value
Primary site of infection (%)			
Bloodstream	29 (18.2%)	8 (30.8%)	0.094
Respiratory	31 (19.5%)	3 (11.5%)	0.573
Gastrointestinal	25 (15.7%)	4 (15.4%)	0.770
Neurological	2 (1.3%)	0 (0.0%)	NA
Genitourinary	39 (24.5%)	6 (23.1%)	1.000
Musculoskeletal	19 (11.9%)	1 (3.8%)	0.476
Other	14 (8.8%)	4 (15.4%)	0.290
Type of organisms (%)			
Gram-negative bacterial infection	66 (41.5%)	11 (42.3%)	
Escherichia coli	30 (18.9%)	5 (19.2%)	1.000
Klebsiella pneumoniae	12 (7.5%)	1 (3.8%)	0.697
Pseudomonas aeruginosa	7 (4.4%)	0 (0.0%)	NA
Gram-positive bacterial infection	32 (20.1%)	6 (23.1%)	
Staphylococcus aureus	14 (8.8%)	4 (15.4%)	0.290
Streptococcus pneumoniae	9 (5.7%)	0 (0.0%)	NA
Streptococcus species	4 (2.5%)	1 (3.8%)	0.535
Polymicrobial infection	20 (12.6%)	4 (15.4%)	0.752
Fungal infection	4 (2.5%)	0 (0.0%)	NA
Not specified	37 (23.3%)	5 (19.2%)	0.803

qSOFA scores were assessed with the most abnormal vital signs taken during the 24-h period before the ICU admission

Bloodstream infection was defined as blood culture-positive infection including infective endocarditis, bacteremia from an unknown origin and catheter-related bacteremia

ICU intensive care unit, *NA* not applicable, *qSOFA* quick Sequential Organ Failure Assessment

in the ward, in-hospital mortality of qSOFA-negative patients was higher (13.6–17.4%) compared to mortality in studies consisting of ER patients [5–9]. Therefore, qSOFA was assumed to have limited performance value in prognosticating high-risk patients. Importantly, qSOFA scores assessed after ICU admission were likely to have been affected with therapeutic interventions such as vasopressors and sedative agents [3, 6]. Therefore, pre-ICU qSOFA scores assessed before ICU admission have been evaluated [21].

We focused on patients with suspected sepsis requiring ICU admission and evaluated pre-ICU qSOFA scores assessed during the 24-h period before ICU admission. Our results raise a question as to why the association between pre-ICU qSOFA-positive and mortality was weaker (HR 1.35, 95% CI 0.56–3.22) than that observed in previous studies [3, 18]. To address this question, it is to be noted, first, that our patients were judged as having a severe infection by treating physicians before enrollment. Physicians detected signs of severe infection based not only on vital sign abnormalities such as qSOFA components but also on clinical diagnosis, primary sites of infection, presumed causative organisms and patient comorbidities [22, 23]. Also, some experts

have questioned the sensitivity of qSOFA because qSOFA would remain negative until life-threatening organ dysfunction has developed [24]. A previous study showed that qSOFA remained negative even at the time of ICU transfer in one-half of infected patients [5]. In our study, the association between qSOFA and mortality became significant only after ICU admission (Pre-ICU qSOFA: crude RR 1.38, 95% CI 0.62–2.74; qSOFA at ICU arrival: crude RR 1.78, 95% CI 1.09–2.89). Physicians might have detected the risk of further clinical deterioration before qSOFA was determined as positive. As a result, the association between pre-ICU qSOFA and mortality would have attenuated. Our results suggested that qSOFA had little additional predictive value for mortality over clinical judgment (Fig. 2, Table 4). Second, we presented 90-day mortality instead of 28-day mortality. Recent studies have shown that patients with sepsis had increasing mortality beyond the standard 28-day mortality and that the use of long-term outcomes had been postulated to infer the full impact of sepsis [25]. Our study represented long-term outcomes of infected patients requiring ICU admission.

In addition to investigating the association between qSOFA-positive and mortality, we described detailed characteristics in qSOFA-negative patients to disclose

Table 4 Performance of qSOFA and SIRS in predicting sepsis and mortality

	Sepsis by Sepsis-3 definition			In-hospital mortality		
	n/N (%)	Crude risk ratio (95% CI)	AUROC	n/N (%)	Crude risk ratio (95% CI)	AUROC
Pre-ICU qSOFA			0.711			0.511
qSOFA-positive (≥ 2)	149/159 (93.7%)	1.16 (0.96–1.41)		48/159 (30.2%)	1.38 (0.62–2.74)	
qSOFA-negative (< 2)	21/26 (80.8%)	1.00 (ref)		6/26 (23.1%)	1.00 (ref)	
Pre-ICU SIRS			0.710			0.521
SIRS-positive (≥ 2)	155/166 (93.4%)	1.18 (0.93–1.50)		48/166 (28.9%)	0.92 (0.45–1.85)	
SIRS-negative (< 2)	15/19 (78.9%)	1.00 (ref)		6/19 (31.6%)	1.00 (ref)	
qSOFA at ICU arrival			0.624			0.586
qSOFA-positive (≥ 2)	92/98 (93.9%)	1.05 (0.96–1.14)		36/98 (36.7%)	1.78 (1.09–2.89)	
qSOFA-negative (< 2)	78/87 (89.7%)	1.00 (ref)		18/87 (20.7%)	1.00 (ref)	
SIRS at ICU arrival			0.709			0.541
SIRS-positive (≥ 2)	133/139 (95.7%)	1.19 (1.03–1.38)		41/139 (29.5%)	1.04 (0.62–1.77)	
SIRS-negative (< 2)	37/46 (80.4%)	1.00 (ref)		13/46 (28.3%)	1.00 (ref)	

Pre-ICU qSOFA and SIRS scores were assessed with the most abnormal vital signs taken during the 24-h period before the ICU admission. qSOFA and SIRS scores at ICU arrival were assessed with the first measurements just after ICU admission

Sepsis was defined according to the Sepsis-3 definition. In-hospital mortality was defined as any cause of death censored at 90 days after the ICU admission

AUROC area under receiver operating characteristics, CI confidence interval, ICU intensive care unit, qSOFA quick Sequential Organ Failure Assessment, SIRS systemic inflammatory response syndrome

features of patients whose risk of mortality was difficult to estimate using qSOFA scores (Table 1, 3). The characteristics, which were more frequently found in qSOFA-negative patients, were hematologic malignancy, immunosuppression, bloodstream infection, and *Staphylococcus aureus* infection. Among 8 bloodstream infections in qSOFA-negative patients, 37.5% (3/8) had chronic dialysis, and 25% (2/8) had hematologic malignancy. We think that the history of comorbidities alerted physicians of further deterioration and prompted physicians to consider ICU transfer before qSOFA scores turned positive. A variety of infections were presented with qSOFA-negative patients in our study. Indeed, we often experienced infective endocarditis, catheter-related bacteremia, pyelonephritis, and bacterial pneumonia in qSOFA-negative patients. Of note, all the patients who died in the qSOFA-negative group had at least one chronic health condition. In these patients, primary sites of infection and comorbidities would be additional useful information for early prognostication.

Our study had several limitations. First, our study was conducted in a single center with a small number of patients. As a result, only 54 in-hospital deaths were observed and the CI for our primary analyses was wide (HR 1.35, 95% CI 0.56–3.22). It is possible that we failed to find an association between pre-ICU qSOFA and in-hospital mortality due to the small sample size. Because no study focused on pre-ICU qSOFA at the time we

planned the study, it was difficult to estimate a priori sample size. Second, because we did not observe all the infected patients presented to the ER or the ward, it is possible that we did not accurately estimate the association between qSOFA and mortality in patients not requiring ICU admission. The generalizability of the result of this study might have been attenuated. Currently, however, only a few studies have focused on pre-ICU qSOFA scores and on qSOFA-negative, infected ICU patients [21]. The results of our study provide an important basis for further prospective studies investigating the role of qSOFA in triage decisions for ICU admission. Third, we did not use uniform criteria for ICU admission. The threshold of ICU transfer in each patient largely depends on physicians and hospital-beds availability. Nevertheless, the median APACHE II scores (21, IQR 17–28), SOFA scores (9, IQR 5–11), and mortality (29.2%) of our patients were higher than those of related studies [3, 6, 18] or than in recent multicenter studies enrolling patients with early septic shock (mortality 18%) [26]. Thus, our results reflected the performance value of qSOFA in high-risk populations. Last, due to the retrospective nature of our study, the frequency of qSOFA variable measurements was not standardized. The pre-ICU qSOFA scores in our study were based on the worst vital signs that were obtainable during the 24-h period before ICU admission. There were no missing data regarding qSOFA scores.

Conclusion

In this observational study, among patients admitted to the ICU with suspected sepsis, we could not find a strong association between pre-ICU qSOFA scores and in-hospital mortality. We described high mortality and bacterial diversity in pre-ICU qSOFA-negative patients. Besides qSOFA scores, primary sites of infection and comorbidities may provide additional useful information for early prognostication in high-risk populations.

Abbreviations

APACHE II: Acute Physiology and Chronic Health Evaluation II; AUROC: area under receiver operating characteristic; CI: confidence interval; ER: emergency room; HR: hazard ratio; ICU: intensive care unit; IQR: interquartile range; qSOFA: quick Sequential Organ Failure Assessment; RR: risk ratio; SIRS: systemic inflammatory response syndrome; SOFA: Sequential Organ Failure Assessment.

Authors' contributions

IN designed the study, analyzed the data, and wrote the first draft of the manuscript. JI reviewed all statistical analyses and critically revised the manuscript. HM extracted the data and critically revised the manuscript. TK supervised the analysis of the data and critically revised the manuscript. JS designed the study and critically revised the manuscript. All the authors read and approved the final manuscript.

Author details

[1] Intensive Care Unit, Department of Internal Medicine, Okinawa Chubu Hospital, 281 Miyazato, Uruma, Okinawa 904-2293, Japan. [2] Intensive Care Unit, Department of Anesthesiology, The Jikei University School of Medicine, 3-19-18 Nishi-Shinbashi, Minato-ku, Tokyo 105-8471, Japan. [3] The Center for Critical Care Nephrology, Clinical Research, Investigation, and Systems Modeling of Acute Illness Center, Department of Critical Care Medicine, University of Pittsburgh School of Medicine, Pittsburgh, PA 15213, USA. [4] Department of Anesthesiology and Critical Care, Jichi Medical University, Saitama Medical Center, 1-847 Amanuma, Oomiya-ku, Saitama, Saitama 330-8503, Japan. [5] Division of Environmental Medicine and Population Sciences, Department of Social and Environmental Medicine, Graduate School of Medicine, Osaka University, 1-1 Yamada-oka, Suita, Osaka 565-0871, Japan.

Acknowledgements

We thank all staff of Okinawa Chubu Hospital. We would like to thank Editage (http://www.editage.jp) for English language editing.

This work was performed at Okinawa Chubu Hospital.

Competing interests

The authors declare that they have no competing interests.

Funding

The authors declare that they have no sources of funding for the research.

References

1. Seymour CW, Gesten F, Prescott HC, Friedrich ME, Iwashyna TJ, Phillips GS, Lemeshow S, Osborn T, Terry KM, Levy MM. Time to treatment and mortality during mandated emergency care for sepsis. N Engl J Med. 2017;376(23):2235–44.
2. Ferrer R, Martin-Loeches I, Phillips G, Osborn TM, Townsend S, Dellinger RP, Artigas A, Schorr C, Levy MM. Empiric antibiotic treatment reduces mortality in severe sepsis and septic shock from the first hour: results from a guideline-based performance improvement program. Crit Care Med. 2014;42(8):1749–55.
3. Seymour CW, Liu VX, Iwashyna TJ, Brunkhorst FM, Rea TD, Scherag A, Rubenfeld G, Kahn JM, Shankar-Hari M, Singer M, et al. Assessment of clinical criteria for sepsis: for the third international consensus definitions for sepsis and septic shock (Sepsis-3). JAMA. 2016;315(8):762–74.
4. Singer M, Deutschman CS, Seymour CW, Shankar-Hari M, Annane D, Bauer M, Bellomo R, Bernard GR, Chiche JD, Coopersmith CM, et al. The third international consensus definitions for sepsis and septic shock (Sepsis-3). JAMA. 2016;315(8):801–10.
5. Churpek MM, Snyder A, Han X, Sokol S, Pettit N, Howell MD, Edelson DP. Quick sepsis-related organ failure assessment, systemic inflammatory response syndrome, and early warning scores for detecting clinical deterioration in infected patients outside the intensive care unit. Am J Respir Crit Care Med. 2017;195(7):906–11.
6. Raith EP, Udy AA, Bailey M, McGloughlin S, MacIsaac C, Bellomo R, Pilcher DV. Prognostic accuracy of the SOFA score, SIRS criteria, and qSOFA score for in-hospital mortality among adults with suspected infection admitted to the intensive care unit. JAMA. 2017;317(3):290–300.
7. Wang JY, Chen YX, Guo SB, Mei X, Yang P. Predictive performance of quick Sepsis-related Organ Failure Assessment for mortality and ICU admission in patients with infection at the ED. Am J Emerg Med. 2016;34(9):1788–93.
8. Giamarellos-Bourboulis EJ, Tsaganos T, Tsangaris I, Lada M, Routsi C, Sinapidis D, Koupetori M, Bristianou M, Adamis G, Mandragos K, et al. Validation of the new Sepsis-3 definitions: proposal for improvement in early risk identification. Clin Microbiol Infect. 2017;23(2):104–9.
9. April MD, Aguirre J, Tannenbaum LI, Moore T, Pingree A, Thaxton RE, Sessions DJ, Lantry JH. Sepsis clinical criteria in emergency department patients admitted to an intensive care unit: an external validation study of quick sequential organ failure assessment. J Emerg Med. 2017;52(5):622–31.
10. Tokuda Y, Miyasato H, Stein GH, Kishaba T. The degree of chills for risk of bacteremia in acute febrile illness. Am J Med. 2005;118(12):1417.
11. Knaus WA, Draper EA, Wagner DP, Zimmerman JE. APACHE II: a severity of disease classification system. Crit Care Med. 1985;13(10):818–29.
12. Ferreira FL, Bota DP, Bross A, Melot C, Vincent JL. Serial evaluation of the SOFA score to predict outcome in critically ill patients. JAMA. 2001;286(14):1754–8.
13. Bone RC, Balk RA, Cerra FB, Dellinger RP, Fein AM, Knaus WA, Schein RM, Sibbald WJ. Definitions for sepsis and organ failure and guidelines for the use of innovative therapies in sepsis. The ACCP/SCCM Consensus Conference Committee. American College of Chest Physicians/Society of Critical Care Medicine. Chest. 1992;101(6):1644–55.
14. Hall KK, Lyman JA. Updated review of blood culture contamination. Clin Microbiol Rev. 2006;19(4):788–802.
15. Chou HL, Han ST, Yeh CF, Tzeng IS, Hsieh TH, Wu CC, Kuan JT, Chen KF. Systemic inflammatory response syndrome is more associated with bacteremia in elderly patients with suspected sepsis in emergency departments. Medicine (Baltimore). 2016;95(49):e5634.
16. Kanda Y. Investigation of the freely available easy-to-use software 'EZR' for medical statistics. Bone Marrow Transpl. 2013;48(3):452–8.
17. Sprung CL, Sakr Y, Vincent JL, Le Gall JR, Reinhart K, Ranieri VM, Gerlach H, Fielden J, Groba CB, Payen D. An evaluation of systemic inflammatory response syndrome signs in the Sepsis Occurrence In Acutely Ill Patients (SOAP) study. Intensive Care Med. 2006;32(3):421–7.
18. Freund Y, Lemachatti N, Krastinova E, Van Laer M, Claessens Y-E, Avondo A, Occelli C, Feral-Pierssens A-L, Truchot J, Ortega M, et al. Prognostic accuracy of Sepsis-3 criteria for in-hospital mortality among patients with suspected infection presenting to the emergency department. JAMA. 2017;317(3):301–8.
19. Singer AJ, Ng J, Thode HC Jr, Spiegel R, Weingart S. Quick SOFA scores predict mortality in adult emergency department patients with and without suspected infection. Ann Emerg Med. 2017;69(4):475–9.
20. Williams JM, Greenslade JH, McKenzie JV, Chu K, Brown AF, Lipman J. Systemic inflammatory response syndrome, quick sequential organ function

assessment, and organ dysfunction: insights from a prospective database of ED patients with infection. Chest. 2017;151(3):586–96.

21. Finkelsztein EJ, Jones DS, Ma KC, Pabon MA, Delgado T, Nakahira K, Arbo JE, Berlin DA, Schenck EJ, Choi AM, et al. Comparison of qSOFA and SIRS for predicting adverse outcomes of patients with suspicion of sepsis outside the intensive care unit. Crit Care. 2017;21(1):73.

22. Vincent JL. The clinical challenge of sepsis identification and monitoring. PLoS Med. 2016;13(5):e1002022.

23. Poeze M, Ramsay G, Gerlach H, Rubulotta F, Levy M. An international sepsis survey: a study of doctors' knowledge and perception about sepsis. Crit Care. 2004;8(6):R409–13.

24. Simpson SQ. New sepsis criteria. Chest. 2016;149(5):1117–8.

25. Winters BD, Eberlein M, Leung J, Needham DM, Pronovost PJ, Sevransky JE. Long-term mortality and quality of life in sepsis: a systematic review. Crit Care Med. 2010;38(5):1276–83.

26. The ARISE Investigators, the ANZICS Clinical Trial Group, Peake SL, Delaney A, Bailey M, Bellomo R, Cameron PA, Cooper DJ, Higgins AM, Holdgate A, et al. Goal-directed resuscitation for patients with early septic shock. N Engl J Med. 2014;371(16):1496–506.

Application of updated guidelines on diastolic dysfunction in patients with severe sepsis and septic shock

David J. Clancy[1], Timothy Scully[1], Michel Slama[2], Stephen Huang[1], Anthony S. McLean[1] and Sam R. Orde[1]*.

Abstract

Background: Left ventricular diastolic dysfunction is suggested to be associated with higher mortality in severe sepsis and septic shock, yet the methods of diagnosis described in the literature are often inconsistent. The recently published 2016 American Society of Echocardiography and European Association of Cardiovascular Imaging (ASE/EACVI) guidelines offer the opportunity to apply a simple pragmatic diagnostic algorithm for the detection of diastolic dysfunction; however, it has not been tested in this cohort.

Aims: We sought to assess the applicability in septic patients of recently published 2016 ASE/EACVI guidelines on diastolic dysfunction compared with the 2009 ASE guidelines. Our hypothesis was that there would be poor agreement in classifying patients.

Methods: Prospective observational study includes patients identified as having severe sepsis and septic shock. Patients underwent transthoracic echocardiography on day 1 and day 3 of their ICU admission. Patients with normal and abnormal (ejection fraction < 52%) systolic function had their diastolic function stratified according to both the 2009 ASE and 2016 ASE/EACVI guidelines.

Results: On day 1 echocardiography, of the 62 patients analysed, 37 (60%) had diastolic dysfunction according to the 2016 ASE/EACVI guideline with a further 23% having indeterminate diastolic function, compared to the 2009 ASE guidelines where only 13 (21%) had confirmed diastolic dysfunction with 46 (74%) having indeterminate diastolic dysfunction. On day 3, of the 55 patients studied, 22 patients (40%) were defined as having diastolic dysfunction, with 6 (11%) having indeterminate diastolic dysfunction according to the 2016 ASE/EACVI guidelines, compared to the 2009 guidelines where 11 (20%) were confirmed to have diastolic dysfunction and 41 (75%) had indeterminate diastolic function. Systolic dysfunction was identified in 18 of 62 patients (29%) on day 1 and 18 of 55 (33%) on day 3. These patients were classified as having abnormal diastolic function in 94 and 89% with the 2016 guidelines on day 1 and day 3, respectively, compared with 50 and 28% using the 2009 guidelines. The 2016 guidelines had less patients with indeterminate diastolic function on days 1 and 3 (11 and 6%) compared to the 2009 guidelines (50 and 72%). Normal systolic function was identified in 44 patients on day 1 and 37 on day 3. In this group, abnormal diastolic function was present in 45 and 54% on days 1 and 3 according to the 2016 ASE/EACVI guidelines, compared with 9 and 16% using the 2009 guidelines, respectively. In those with normal systolic function, the 2016 guidelines had less indeterminate patients with 30 and 16% on days 1 and 3, respectively, compared to 84 and 76% in the 2009 guidelines.

Conclusion: The 2016 ASE/EACVI diastolic function guidelines identify a significantly higher incidence of dysfunction in patients with severe sepsis and septic shock compared to the previous 2009 guidelines. Although the new guidelines seem to be an improvement, issues remain with the application of guidelines using traditional measures of diastolic dysfunction in this cohort.

*Correspondence: sam.orde@health.nsw.gov.au
[1] ICU, Nepean Hospital, Kingswood, NSW 2747, Australia
Full list of author information is available at the end of the article

Keywords: Sepsis, Diastolic function, Systolic function

Background

Systolic and diastolic dysfunction occur frequently in severe sepsis and septic shock [1]. Whilst systolic dysfunction has been suggested not to be associated with mortality [2], there is conflicting evidence in regard to diastolic dysfunction and its effect on mortality in sepsis [3–12]. One of the major issues in research in this field to date is the large variation in diagnostic criteria used to define diastolic dysfunction [7, 8, 11, 13], which limits the interpretation of subsequent analyses [4]. Previous guidelines from the American Society of Echocardiography (ASE) [14] have been limited by several factors, for example the mandatory inclusion of left atrial size that is assumed to increase in response to raised left atrial pressures [13, 15]. This may not be the case in the acute situation. The most recent recommendations from the ASE and the European Association of Cardiovascular Imaging (ASE/EACVI) published in 2016 [16] have significant advantages, including increased flexibility, with recognition that not all parameters (i.e. left atrial size) are abnormal in diastolic dysfunction. Furthermore, they recognize that given the relationship between systolic function and myocardial relaxation that patients with abnormal systolic function or structural abnormalities must automatically have a degree of impaired diastolic function. Hence, they have prescribed an approach whereby those with normal systolic function need to have impairment of diastolic function detected before subsequent grading of severity, whereas those with abnormal systolic function or structural issues must have impaired relaxation and subsequently can proceed to grading of their diastolic dysfunction. The parameters used in the algorithms have been simplified, with less importance placed on parameters that are difficult to measure in the intensive care unit. The authors of these guidelines note that they are applicable to the general population seen in an ambulant setting, but not in children or in the peri-operative setting. In the absence of an accepted gold standard for diastolic dysfunction, these same guidelines are utilized to make the diagnosis of diastolic dysfunction in the critically ill population. However, despite improvements made in defining diastolic dysfunction, caveats remain with each parameter that can make the recognition of impaired relaxation difficult in the critically ill patients.

We sought to compare the 2009 ASE and the recent 2016 ASE/EACVI algorithms for diagnosing diastolic dysfunction in a population with severe sepsis and septic shock to assess and compare their ability to detect and differentiate grades of diastolic dysfunction. Our hypothesis was that there would be poor agreement in classifying patients with diastolic dysfunction between the 2009 and 2016 guidelines for diastolic dysfunction.

Methods

We conducted a prospective, observational cohort study at the Nepean Hospital Intensive Care Unit, Sydney, NSW, from September 2014 to February 2016. The study was approved by the Nepean Blue Mountains Local Health District Research Governance Office (14/35-LR/14/Nepean/70). As echocardiography is a standard procedure in critically ill patients in our unit, consent was waived. Inclusion criteria were: adult patients (> 18 years) admitted to Nepean ICU with severe sepsis or septic shock based on the previous 2012 Surviving Sepsis guidelines that were current at the time of data collection. Severe sepsis was defined as having a documented or strong suspicion of infection, with at least 2 of 4 clinical signs of inflammation (temperature > 38 or < 36 °C, heart rate > 90 bpm, white blood cell count < 4 or > 12×10^9/L, respiratory rate > 20/min or $PaCO_2$ < 32 mmHg) with additional evidence of organ dysfunction. Septic shock is defined as sepsis with refractory hypotension requiring vasoactive treatment [17]. The authors recognize that since completion of enrolment in this study the definition of sepsis and septic shock has changed [18]. Exclusion criteria included: pregnancy, congenital heart disease, artificial valve prosthesis, severe mitral pathology and inadequate image quality.

Patient data collected included: demographic and physiological data, SOFA scores, fluid balances, inotropic use and mechanical ventilation parameters. Previous echo reports (including diastolic dysfunction) when available were acquired, although the grading of diastolic dysfunction for these studies was not based on the 2016 ASE/EACI guidelines. SOFA scores were retrospectively calculated at the time of the echo studies. Current rates of noradrenaline infusion and total volume of noradrenaline infused were also recorded to the nearest hour.

Echocardiography

A baseline, comprehensive echocardiogram was performed by sonographers or S.O. (intensive care and echocardiography specialist) at the earliest opportunity following admission (day 1). Parameters measured were in accordance with current practice and included: LV size, LV ejection fraction, left atrial volume, mitral inflow velocity, septal and lateral annulus tissue Doppler, tricuspid regurgitation (TR) velocity and cardiac output. Ejection fraction and left atrial volume were measured with Simpson's biplane technique. Measurements were averaged from 3 cardiac cycles if the patient was in sinus rhythm and 5 cardiac cycles in those with atrial fibrillation. Tissue Doppler measurements were taken from the modal velocity (or peak intensity of the Doppler signal) rather than the peak of the waves, given the variable accuracy of peak tissue Doppler measurements in various machines [19]. A repeat study was performed as soon as feasible from day 3 of admission.

Systolic dysfunction was defined as those with a calculated ejection fraction (EF) (using Simpson's biplane method) < 52%. Diastolic dysfunction was classified according to both the 2009 ASE and 2016 ASE/EACVI guidelines (see Fig. 1 for summary of diagnostic algorithms). In regard to the 2009 ASE guidelines, deceleration time was excluded given its limitation in fusion of the *E* and *A* waves due to tachycardia and Valsalva manoeuvres were not performed due to difficulty in performing in the critically ill. Pulmonary venous Doppler parameters were sought if available to aid in the diagnosis, but only to be used if the sample was adequate. The $E:e'$ was calculated based on an average of the medial and lateral e' values. Left atrial volume was indexed for body surface area and considered increased if > 34 ml/m^2. If height and

weight data were not available, left atrial volume was considered increased if > 52 ml (for females) and > 58 ml (for males). For the 2016 guidelines, if patients had normal systolic function and no obvious structural abnormalities, they were first screened for diastolic dysfunction via a separate algorithm before subsequent grading, requiring at least 3 of the 4 prescribed parameters to be positive. Those with structural abnormalities, known ischaemic heart disease or abnormal systolic function, given that they will have impaired myocardial relaxation, proceeded directly to grading of diastolic dysfunction.

Data and statistical analysis

Statistical analysis was performed with the software program JMP version 11 (SAS, Cary, North Carolina, USA). Cohen's kappa analysis was performed to assess the level of agreement of the 2009 and 2016 guidelines, with the null hypothesis accepted if kappa was greater than 0.7 (considered reasonable agreement) and rejected if kappa was less than 0.4 (considered poor agreement). Using a significance level of 0.05, a sample size of 44 was required to give 90% power of detecting a true difference [20]. Given the risk of missing

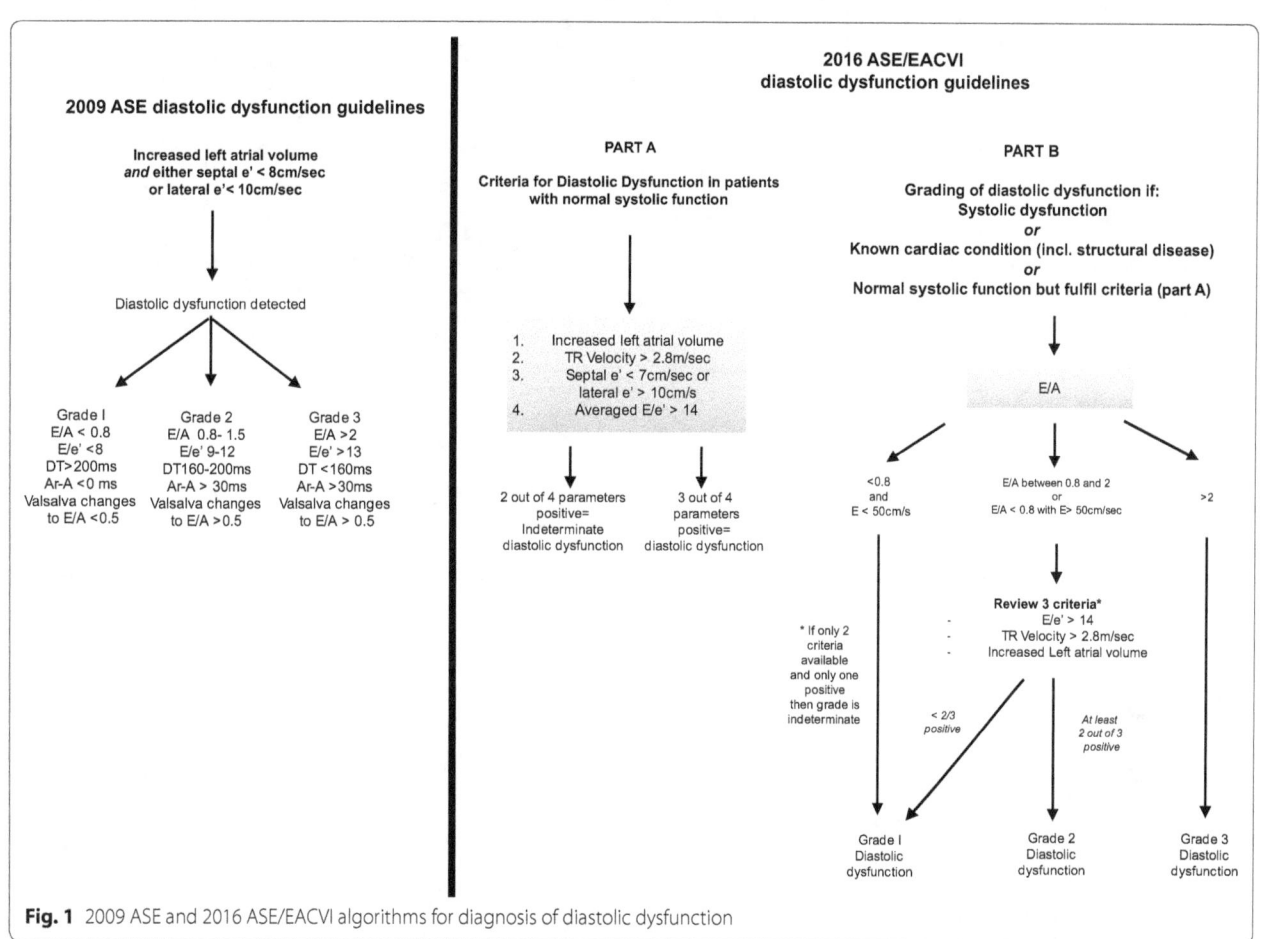

Fig. 1 2009 ASE and 2016 ASE/EACVI algorithms for diagnosis of diastolic dysfunction

data or insufficient image quality, this sample size was extended to at least 60 patients. Continuous variables are reported as mean ± standard deviation (SD) or median ± interquartile range (IQR) and are analysed between groups using analysis of variance, and if a significant difference found, individual group analysis was performed by Tukey's HSD test. Categorical variables are expressed as number of patients and percentage of group, with comparisons made by Pearson's Chi-squared test or Fisher's exact test if less than 5 patients were in a specific group. For unadjusted comparisons between groups, a Student's t test was used for normally distributed data and a Wilcoxon signed-rank test for non-normally distributed data. Probability values are considered two-sided, and a p value < 0.05 was considered significant. All echocardiograms were reviewed by two different examiners (T.S and D.C) who were blinded to each other's findings. Measurements taken were in keeping with recommendations from the ASE [16, 21] and as such are reproducible. Grading of diastolic dysfunction was performed by two examiners (M.S and D.C). Any discrepancies were resolved by consensus in the presence of an adjudicator (S.O).

Results

Sixty-eight patients were included in the study (see Fig. 2). Six were lost to follow-up or had insufficient imaging and were excluded from analysis. A further seven patients (11%) died before repeat echocardiography. In total, 15 (24%) patients died in the ICU, with a total of 20 (32%) dying in hospital. Baseline demographics of all patients are included (Table 1). The median time to first echocardiograph was 19 h from admission (IQR 11.5, 31.5) and 90 h (IQR 68, 108) for the repeat echocardiograph.

On day 1 echocardiography, of the 62 patients analysed 37 (60%) had diastolic dysfunction according to the 2016 ASE/EACVI guideline with a further 23% having indeterminate diastolic function, compared to the 2009 ASE guidelines where only 13 (21%) had confirmed diastolic dysfunction with 46 (74%) having indeterminate diastolic dysfunction. The degree of agreement between the two guidelines on day 1 was poor, with Kappa being 0.24

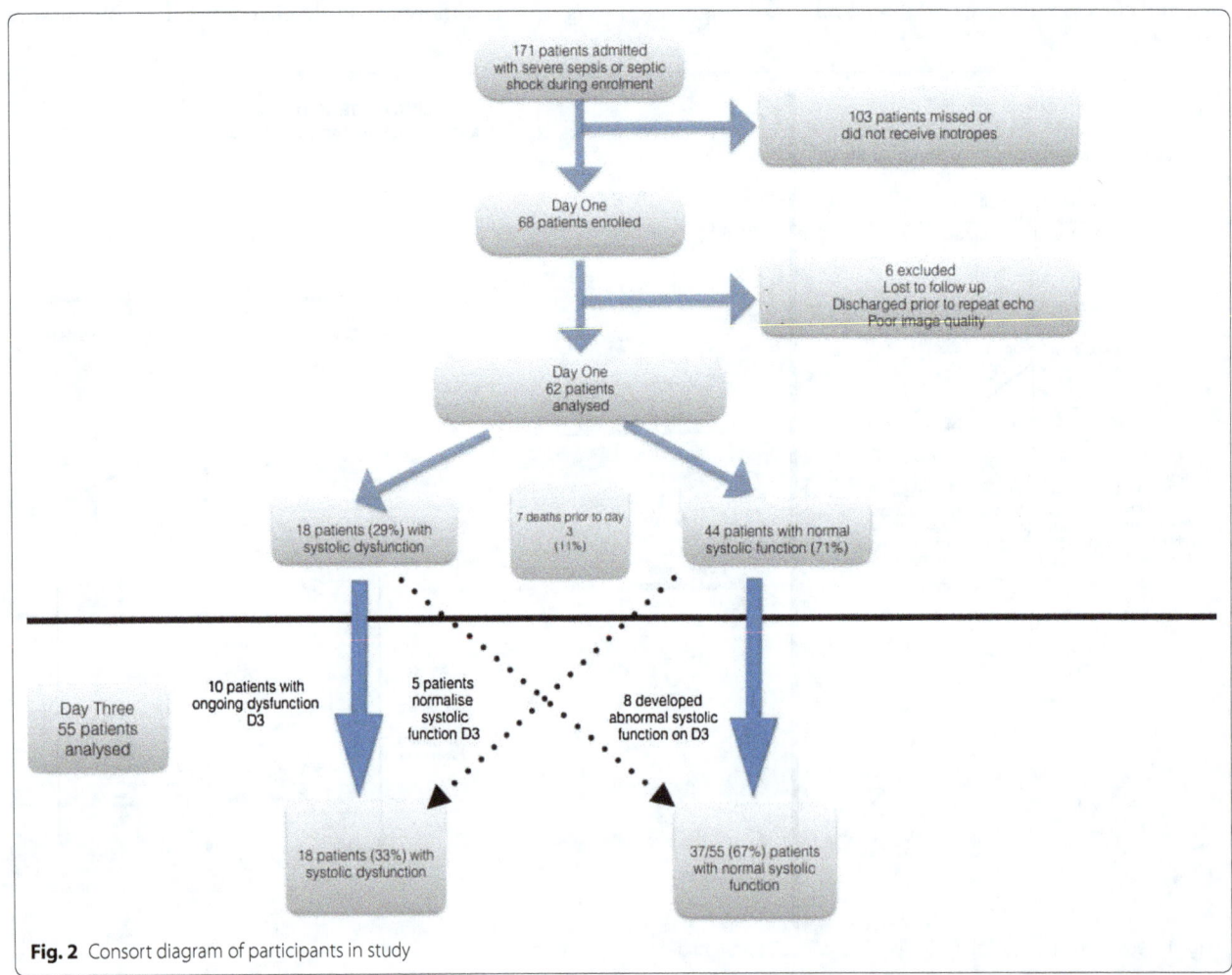

Fig. 2 Consort diagram of participants in study

Table 1 Baseline demographics of all patients and those with normal systolic function on day 1

Variable	All patients (62)	Normal ejection fraction on day 1 N = 44 (71%)		
		Normal diastolic function (n = 11)	Abnormal diastolic dysfunction (n = 20)	Indeterminate diastolic function (n = 13)
Demographics				
Age	63.1 ± 12.4	55 ± 14	67 ± 8*	62 ± 12
Sex (M)	35 (56%)	6 (55%)	6 (30%)	6 (46%)
Past medical history				
IHD	19 (31%)	0	3 (15%)	5 (38%)
Diabetes	20 (32%)	3 (27%)	5 (25%)	4 (31%)
HTN	37 (60%)	4 (36%)	6 (30%)	6 (46%)
Previous documented diastolic dysfunction	6 (10%)	0	3 (15%)	2 (15%)
Previous documented systolic dysfunction	5 (8%)	1 (9%)	0	0
CRF	11 (18%)	0	5 (25%)	3 (23%)**
Clinical data				
Mechanical ventilation D1 (n)	44 (71%)	7 (64%)	13 (65%)	9 (69%)
Mechanical ventilation D3	32 (52%)	6 (55%)	8 (40%)	9 (69%)
Total noradrenaline at first echo (ml)	155 (51, 330)	49 (15, 162)	129 (47, 330)	202 (111,573)
HR day 1	97 ± 21	97 ± 25	91 ± 17	101 ± 14
Arrhythmia D1	13 (21%)	2 (18%)	4 (20%)	2 (15%)
SOFA D1	10 ± 3.7	9.5 ± 4	9.9 ± 3.9	9.1 ± 3.7
PEEP D1	8 (5, 10)	10 (5, 14)	8 (6, 10)	8 (5,9)

Diastolic dysfunction assessed by 2016 ASE/EACVI guidelines

p values not given unless significant, *$p < 0.018$; **$p < 0.021$

($p = 0.0002$). On day 3, of the 55 patients studied, 22 patients (40%) were defined as having diastolic dysfunction, with 6 (11%) having indeterminate diastolic dysfunction according to the 2016 ASE/EACVI guidelines, compared to the 2009 guidelines where 11 (20%) were diagnosed to have diastolic dysfunction and 41 (75%) had indeterminate diastolic function. Again agreement was poor (Kappa 0.13, $p = 0.03$). The details of the abnormal parameters with respect to the 2009 and 2016 grading of diastolic dysfunction for days 1 and 3 are included (see Additional files 1 and 2).

Systolic dysfunction was identified in 18 patients (29%) on day 1 and 18 of 55 (33%) on day 3 (see Additional file 3). These patients were able to be classified as having abnormal diastolic function in 94 and 89% on day 1 and day 3 with the 2016 guidelines, compared with 50 and 28% with the 2009 guidelines, with the remainder being indeterminate (see Fig. 3). This demonstrates poor agreement between the two guidelines with the kappa coefficient on day 1 of 0.26 ($p = 0.004$) and 0.07 on day 3 ($p = 0.34$).

There were 44 patients on day 1 with a normal ejection fraction. Using the 2016 ASE/EACVI guidelines, 11 (25%) patients had normal diastolic function, with 20

(45%) having diastolic dysfunction and 13 (30%) unable to be determined, whereas using the 2009 guidelines 7% were normal, 9% had diastolic dysfunction and 84% were indeterminate (see Fig. 4). There was poor agreement between the 2009 and 2016 diastolic dysfunction guidelines (kappa coefficient 0.18, $p = 0.004$).

Of those with normal diastolic function on day 1 according to the 2016 guidelines, 3 proceeded to diastolic dysfunction on day 3, with another 2 having indeterminate diastolic function. Seven of the indeterminate patients on day 1 progressed to definite diastolic dysfunction, with 5 having evidence of raised left atrial pressure (grade 2 or 3) on day 3.

On day 3, out of the 37 patients with normal systolic function, 11 (30%) had normal diastolic function, 20 (54%) had diastolic dysfunction and 6 (16%) were indeterminate according to the 2016 guidelines, compared to 8% normal, 16% with diastolic dysfunction and 76% indeterminate using the 2009 guidelines (Fig. 4). Again, this demonstrated poor agreement between the two guidelines (kappa coefficient 0.13, $p = 0.005$). Those with normal systolic function but abnormal diastolic dysfunction tended to be older compared with patients with normal

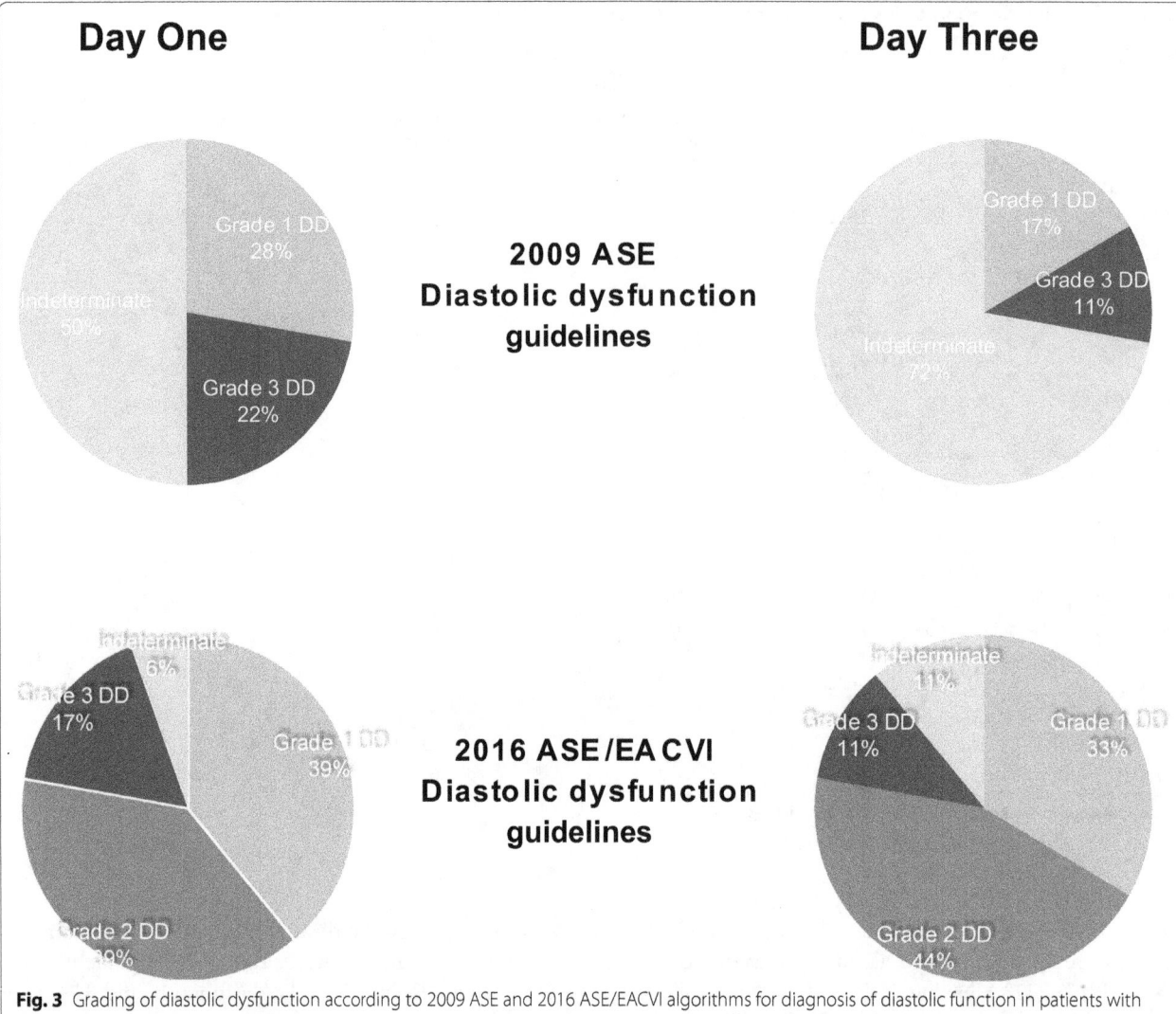

Fig. 3 Grading of diastolic dysfunction according to 2009 ASE and 2016 ASE/EACVI algorithms for diagnosis of diastolic function in patients with abnormal systolic function on day 1 and day 3

diastolic function on both days. There was no significant difference in noradrenaline requirements, heart rates, SOFA scores, PEEP, or mechanical ventilation on either day 1 (see Table 1) or day 3. Echocardiography parameters for patients with normal systolic function on day 1 are included in Table 2.

Discussion

Our results demonstrate an increased detection of diastolic dysfunction in patients with severe sepsis and septic shock using more recent 2016 ASE/EACVI guidelines as compared with the 2009 ASE version. In the absence of a gold standard for diastolic dysfunction, it is unknown whether this is a true reflection of the patient's diastolic function. However, given the 2009 ASE guidelines have a significant higher percentage of patients with

indeterminate diastolic dysfunction compared to the 2016 guidelines, the new guidelines appear to have an improved clinical applicability and should form the reference standard for use in this cohort and in further research in this field. The limitations of the 2009 guidelines are supported by prior studies [13] [7].

There are several advantages in the current guidelines that increase their ability to be applied to patients with severe sepsis and septic shock. Firstly, the recognition that those with systolic dysfunction must have impaired relaxation is an important distinction backed up with long-standing evidence [22]. Previous research regarding diastolic dysfunction in severe sepsis and septic shock has not made this important distinction. Secondly, there is increased flexibility in recognizing that not all parameters may be present in any one patient, which

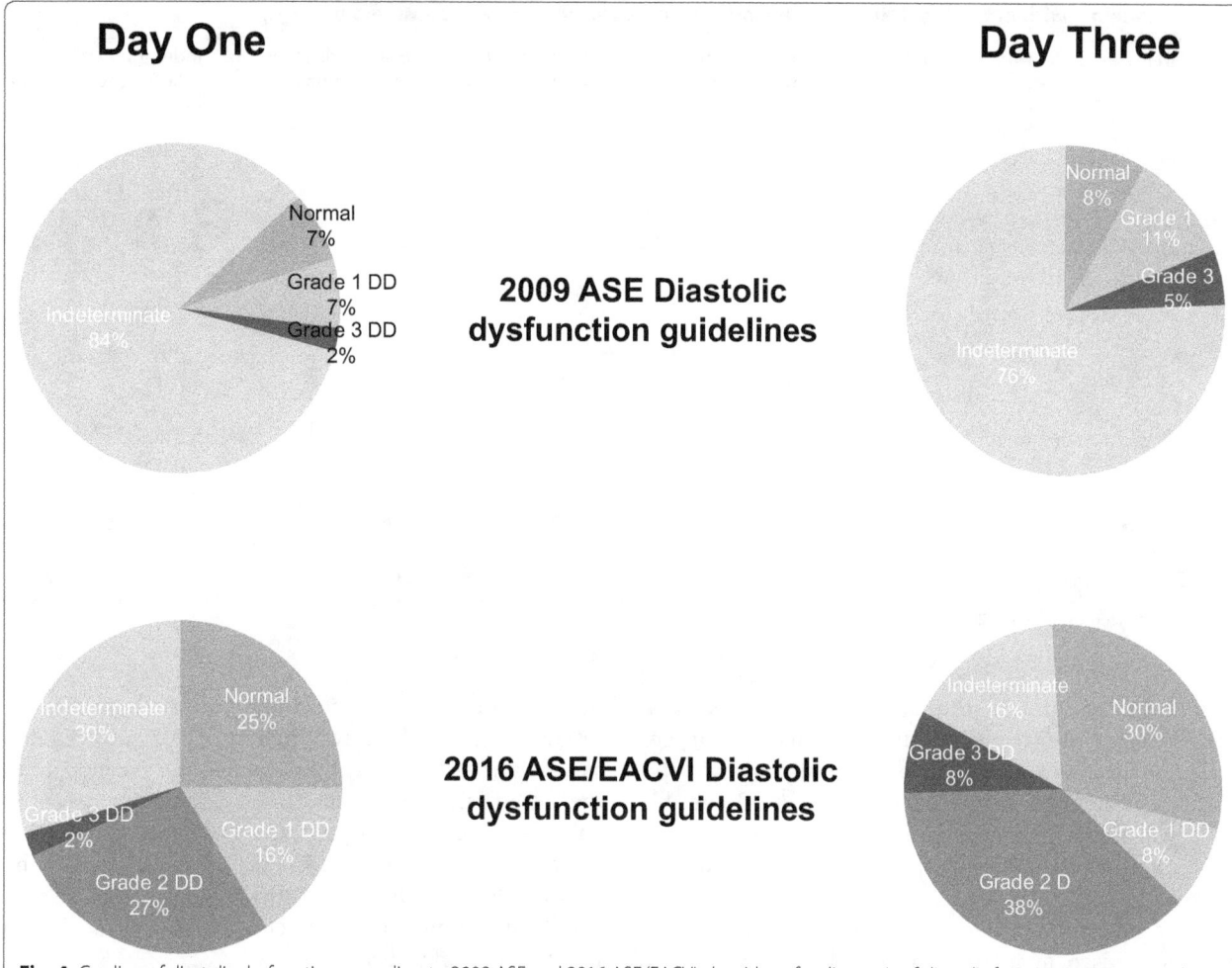

Fig. 4 Grading of diastolic dysfunction according to 2009 ASE and 2016 ASE/EACVI algorithms for diagnosis of diastolic function in patients with normal systolic function on days 1 and 3

is particularly important when applying the criteria to acute situations. Finally, we note that all of the parameters in this guideline are relatively easy to measure if the clinician is aware of the pitfalls and maintains due diligence with measurements as part of the rigour required for accurately assessing diastolic function. Subsequently, there is less emphasis on parameters that may be difficult to perform in the critically ill or have significant caveats (Valsalva manoeuvres, pulmonary venous Doppler, deceleration time) when compared to the 2009 guidelines.

The presence of diastolic dysfunction in severe sepsis and septic shock has significant clinical implications and hence the importance of a structured diagnostic algorithm as provided by the 2016 ASE/EACVI guidelines. Several studies and a subsequent meta-analysis [4] have indicated an increase in mortality in those patients with diastolic dysfunction, although the current study raises questions about the manner of diagnosis leading to such a conclusion in these studies. One of the many

hypotheses surrounding the improved outcomes in the use of beta blockade and noradrenergic sparing agents (i.e. vasopressin) in severe sepsis is that lowering the heart rate may improve diastolic function [23–25]. This may be important as the proposed increased efficiency of diastolic filling in tachycardia (frequency-dependent acceleration of relaxation) is limited in sepsis [26]. One of the largest studies to date highlighted that left ventricular diastolic dysfunction (but not systolic function) had a significant correlation with raised troponins in severe sepsis, which is known to be a predictor of mortality [3]. This relationship of raised troponins and diastolic dysfunction may reflect impaired myocardial relaxation from myocardial oxygen supply demand imbalance, which in turn may be a function of excessive catecholamines, tachycardia or microvascular dysfunction. This potential ischaemia resulting in diastolic dysfunction makes it imperative that myocardial work and oxygen demand are reduced. However, we feel the research to date is significantly impaired

Table 2 Patients with normal systolic function and their echocardiographic parameters on day 1

Echo parameter	Normal diastolic function $n = 11$ (25%)	Grade I diastolic dysfunction $n = 7$ (16%)	Grade 2 diastolic dysfunction $n = 12$ (27%)	Grade 3 diastolic dysfunction ($n = 1$) (2%)	Indeterminate diastolic function ($n = 13$) (30%)
Septal hypertrophy	0	7 (100%)	5 (42%)	0	4 (31%)
$E/e' > 14$	0	0	8 (67%)	1 (100%)	3 (23%)
Mean E/e'	9.5 ± 2.4	10 ± 2.3	15.6 ± 4.6	22.4	13 ± 4.9
Septal $e' < 7$ cm/s (n)	6 (55%)	5 (71%)	10 (83%)	1	10 (77%)
Septal e' (cm/s)	0.08 ± 0.02	0.06 ± 0.02	0.055 ± 0.01	0.03	0.055 ± 0.01
Lateral $e' < 10$ cm/s (n)	5 (45%)	4 (57%)	11 (92%)	1	10 (77%)
Mean lateral e' (cm/s)	0.09 ± 0.03	0.08 ± 0.03	0.08 ± 0.02	0.07	0.085 ± 0.02
Increased left atrial volume (n)	3 (27%)	3 (43%)	11 (92%)	1	8 (67%)
Mean left atrial volume (ml)	51 ± 12	52 ± 20	87.5 ± 29	111	56 ± 15
TR velocity > 2.8 (n)	1 (9%)	0 (0%)	9 (75%)	1	0
TR velocity average (m/s)	2.43 (1.97,2.67)	2.4 (1.6, 2.74)	2.96 (2.8, 3.22)	3.29	2.35 (2.2, 2.52)
Cardiac output (L/min)	5.5 ± 1.5	6.9 ± 2.6	6.2 ± 1.65	N/A	6.05 ± 1.2

Diastolic dysfunction assessed by 2016 ASE/EACVI guidelines

due to the lack of a uniform approach to the detection and diagnosis of diastolic dysfunction, which is particularly evident in the meta-analysis by Sanfilippo et al. [4].

It is important for the critical care physician to be able to detect diastolic dysfunction in patients with severe sepsis and septic shock. Despite the relative improved diagnostic capabilities of the 2016 ASE/EACVI guidelines, significant challenges still remain. Firstly, each parameter used in the current guidelines is subject to several caveats. Examples of this include preload dependence [27], the effects of positive pressure ventilation [28] on mitral inflow velocity, and the angle dependence of tissue Doppler [29]. Secondly, several of the parameters are surrogate markers of left atrial pressure, which may not increase acutely in the setting of impaired myocardial relaxation, particularly in sepsis where cardiac dysfunction may exist in the absence of raised filling pressures. For example, there is little known regarding the ability of the left atrium to increase its volume in response to acute changes in pressure due to varying atrial compliance. This is not to discount the value of left atrial volume from the algorithm, as a raised left atrial volume is important if present in differentiating diastolic dysfunction from indeterminate diastolic function. Features of raised left atrial pressure may not be present early in the setting of de novo impaired myocardial relaxation. Herein lies one of the issues when detecting diastolic dysfunction in the critically ill: are we concerned with features of left atrial pressure (which in itself is different to left ventricular end diastolic pressure) which may not be demonstrated early in the patient with de novo diastolic dysfunction

due to sepsis, or is the detection of impaired myocardial relaxation (as in e') more important [12]? Furthermore, as recognized by the authors of the current guidelines the cut-off values of parameters used, including that of e', have been validated in patients who are at rest and are not currently under stressed states, as may be seen in the critically ill [16]. Detecting impaired myocardial relaxation in the hyperdynamic circulation is difficult due to the strict cut-off values.

Myocardial relaxation and diastolic function will be abnormal in the setting of systolic dysfunction. This is evident with only 6 and 11% of patients with abnormal systolic function on day 1 and day 3, respectively, having indeterminate diastolic dysfunction (per the 2016 guidelines). Issues may arise, however, when trying to assess the patient with normal systolic function, as noted by the increased proportion of patients with indeterminate diastolic dysfunction in this cohort. Despite the aforementioned limitations, it is the opinion of the authors that future research in this field could use the 2016 ASE/EACVI guidelines as a reference standard for the diagnosis and detection of diastolic dysfunction. By having a consistent framework for the definition of diastolic dysfunction, further research will be strengthened. Such research may revolve around the association with mortality (particularly those with normal systolic function), the impact of fluid balances, ventilation, beta blockade therapy and the comparative use of novel modalities for detecting diastolic dysfunction.

Our study has several limitations. This is a single-centre study and although performed in a unit with an active echocardiographic service, it was not always possible to recruit suitable study patients. A significant proportion of patients with indeterminate diastolic dysfunction based on the 2016 guidelines on day 3 had missing data, which may have changed their grading. Further, a significant proportion of those with normal systolic function had increased myocardial wall thickness, indicating that they would likely have had diastolic dysfunction prior to their ICU presentation. Attempts to clarify pre-existing diastolic dysfunction by searching through patient's history revealed limited documentation of pre-existing diastolic dysfunction. The authors have not performed a comparison of the two guidelines in ability to predict mortality as firstly, the sample size is too small and secondly the impetus was to focus on how diastolic dysfunction is defined in this cohort, something which is a significant limitation of previous research. Based on our findings, the 2016 ASE/EACVI guidelines could be used in further research to detect if diastolic dysfunction does affect prognosis in severe sepsis and septic shock.

Conclusion

The 2016 ASE/EACVI guidelines on assessing diastolic function identify a significantly higher incidence of dysfunction in patients with severe sepsis and septic shock compared to the previous 2009 guidelines. Despite limitations, the 2016 ASE/EACVI recommendations appear to have an improved clinical applicability in septic patients relative to the 2009 ASE guidelines. Difficulties remain with recognition of impaired diastolic function in this cohort, particularly those with normal systolic function. Previously published prognostic studies based on diastolic dysfunction in septic patients need to be interpreted with the above findings in mind.

Abbreviations

A: late diastolic velocity of mitral inflow; Ar-a: difference between duration of atrial wave on pulmonary venous Doppler and at mitral annulus; ASE: American Society of Echocardiography; ASE/EACVI: American Society of Echocardiography/European Association of Cardiovascular Imaging; CI: confidence interval; DT: deceleration time; *E*: early diastolic velocity of mitral inflow; *e'*: early diastolic myocardial tissue velocity; *E/A*: ratio of early to late diastolic velocity of mitral inflow; *s'*: peak systolic myocardial velocity; *E/e'*: ratio of early diastolic mitral inflow velocity to early diastolic myocardial tissue velocity; EF: ejection fraction; LA: left atrium; LV: left ventricle; IQR: interquartile range; PEEP: positive end expiratory pressure; SD: standard deviation; SOFA: sepsis-relating organ failure assessment; TDI: tissue Doppler imaging; TR: tricuspid regurgitation.

Authors' contributions

DC made contributions to conception, design, statistical analysis and interpretation of data and prepared the manuscript. TS contributed to the data collation and interpretation and the drafting of the manuscript. MS assisted with data interpretation and drafting of the manuscript. SH assisted with statistical analysis and drafting of the manuscript. AM made contributions to the conception and design of the study and made significant contributions to the drafting and revision of the manuscript. SO designed and conceived of the study, acquired data including performing echocardiographs, analysis of the data and preparation of the manuscript. All authors read and approved the final manuscript.

Author details
[1] ICU, Nepean Hospital, Kingswood, NSW 2747, Australia. [2] Medical ICU, Amiens University Hospital, Amiens, France.

Acknowledgements
The authors would like to acknowledge Ms. Iris Ting, Ms. Louise Smith and Ms. Euguenia Kholodniak of the Nepean Intensive Care Cardiovascular Ultrasound Laboratory for their expertise and skill in assisting in acquiring echocardiography studies.

Competing interests
The authors declare that they have no competing interests.

Funding
Not applicable.

References

1. Pulido JN, Afessa B, Masaki M, Yuasa T, Gillespie S, Herasevich V, et al. Clinical spectrum, frequency, and significance of myocardial dysfunction in severe sepsis and septic shock. JMCP. 2012;87(7):620–8.
2. Huang SJ, Nalos M, McLean AS. Is early ventricular dysfunction or dilatation associated with lower mortality rate in adult severe sepsis and septic shock? A meta-analysis. Crit Care. 2013;17(3):R96.
3. Landesberg G, Jaffe AS, Gilon D, Levin PD, Goodman S, Abu-Baih A, et al. Troponin elevation in severe sepsis and septic shock. Crit Care Med. 2014;42(4):790–800.
4. Sanfilippo F, Corredor C, Fletcher N, Landesberg G, Benedetto U, Foex P, et al. Diastolic dysfunction and mortality in septic patients: a systematic review and meta-analysis. Intensive Care Med. 2015;41:1004–13.
5. Munt B, Jue J, Gin K, Fenwick J, Tweeddale M. Diastolic filling in human severe sepsis: an echocardiographic study. Crit Care Med. 1998;26(11):1829–33.
6. Rolando G, Espinoza EDV, Avid E, Welsh S, Pozo JD, Vazquez AR, et al. Prognostic value of ventricular diastolic dysfunction in patients with severe sepsis and septic shock. Revista Brasileira de Terapia Intensiva. 2015;27(4):1–7.
7. Brown SM, Pittman JE, Hirshberg EL, Jones JP, Lanspa MJ, Kuttler KG, et al. Diastolic dysfunction and mortality in early severe sepsis and septic shock: a prospective, observational echocardiography study. Crit Ultrasound J. 2012;4(1):1.
8. Bouhemad B, Nicolas-Robin A, Arbelot C, Arthaud M, Féger F, Rouby J-J. Isolated and reversible impairment of ventricular relaxation in patients with septic shock. Crit Care Med. 2008;36(3):766–74.
9. De Geer L, Engvall J, Oscarsson A. Strain echocardiography in septic shock - a comparison with systolic and diastolic function parameters, cardiac biomarkers and outcome. Crit Care. 2015;19:122.
10. Mourad M, Chow-Chine L, Faucher M, Sannini A, Brun JP, de Guibert JM, et al. Early diastolic dysfunction is associated with intensive care unit mortality in cancer patients presenting with septic shock. Br J Anaesth. 2013;112(1):102–9.
11. Sturgess DJ, Marwick TH, Joyce C, Jenkins C, Jones M, Masci P, et al. Prediction of hospital outcome in septic shock: a prospective comparison of tissue Doppler and cardiac biomarkers. Crit Care. 2010;14(2):R44-11.
12. Sanfilippo F, Corredor C, Arcadipane A, Landesberg G, Vieillard-Baron A, Cecconi M, et al. Tissue Doppler assessment of diastolic function and rela-

tionship with mortality in critically ill septic patients: a systematic review and meta-analysis. Br J Anaesth. 2017;119(4):583–94.

13. Lanspa MJ, Gutsche AR, Wilson EL, Olsen TD, Hirshberg EL, Knox DB, et al. Application of a simplified definition of diastolic function in severe sepsis and septic shock. Crit Care. 2016;20(1):243.

14. Nagueh SF, Appleton CP, Gillebert TC, Marino PN, Oh JK, Smiseth OA, et al. Recommendations for the evaluation of left ventricular diastolic function by echocardiography. J Am Soc Echocardiogr. 2009;22(2):107–33.

15. Pritchett AM, Mahoney DW, Jacobsen SJ, Rodeheffer RJ, Karon BL, Redfield MM. Diastolic dysfunction and left atrial volume: a population-based study. JAC. 2005;45(1):87–92.

16. Nagueh S, Smiseth O, Appleton C, Byrd B, Dokainish H, Edvardsen T, et al. Recommendations for the evaluation of left ventricular diastolic function by echocardiography: an update from the American Society of Echocardiography and the European Association of Cardiovascular Imaging. J Am Soc Echocardiogr. 2016;29(4):277–314.

17. Dellinger RP, Levy MM, Rhodes A, Annane D, Gerlach H, Opal SM, et al. Surviving sepsis campaign: international guidelines for management of severe sepsis and septic shock, 2012. Intensive Care Med. 2013;41(2):580–637.

18. Shankar-Hari M, Phillips GS, Levy ML, Seymour CW, Liu VX, Deutschman CS, et al. Developing a new definition and assessing new clinical criteria for septic shock: for the third international consensus definitions for sepsis and septic shock (sepsis-3). JAMA. 2016;315(8):775–87.

19. Dhutia NM, Zolgharni M, Willson K, Cole G, Nowbar AN, Dawson D, et al. Guidance for accurate and consistent tissue Doppler velocity measurement: comparison of echocardiographic methods using a simple vendor-independent method for local validation. Eur Heart J Cardiovasc Imaging. 2014;15(7):817–27.

20. Flack VF, Afifi AA. Sample size determinations for the two rater kappa statistic. Psychometrika. 1988;53:321–5.

21. Lang R, Badano L, Mor-Avi V, Afilalo J, Armstrong A, Ernande E, et al. Recommendations for cardiac chamber quantification by echocardiography in adults: an update from the American Society of Echocardiography and the European Association of Cardiovascular Imaging. J Am Soc Echocardiogr. 2015. https://doi.org/10.1016/j.echo.2014.10.003.21.

22. Papapietro S, Coghlan C. Impaired maximal rate of left ventricular relaxation in patients with coronary artery disease and left ventricular dysfunction. Circulation. 1979;59(5):984–91.

23. Russell J, Walley K, Singer J, Gordon A, Hebert P, Cooper J, et al. Vasopressin versus norepinephrine infusion in patients with septic shock. NEJM. 2008;358:877–87.

24. Morelli A, Ertmer C, Westphal M, Rehberg S, Kampmeier T, Ligges S, et al. Effect of heart rate control with esmolol on hemodynamic and clinical outcomes in patients with septic shock. JAMA. 2013;310(16):1683–9.

25. Astuto M. Sepsis and beta-blockade: a look into diastolic function. Curr Med Res Opin. 2015;31(10):1827–8.

26. Joulin O, Marechaux S, Hassoun S, Montaigne D, Lancel S, Neviere R. Cardiac force-frequency relationship and frequency-dependent acceleration of relaxation are impaired in LPS-treated rats. Crit Care. 2009;13(1):R14.

27. Vignon P, Allot V, Lesage J, Martaillé J-F, Aldigier J-C, François B, et al. Diagnosis of left ventricular diastolic dysfunction in the setting of acute changes in loading conditions. Crit Care. 2007;11(2):R43.

28. Faehnrich JA, Noone RB, White WD, Leone BJ, Hilton AK, Sreeram GM, et al. Effects of positive-pressure ventilation, pericardial effusion, and cardiac tamponade on respiratory variation in transmitral flow velocities. YJCAN. 2003;17(1):45–50.

29. Storaa C, Aberg P, Lind B, Brodin L-A. Effect of angular error on tissue Doppler velocities and strain. Echocardiography. 2003;20(7):581–7.

4

Acute kidney injury in major abdominal surgery: incidence, risk factors, pathogenesis and outcomes

Joana Gameiro*, José Agapito Fonseca, Marta Neves, Sofia Jorge and José António Lopes

Abstract

Acute kidney injury (AKI) is a common complication in patients undergoing major abdominal surgery. Various recent studies using modern standardized classifications for AKI reported a variable incidence of AKI after major abdominal surgery ranging from 3 to 35%. Several patient-related, procedure-related factors and postoperative complications were identified as risk factors for AKI in this setting. AKI following major abdominal surgery has been shown to be associated with poor short- and long-term outcomes. Herein, we provide a contemporary and critical review of AKI after major abdominal surgery focusing on its incidence, risk factors, pathogeny and outcomes.

Keywords: Acute kidney injury, Postoperative, Incidence, Prognosis, Risk factors, Pathogenesis

Background

Acute kidney injury (AKI) is a common occurrence in hospitalized patients and it has a detrimental effect on patient outcome. Indeed, AKI is associated with increased costs, length of hospital stay and in-hospital mortality [1–3]. Postoperative AKI has been associated with higher risk of developing chronic kidney disease (CKD) [4, 5] and increased early [6–17] and long-term mortality [10–22], comparable to the consequences of AKI facing critically ill patients. Postoperative AKI is hence of particular interest, serving as a measurable indicator of perioperative harm and an important potential target for intervention [23].

The clinical characteristics and the impact of AKI in cardiac surgery have been extensively studied [24, 25], and most of the published data regarding AKI in the non-cardiac surgery population are limited to high-risk aortic procedures [26–31]. Abdominal surgery is frequently associated with AKI. Recently, a number of studies have addressed AKI following major abdominal surgery [11, 19, 32, 33], especially since it shows a pathophysiology that is distinct from that of cardiac and vascular surgery. Therefore, it is unsuitable to assume that the risk factors for AKI after abdominal surgery are the same as those after cardiac and vascular surgery. The purpose of this review is therefore to perform a critical and contemporary review of the incidence, risk factors, pathogenesis and outcome of AKI in patients undergoing major non-vascular abdominal surgery.

Incidence, risk factors and pathogenesis

Incidence

Over the last decade, the definition of AKI has evolved from the former term acute renal failure to a set of uniform criteria combining small changes in creatinine and urine output ultimately defining AKI [34]. The first definition of AKI, the Risk, Injury, Failure, Loss of kidney function and End-stage kidney disease (RIFLE) classification, was published in 2004 [35]. In 2007, the Acute Kidney Injury Network (AKIN) classification, also known as 'modified RIFLE', was published [36]. In recent times, the RIFLE and AKIN classifications have been merged into the Kidney Disease: Improving Global Outcomes (KDIGO) classification in order to provide simpler and more integrated criteria applicable in clinical activity, research, and public health surveillance. (Table 1) [37] AKI is thus defined as an increase in serum creatinine

*Correspondence: joana.estrelagameiro@gmail.com
Division of Nephrology and Renal Transplantation, Department of Medicine, Centro Hospitalar Lisboa Norte, EPE, Av. Prof. Egas Moniz, 1649-035 Lisbon, Portugal

Table 1 Risk, Injury, Failure, Loss of kidney function, End-stage kidney disease (RIFLE) [35], Acute Kidney Injury Network (AKIN) [36], and kidney disease improving global outcomes (KDIGO) [37] classifications

Class/stage	SCr/GFR			UO		
	RIFLE	AKIN	KDIGO	RIFLE	AKIN	KDIGO
Risk/1[a]	↑ SCr × 1.5 or ↓ GFR > 25%	↑ SCr ≥ 26.5 μmol/l (≥ 0.3 mg/dl) or ↑ SCr ≥ 150–200% (1.5–2X)	↑ SCr ≥ 26.5 μmol/l (≥ 0.3 mg/dl) or ↑ SCr ≥ 150–200% (1.5–2X)	<0.5 ml/kg/h (> 6 h)	<0.5 ml/kg/h (> 6 h)	<0.5 ml/kg/h (> 6 h)
Injury/2[a]	↑ SCr X 2 or ↓ GFR > 50%	↑ SCr > 200–300% (> 2–3X)	↑ SCr > 200–300% (> 2–3X)	<0.5 ml/kg/h (> 12 h)	<0.5 ml/kg/h (> 12 h)	<0.5 ml/kg/h (> 12 h)
Failure/3[a]	↑ SCr X 3 or ↓ GFR > 75% or if baseline SCr ≥ 353.6 μmol/l (≥ 4 mg/dl) ↑ SCr > 44.2 μmol/l (> 0.5 mg/dl)	↑ SCr > 300% (> 3X) or if baseline SCr ≥ 353.6 μmol/l (≥ 4 mg/dl) ↑ SCr ≥ 44.2 μmol/l (≥ 0.5 mg/dl) or initiation of renal replacement therapy	↑ SCr > 300% (> 3X) or ↑ SCr to ≥ 353.6 μmol/l (≥ 4 mg/dl) or initiation of renal replacement therapy	<0.3 ml/kg/h (> 24 h) or anuria (> 12 h)	<0.3 ml/kg/h (24 h) or anuria (12 h)	<0.3 ml/kg/h (24 h) or anuria (12 h)

SCr serum creatinine, *GFR* glomerular filtration rate, *UO* urine output, *RIFLE* Risk, Injury, Failure, Loss of kidney function (dialysis dependence for at least 4 weeks), End-stage kidney disease (dialysis dependence for at least 3 months), *AKIN* Acute Kidney Injury Network, *KDIGO* kidney disease improving global outcomes

[a] Risk class (RIFLE) corresponds to stage 1 (AKIN and KDIGO), injury class (RIFLE) corresponds to stage 2 (AKIN and KDIGO), and failure class (RIFLE) corresponds to stage 3 (AKIN and KDIGO)

(SCr) by $\geq$ 0.3 mg/dl ($\geq$ 26.5 µmol/l) within 48 h; or an increase in SCr to $\geq$ 1.5 times the baseline value, which is known or presumed to have occurred within the prior 7 days; or urine volume < 0.5 ml/kg/h for 6 h [38]. These classifications also categorize patients according to the severity of AKI [38].

In the past decades, the incidence of AKI has suffered an increase and has been related to multiple factors such as an increasingly aging population, increasing number of comorbidities of the hospitalized population, increased prevalence of chronic kidney disease and diabetes, and the liberal use of intravenous contrast agents for imaging and cardiovascular intervention procedures [39].

Additionally, mortality has been trending downwards despite the reported modifications in the clinical profile and characteristics of patients with AKI [40, 41]. Nonetheless, it is not clear if this fact can be credited to an improvement in patient care or to specific interventions or therapies directed at those with AKI [42, 43].

Depending on the classification system employed in the studies, the reported incidence of AKI varies from 5.0 to 7.5% in hospitalized patients, reaching up to 50–60% in critically ill patients [2, 44–46].

Surgery remains a leading cause of AKI in hospitalized patients, accounting for up to 40% of in-hospital AKI cases. The incidence of AKI in this group of patients is variable, depending on the surgical setting and the AKI definition used, with the highest rates found after cardiac (18.7%), general (13.2%), and thoracic (12.0%) surgeries [47, 48].

A considerable heterogeneity regarding the rate of AKI reported has been shown in recent studies of AKI following major abdominal surgery. (Table 2) The incidence varied between 3.1 and 35.3%, with the majority of patients in all studies placing in the less severe stage of AKI (Risk or Stage 1). One of the major limitations of these studies is that, only three evaluated simultaneously serum creatinine and urine output to define and categorize AKI, as recommended [35].

Urine output (UO) is a sensitive and early marker for AKI, independent of serum creatinine, thereby included as a criterion to diagnose AKI [49, 50]. However, recent literature reports that there is a physiologic reduction in UO as a result from hypovolemia, anesthesia and release of aldosterone and vasopressin in response to stress, which raises the hypothesis that UO may not be a reliable criterion for postoperative AKI, or that the threshold for AKI diagnosis with UO should be lower [51–53].

Research has focused on serum and urine biomarkers that could predict AKI before functional damage occurs [54]. This has been investigated mainly in cardiac procedures, with the most promising marker being plasma and urinary neutrophil gelatinase-associated lipocalin (NGAL) [54]. Also, the combination of urinary Kidney Injury Molecule-1 (KIM-1), N-acetyl-beta-D-glucosaminidase, and NGAL improved the sensitivity of early recognition of postoperative AKI when compared with individual biomarkers [55]. Recently, tissue inhibitor of metalloproteinases-2 (TIMP-2) and insulin-like growth factor binding protein 7 (IGFBP7) have been validated as risk predictors for AKI [56].

According to a recently published meta-analysis of 19 studies representing 82,514 patients undergoing abdominal surgery, the pooled incidence of AKI was 13.4% [23]. However, the incidence did not significantly vary by AKI definition, surgical category or inclusion or exclusion of preexisting CKD, demonstrating that other factors are probably also implied, such as the different surgical settings and baseline patient characteristics between individual studies [23].

Risk factors

A number of studies have investigated and identified patient- and procedure-related risk factors associated with the development of AKI, namely older age, African American race, hypertension, diabetes mellitus and CKD [20, 48]. Patient-related factors are often more strongly associated with postoperative mortality than surgical factors [57].

Focusing on major abdominal surgery, demographic patient characteristics such as male gender, older age, and higher body mass index, as well as preexisting CKD, hypertension, cardiovascular disease, diabetes, chronic obstructive pulmonary disease, metastatic cancer, hypoalbuminemia, use of angiotensin-converting enzyme inhibitors (ACEI) or angiotensin-receptor blockers have been implicated as predisposing to AKI [8, 9, 58–65].

Additionally, several risk assessment scores have been associated with higher incidence of AKI. A higher MELD score, which predicts liver failure progression; a higher Revised Cardiac Index score, developed to predict cardiac complications and mortality after major noncardiac surgery; and higher SAPS II score, used to evaluate disease severity, have all been independently associated with AKI [8, 63, 65, 66].

Numerous studies have established the negative bearing of surgery or procedure-related factors in AKI in major abdominal surgery, specifically the use of intravenous contrast for vascular imaging and intervention, the use of diuretics and vasopressors, more invasive procedures, episodes of intraoperative hemodynamic instability, need for intraoperative blood transfusions, large colloid infusion during surgery, epidural anesthesia in liver resections and cases of emergent surgery [8, 9, 58, 60–63, 65, 67–69].

Table 2 Incidence and categorization of AKI and its association with mortality after major abdominal surgery

Study	Design	Setting	Criteria	AKI definition	N	Incidence	Mortality	AUROC
Armstrong et al. [59]	Retrospective, single center	HBP	SCr	AKIN	1535	5.10% 1-4.0% 2-0.8% 3-0.3%	1.7% AKI versus 3.4% non-AKI, $P = 0.21$	NA
Bell et al. [58]	Interrupted time series analysis	MA/GI	SCr	KDIGO	3271	9.80%	NA	NA
Bihorac et al. [20]	Retrospective, single center	MA/GI	SCr	RIFLE	2337	39.3%	NA	NA
Biteker et al. [12]	Prospective, single center	MA/GI	SCr	RIFLE	510	6.7%	6.1% AKI versus 0.9% non-AKI, $P = 0.003$	NA
Brunelli et al. (2012)	Retrospective, single center	MA/GI	SCr	AKIN/RIFLE	1912	26.80%	NA	NA
Causey et al. [32]	Retrospective, single center	Colorectal	SCr	RIFLE	339	11.8%	6.30% AKI versus 0.9%, $P = 0.065$	NA
Chao et al. (2013)	Prospective, multicenter	MA/GI	SCr	AKIN	4240	23.1% 1-13.7% 2-1.8% 3-7.6%	28.40% 1-16% 2-29.7% 3-48.3% (HR 3.19, 95% CI 2.16-4.71; $P < 0.001$)	0.728
Cho et al. [4]	Prospective, single center	HBP	SCr, UO	AKIN	131	7.6% 1-3.8% 2-1.5% 3-2.3%	7.10% AKI versus 2.5% non-AKI, $P > 0.05$	NA
Coca et al. [98]	Retrospective, multicenter	Non cardiac surgery	SCr	AKIN	11.460	18.9% 1-5.2% 2-2.5% 3-1.2%	NA	NA
Correa-Gallego et al. [60]	Retrospective, single center	HBP	SCr	RIFLE	2166	15.5% R 12.8% I 2.3% F 0.4%	1% AKI versus 2% non-AKI, $P = 0.5$	NA
Grams et al. [89]	Retrospective, single center	MA/GI	SCr	KDIGO	44.597	13.2% 1-9.4% 2-2.2% 3-1.5%	IRR 6.40 (95% CI, 5.75, 7.12) $P < 0.05$)	NA
Kambakamba et al. [67]	Retrospective, single center	HBP	SCr	AKIN	829	8.2%	21% AKI versus 0.3% non-AKI, $P < 0.001$	0.765
Kim et al. [68]	Retrospective, single center	UGI	SCr	KDIGO	4718	14.4% 1-12.5% 2-1.3% 3-0.6%	3.8% AKI versus 0.3% non-AKI, $P < 0.001$ (OR, 8.75; 95% CI, 3.98-19.27; $P < 0.001$)	NA
Lee et al. [62]	Retrospective, single center	UGI	SCr	AKIN	595	35.3% 1-30.3% 2-2.7% 3-4.2%	4.80% AKI versus 2.1% non-AKI, $P = 0.115$	NA

Table 2 continued

Study	Design	Setting	Criteria	AKI definition	N	Incidence	Mortality	AUROC
Slankamenac et al. [64]	Retrospective, single center	HBP	SCr, UO	RIFLE	569	15.1%	22.5% AKI versus 0.8% non-AKI, $P < 0.001$	0.75
Sun et al. [69]	Retrospective, single center	GYN	SCr	AKIN	863	3.1%	NA	NA
Sun et al. [69]	Retrospective, single center	MA/GI	SCr	AKIN	1351	9.6%	NA	NA
Teixeira et al. [8]	Retrospective, single center	MA/GI	SCr, UO	KDIGO	450	22.4% 1–63.4% 2–19.8% 3–16.8%	20.8% AKI versus 2.3% non-AKI, $P < 0.001$; OR 3.7, 95% CI 1.2–11.7, $P = 0.024$	NA
Tomozawa et al. [65]	Retrospective, single center	HBP	SCr	AKIN	642	12.1% 1–9.8% 2–2.0% 3–0.3%	14.1% AKI versus 2.3% non-AKI, $P < 0.0001$	NA
Vaught et al. [9]	Retrospective, single center	GYN	SCr	RIFLE	2341	12.6% R–7.9% I–2.7% F–1.9%	10% AKI versus 0.5% non-AKI, $P < 0.0083$	0.88

GI gastrointestinal, HPB hepato-biliary, RIFLE risk, injury failure, loss, end stage, AKIN Acute Kidney Injury Network, KDIGO Kidney Disease Improving Global Outcomes, MA major abdominal, GYN gynecological, SCr serum creatinine, UO urinary output, IRR incidence rate ratio, NA not available

Nevertheless, the impact of the urgency of surgery has not been consensual in all studies. For instance, urgent surgery was not associated with an increased risk of postoperative AKI in a recent study by Teixeira et al. [8], despite the higher incidence of risk factors for AKI in these patients.

The role of laparoscopy has also been studied as the creation of a pneumoperitoneum is concomitant to increased intraabdominal pressure and the associated hormonal modifications that have been associated with decreased renal blood flow and could be linked to AKI [8]. Nevertheless, Teixeira et al. [8] demonstrated no difference in AKI between patients undergoing laparoscopy versus laparotomy.

O'Connor et al. [23] essayed to determine AKI incidence in different surgical settings, namely gastrointestinal, upper gastrointestinal, hepato-biliary, colorectal and major gynecological surgeries, however they were not able to demonstrate a significant difference in pooled AKI between these subgroups due to substantial heterogeneity between the studies. Similarly, in the study by Teixeira et al., colorectal surgery had an increased rate of AKI, which was not evidenced in other surgery types such as gastric, hepato-biliary and pancreatic, small bowel and esophageal. However, this finding was not independently associated with a higher risk of postoperative AKI [8]. These studies did not analyze the incidence of AKI after liver transplant surgery which can reach up to 70%, as it includes several specific risk factors in its pathogenesis, namely those related to the recipient and graft [70, 71]. Also important to consider, with the increasing prevalence of obesity in the global population, the prevalence of bariatric surgery has risen in the past decades and AKI has also been reported in 5–10% of these patients [72, 73].

Growing evidence has demonstrated that the need for intraoperative blood transfusions may contribute to organ injury in susceptible patients by promoting a pro-inflammatory state, exacerbating tissue oxidative stress, and activating leukocytes and the coagulation cascade, thus impairing oxygen delivery paradoxically [74–76].

Colloids have been used for acute fluid resuscitation in trauma, perioperatively and in critically ill patients, due to their longer intravascular persistence. Recent studies have shown no evidence of a significant mortality benefit from resuscitation with colloids [77–81]. In critically ill patients, the use of hydroxyethyl starch has been associated with AKI [77, 82]. However, this association has not been demonstrated in the surgical setting, namely after living donor hepatectomy, cardiac surgery, or gastroenterological surgery [83–85].

Furthermore, patients who developed significant postoperative complications, such as leak, respiratory failure and sepsis, also have an increased rate of AKI [58, 59, 61, 62] (Fig. 1).

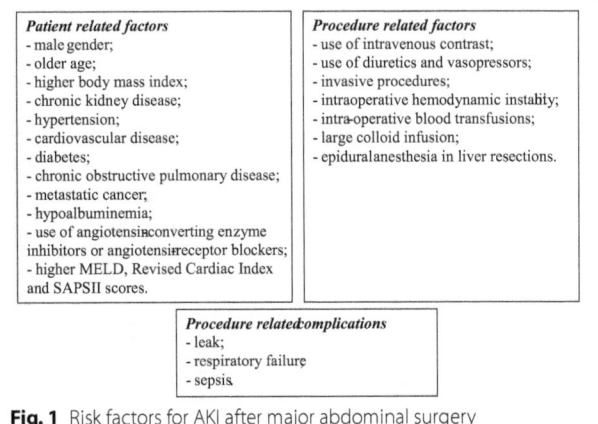

Patient related factors	Procedure related factors
- male gender; - older age; - higher body mass index; - chronic kidney disease; - hypertension; - cardiovascular disease; - diabetes; - chronic obstructive pulmonary disease; - metastatic cancer; - hypoalbuminemia; - use of angiotensin converting enzyme inhibitors or angiotensin receptor blockers; - higher MELD, Revised Cardiac Index and SAPSII scores.	- use of intravenous contrast; - use of diuretics and vasopressors; - invasive procedures; - intraoperative hemodynamic instability; - intra-operative blood transfusions; - large colloid infusion; - epidural anesthesia in liver resections.

Procedure related complications
- leak;
- respiratory failure
- sepsis.

Fig. 1 Risk factors for AKI after major abdominal surgery

Pathogenesis

The pathogenesis of postoperative AKI is complex and multifactorial. In this setting, we must consider not only the effects of fluid depletion, but also the neuroendocrine response to anesthesia and surgery itself [86, 87].

Fluid depletion includes the preoperative period as a result of the routine nil-by mouth regimens and the loss of fluid through concomitant pathology, and the perioperative period resulting from blood and intravascular fluid losses, insensible losses, and the so-called third space effect, through extravasation of fluid out of the vascular compartment. Mechanical ventilation of the intubated patient constitutes an additional mechanism for increased fluid loss during general anesthesia. The perioperative fluid requirements vary according to the extent of the surgical insult [86].

The renal response to hypoperfusion is afferent arteriole dilation and efferent arteriole vasoconstriction to maintain glomerular filtration in addition to neurohormonal responses as a means to expand the intravascular volume [57, 86, 87]. The increases in sympathomimetic hormones lead to renal cortical vasoconstriction, which is a compensatory attempt to redistribute blood flow to the renal medulla, but in fact causes ischemia of the medulla which is particularly vulnerable due to its elevated metabolic demand [57, 86, 87].

Most anesthetics cause peripheral vasodilatation and myocardial depression, also impairing kidney perfusion [86, 87]. The effect of the surgery results in both an increase in catabolic hormones and cytokines, leading to increased secretion of antidiuretic hormone, which will result in water retention. Increases in aldosterone, through activation of the renin–angiotensin system, associated with increased glucocorticoids cause sodium and water retention and potassium loss. Plasma renin activity is also elevated as a result of a decrease in circulating blood volume. Thus, adjustments in overall fluid and electrolyte homeostasis occur on account of impaired water excretion, impaired sodium excretion, and increased excretion of potassium [86].

Patients with long-term ACEI therapy have higher risk of postoperative renal dysfunction as a result of a loss of ability of the renin–angiotensin system to compensate for decreases in renal perfusion [86, 87].

Ischemic kidneys are more susceptible to continuing detrimental insults, such as, nephrotoxins and sepsis [86]. Nephrotoxins such as contrast media increase intrarenal vasoconstriction, decrease medullary blood supply and present the medullary nephrons with an increased osmotic load leading to an increased oxygen requirement in the presence of an already low tissue oxygen tension [88].

Nevertheless, in most cases, hemodynamic or toxic actions seem to be insufficient in the pathogenesis of AKI [89]. The role of nonhemodynamic factors, such as dysfunctional inflammatory cascades, oxidative stress, activation of proapoptotic pathways, differential molecular expression, and leukocyte trafficking, in AKI has been increasingly recognized [89, 90]. During abdominal surgery, a pro-inflammatory response is activated by the released endotoxin load from gut ischemia, impaired visceral perfusion, and portal endotoxaemia [91]. Furthermore, in the postischemic or reperfusion period there is further tubular injury caused by reactive oxygen species and tissue inflammation [90, 92]. The immune activation following AKI appears to negatively impact other organs [89].

Outcomes

Various studies have verified the deleterious impact of AKI on the early outcomes of patients, namely longer lengths of hospital stay, increased healthcare costs, increased mortality and an increased likelihood of discharge to an extended care facility [46, 93–97]. Granting that AKI patients may have more comorbidities than non-AKI patients, these do not appear to account for all of the increased early mortality associated with AKI [3, 46, 97, 98]. Other factors should perhaps be regarded since even increases in SCr considered as minor lead to worse outcomes [88, 97, 98]. Accordingly, AKI has been progressively more thought of as part of a systemic disease with underlying mechanisms that cause multiorgan dysfunction including the kidney, which could help explain the decreased survival observed in AKI patients [87, 99].

An observational study by Grams et al. demonstrated an association between postoperative AKI after major surgery and longer lengths of stay (15.8 vs 8.6 days) and higher rates of 30-day hospital readmission (21 vs 13%) [48].

The association between a higher incidence of other postoperative complications, increased length of stay, higher healthcare costs and increased hospital readmissions and postoperative AKI related to major abdominal surgery has also been widely described. Lee et al. performed a retrospective analysis of 595 esophageal cancer surgery patients and established that the extent of hospital stay was significantly longer in patients with AKI [62]. In a retrospective review of 339 colectomies by Causey et al., AKI development was associated with a 5-day increase in hospital length of stay and nearly doubled the rate of other infectious complications (56 vs 30%) [61]. Tomozawa et al. reported that AKI after liver resection surgery was correlated with prolonged length of stay, and increased rates of artificial ventilation, need for reintubation, and requirement for renal replacement therapy [65]. In a retrospective study by Kim et al. gastric surgery patients with AKI had significantly longer hospital stay and higher prevalence of intensive care unit (ICU) admission after the operation (mean 18.7 vs 12.0 days, $P < 0.001$; 9.1 vs 1.2%, $P < 0.001$, respectively) [67].

The influence of postoperative AKI on higher in-hospital and 30-day mortality has also been demonstrated after major abdominal surgery. Kim et al. conducted a retrospective study of 4718 gastric surgery patients and reported that the in-hospital and 3-month mortality for patients with AKI were significantly higher than those for patients without AKI (3.5 vs 0.2%, $P < 0.001$; 3.8 vs 0.3%, $P < 0.001$, respectively), and moreover that the rate of in-hospital and 3-month mortality increased with the advancement in the stage of AKI, in a stepwise manner [67]. In a retrospective analysis of 642 liver resection patients by Tomozawa et al., AKI was associated with increased mortality (14.1 vs 2.3%, $P < 0.0001$) [65]. In a study by Teixeira, et al., 450 major abdominal surgery patients were retrospectively studied and postoperative AKI was independently associated with increased in-hospital mortality (20.8 vs 2.3%, $P < .0001$; unadjusted OR 11.2, 95% CI 4.8–26.2, $P < .0001$; adjusted OR 3.7, 95% CI 1.2–11.7, $P = 0.024$), furthermore there was a direct relationship between more severe AKI and increased in-hospital mortality [8]. O'Connor has also recently reported a 12.6-fold relative mortality risk in patients with postoperative AKI after major abdominal surgery [23].

Additionally, it is known that the detrimental effects of AKI persist after hospitalization, with greater risk of developing CKD and increased long-term mortality in AKI patients [20, 100, 101]. Progression to CKD results from an inadequate resolution of the acute insult following AKI, with persistent inflammation, increased transformation of pericytes into myofibroblasts in response to tubular injury, and consequent build-up of extracellular matrix and vascular rarefaction, leading to permanent scarring in renal structure and changes in renal function [102]. The risk of development or progression of CKD occurs in proportion to the severity of AKI [103]. The increased risk of proteinuria and hypertension and GFR decline described after AKI are known risk factors for cardiovascular disease, and may contribute to the decrement in survival observed among AKI survivors [104–107].

The long-term effect of AKI in postoperative patients has also been described. In a retrospective cohort study of 10,518 patients with AKI discharged after a major surgery, Bihorac et al. [20] reported that even small changes in creatinine level during hospitalization were associated with an independent long-term risk of death. Also, Grams et al. [48] performed an observational study of 3.6 million veterans submitted to major surgery and described an association between postoperative AKI and 1-year end-stage renal disease (0.94 vs 0.05%), and mortality (19 vs 8%), with more severe stage of AKI relating to poorer outcomes.

In a retrospective cohort of 390 major abdominal surgery patients, Gameiro et al. [108] demonstrated that AKI was independently associated with worse renal outcomes, comprising renal function decline and/or long-term need for dialysis (47.2 vs 22.0%, $P < 0.0001$), as well as with mortality after hospital discharge (47.2 vs 20.5%, $P < 0.0001$).

Conclusion
AKI is a frequent occurrence following major abdominal surgery and is independently associated with both in-hospital and long-term mortality, as well as with a higher risk of progressing to CKD. Preventive strategies such as hemodynamics stabilization, fluid balance control, evasion of nephrotoxins, improved preoperative patient management (body weight reduction, hypertension, diabetes, cardiovascular and pulmonary disease control) and prevention/treatment of any postoperative complications encountered could potentially reduce postoperative AKI and thereby improve patient outcomes.

Abbreviations
AKI: acute kidney injury; CKD: chronic kidney disease; RIFLE: Risk, Injury, Failure, Loss of kidney function and End-stage kidney disease; AKIN: Acute Kidney Injury Network; KDIGO: Kidney Disease: Improving Global Outcomes; SCr: serum creatinine; UO: urine output; ACEI: angiotensin-converting enzyme inhibitors; MELD: Model for end-stage liver disease; SAPS II: Simplified Acute Physiology Score; ICU: intensive care unit; KIM-1: kidney injury molecule-1; NGAL: neutrophil gelatinase-associated lipocalin.

Authors' contributions
The authors participated as follows: JG and JAF drafted the article, SJ and MN revised the article, JAL revised the article and approved the final version to be submitted for publication. All authors read and approved the final manuscript.

Acknowledgements
None.

Competing interests
The authors declare that they have no competing interests.

References
1. Chertow G, Burdick E, Honour M, Bonventre J, Bates D. Acute kidney injury, mortality, length of stay, and costs in hospitalized patients. J Am Soc Nephrol. 2005;16(11):3365–70.
2. Uchino S, Kellum JA, Bellomo R, et al. Beginning and Ending Supportive Therapy for the Kidney (BEST Kidney) Investigators. Acute renal failure in critically ill patients: a multinational, multicenter study. JAMA. 2005;294(7):813–8.
3. Barrantes F, Tian J, Vazquez R, Amoateng-Adjepong Y, Manthous CA. Acute kidney injury criteria predict outcomes of critically ill patients. Crit Care Med. 2008;36:1397–403.
4. Cho E, Kim SC, Kim MG, Jo S-K, Cho W-Y, Kim H-K. The incidence and risk factors of acute kidney injury after hepatobiliary surgery: a prospective observational study. BMC Nephrol. 2014;15:169.
5. Ryden L, Sartipy U, Evans M, Holzmann MJ. Acute kidney injury after coronary artery bypass grafting and long-term risk of end-stage renal disease. Circulation. 2014;130:2005–11.
6. Elmistekawy E, McDonald B, Hudson C, et al. Clinical impact of mild acute kidney injury after cardiac surgery. Ann Thorac Surg. 2014;98:815–22.
7. Hobson C, Ozrazgat-Baslanti T, Kuxhausen A, et al. Cost and mortality associated with postoperative acute kidney injury. Ann Surg. 2015;261:1207–14.
8. Teixeira C, Rosa R, Rodrigues N, et al. Acute kidney injury after major abdominal surgery: a retrospective cohort analysis. Crit Care Res Pract. 2014;2014:132175.
9. Vaught A, Ozrazgat-Baslanti T, Javed A, et al. Acute kidney injury in major gynaecological surgery: an observational study. BJOG. 2015;122:1340–8.
10. Harris DG, Koo G, McCrone MP, et al. Acute kidney injury in critically ill vascular surgery patients is common and associated with increased mortality. Front Surg. 2015;2:8.
11. Abelha FJ, Botelho M, Fernandes V, et al. Determinants of post-operative acute kidney injury. Crit Care. 2009;13:R79.
12. Biteker M, Dayan A, Tekkesin AI, et al. Incidence, risk factors, and outcomes of perioperative acute kidney injury in noncardiac and nonvascular surgery. Am J Surg. 2014;207:53–9.
13. Drews JD, Patel HJ, Williams DM, et al. The impact of acute renal failure on early and late outcomes after thoracic aortic endovascular repair. Ann Thorac Surg. 2014;97:2027–33 (discussion 2033).
14. Kandler K, Jensen ME, Nilsson JC, et al. Acute kidney injury is independently associated with higher mortality after cardiac surgery. J Cardiothorac Vasc Anesth. 2014;28:1448–52.
15. Munoz-Garcia AJ, Munoz-Garcia E, Jimenez-Navarro MF, et al. Clinical impact of acute kidney injury on short- and long-term outcomes after transcatheter aortic valve implantation with the CoreValve prosthesis. J Cardiol. 2015;66:46–9.
16. Zhu JC, Chen SL, Jin GZ, et al. Acute renal injury after thoracic endovascular aortic repair of Stanford type B aortic dissection: incidence, risk factors, and prognosis. J Formos Med Assoc. 2014;113:612–9.
17. Pickering JW, James MT, Palmer SC. Acute kidney injury and prognosis after cardiopulmonary bypass: a meta-analysis of cohort studies. Am J Kidney Dis. 2015;65:283–93.

18. Adalbert S, Adelina M, Romulus T, et al. Acute kidney injury in peripheral arterial surgery patients: a cohort study. Ren Fail. 2013;35:1236–9.

19. Kheterpal S, Tremper KK, Englesbe MJ, et al. Predictors of post-operative acute renal failure after noncardiac surgery in patients with previously normal renal function. Anesthesiology. 2007;107:892–902.

20. Bihorac A, Yavas S, Subbiah S, et al. Long-term risk of mortality and acute kidney injury during hospitalization after major surgery. Ann Surg. 2009;249:851–8.

21. Hobson CE, Yavas S, Segal MS, et al. Acute kidney injury is associated with increased long-term mortality after cardiothoracic surgery. Circulation. 2009;119:2444–53.

22. Hansen MK, Gammelager H, Mikkelsen MM, et al. Postoperative acute kidney injury and five-year risk of death, myocardial infarction, and stroke among elective cardiac surgical patients: a cohort study. Crit Care. 2013;17:R292.

23. O'Connor M, Kirwan C, Pearse R, Prowle JR. Incidence and associations of acute kidney injury after major abdominal surgery. Intensive Care Med. 2016;42(4):521–30.

24. Sirvinskas E, Andrejaitiene J, Raliene L, et al. Cardiopulmonary bypass management and acute renal failure: risk factors and prognosis. Perfusion. 2008;23(6):323–7.

25. De Santo LS, Romano G, Galdieri N, et al. RIFLE criteria for acute kidney injury in valvular surgery. J Heart Valve Dis. 2010;19(1):139–47 **(discussion 148)**.

26. Svensson L, Crawford E, Hess K, Coselli J, Safi H. Experience with 1509 patients undergoing thoracoabdominal aortic operations. J Vasc Surg. 1993;17(2):357–68 **(discussion 368–70)**.

27. Svensson L, Coselli J, Safi H, Hess K, Crawford E. Appraisal of adjuncts to prevent acute renal failure after surgery on the thoracic or thoracoabdominal aorta. J Vasc Surg. 1989;10(3):230–9.

28. Wald R, Waikar S, Liangos O, Pereira B, Chertow G, Jaber B. Acute renal failure after endovascular vs open repair of abdominal aortic aneurysm. J Vasc Surg. 2006;43(3):460–6 **(discussion 466)**.

29. Tallgren M, Niemi T, Pöyhiä R, et al. Acute renal injury and dysfunction following elective abdominal aortic surgery. Eur J Vasc Endovasc Surg. 2007;33(5):550–5.

30. Arnaoutakis G, Bihorac A, Martin T, et al. RIFLE criteria for acute kidney injury in aortic arch surgery. J Thorac Cardiovasc Surg. 2007;134(6):1554–60 **(discussion 1560–1)**.

31. Mori Y, Sato N, Kobayashi Y, Ochiai R. Acute kidney injury during aortic arch surgery under deep hypothermic circulatory arrest. J Anesth. 2011;25(6):799–804.

32. Causey M, Maykel J, Hatch Q, Miller S, Steele S. Identifying risk factors for renal failure and myocardial infarction following colorectal surgery. J Surg Res. 2011;170(1):32–7.

33. Cho A, Lee J, Kwon G, et al. Post-operative acute kidney injury in patients with renal cell carcinoma is a potent risk factor for new-onset chronic kidney disease after radical nephrectomy. Nephrol Dial Transplant. 2011;26(11):3496–501.

34. Sawhney S, Fraser SD. Epidemiology of AKI: utilizing large databases to determine the burden of AKI. Adv Chronic Kidney Dis. 2017;24(4):194–204.

35. Bellomo R, Ronco C, Kellum JA, et al. Acute renal failure—definition, outcome measures, animal models, fluid therapy and information technology needs: the Second International Consensus Conference of the Acute Dialysis Quality Initiative (ADQI) Group. Crit Care. 2004;8:R204–12.

36. Mehta RL, Kellum JA, Shah SV, et al. Acute Kidney Injury Network: report of an initiative to improve outcomes in acute kidney injury. Crit Care. 2007;11(2):R31.

37. Kidney Disease: Improving Global Outcomes (KDIGO) Acute Kidney Injury Work Group. KDIGO clinical practice guideline for acute kidney injury. Kidney Int Suppl. 2012;2:S1–138.

38. Kellum JA, Lameire N, KDIGO AKI Guideline Work Group. Diagnosis, evaluation, and management of acute kidney injury: a KDIGO summary (Part 1). Crit Care. 2013;17(1):204.

39. Lameire N, Van Biesen W, Vanholder R. The changing epidemiology of acute renal failure. Nat Clin Nephrol. 2006;2:364–77.

40. Brown J, Rezaee M, Marshall E, Matheny M. Hospital mortality in the United States following acute kidney injury. Biomed Res Int. 2016;2016:4278579.

41. Ympa YP, Sakr Y, Reinhart K, Vincent JL. Has mortality from acute renal failure decreased? A systematic review of the literature. Am J Med. 2005;118:827–32.

42. Liaño F, Junco E, Pascual J, Madero R, Verde E. The spectrum of acute renal failure in the intensive care unit compared with that seen in other settings. The Madrid Acute Renal Failure Study Group. Kidney Int Suppl. 1998;66:S16–24.

43. Bellomo R. The epidemiology of acute renal failure: 1975 versus 2005. Curr Opin Crit Care. 2006;12:557–60.

44. Thakar CV, Christianson A, Freyberg R, Almenoff P, Render ML. Incidence and outcomes of acute kidney injury in intensive care units: a Veterans Administration study. Crit Care Med. 2009;37(9):2552–8.

45. Case J, Khan S, Khalid R, Khan A. Epidemiology of acute kidney injury in the intensive care unit. Crit Care Res Pract. 2013;2013:479730.

46. Hoste EA, Clermont G, Kersten A, et al. RIFLE criteria for acute kidney injury are associated with hospital mortality in critically ill patients: a cohort analysis. Crit Care. 2006;10(3):R73.

47. Thakar CV. Perioperative acute kidney injury. Adv Chronic Kidney Dis. 2013;20:67–75.

48. Grams ME, Sang Y, Coresh J, et al. Acute kidney injury after major surgery: a retrospective analysis of veteran's health administration data. Am J Kidney Dis. 2016;67(6):872–80.

49. Macedo E. Urine output assessment as a clinical quality measure. Nephron. 2015;131:252–4.

50. Macedo E, Malhotra R, Bouchard J, Wynn S, Mehta R. Oliguria is an early predictor of higher mortality in critically ill patients. Kidney Int. 2011;80(7):760–7.

51. Alpert RA, Roizen MF, Hamilton WK, et al. Intraoperative urinary output does not predict postoperative renal function in patients undergoing abdominal aortic revascularization. Surgery. 1984;95:707–11.

52. Hahn RG. Volume kinetics for infusion fluids. Anesthesiology. 2010;113(2):470–81.

53. Goren O, Matot I. Perioperative acute kidney injury. Br J Anaesth. 2015;115(Suppl 2):ii3–14.

54. Koyner JL, Parikh CR. Clinical utility of biomarkers of AKI in cardiac surgery and critical illness. Clin J Am Soc Nephrol. 2013;8(6):1034–42.

55. Han WK, Wagener G, Zhu Y, Wang S, Lee HT. Urinary biomarkers in the early detection of acute kidney injury after cardiac surgery. Clin J Am Soc Nephrol. 2009;4(5):873–82.

56. Meersch M, Schmidt C, Van Aken H, et al. Urinary TIMP-2 and IGFBP7 as early biomarkers of acute kidney injury and renal recovery following cardiac surgery. PLoS ONE. 2014;9(3):e93460.

57. Calvert S, Shaw A. Perioperative acute kidney injury. Perioper Med. 2012;4(1):6.

58. Bell S, Davey P, Nathwani D, et al. Risk of AKI with gentamicin as surgical prophylaxis. J Am Soc Nephrol. 2014;25(11):2625–32.

59. Armstrong T, Welsh FK, Wells J, Chandrakumaran K, John TG, Rees M. The impact of pre-operative serum creatinine on short-term outcomes after liver resection. HPB (Oxford). 2009;11:622–8.

60. Correa-Gallego C, Berman A, Denis SC, et al. Renal function after low central venous pressure-assisted liver resection: assessment of 2116 cases. HPB (Oxford). 2015;17:258–64.

61. Causey MW, Maykel JA, Hatch Q, Miller S, Steele SR. Identifying risk factors for renal failure and myocardial infarction following colorectal surgery. J Surg Res. 2011;170:32–7.

62. Lee EH, Kim HR, Baek SH, et al. Risk factors of postoperative acute kidney injury in patients undergoing esophageal cancer surgery. J Cardiothorac Vasc Anesth. 2014;28:948–54.

63. Bredt L, Peres L. Risk factors for acute kidney injury after partial hepatectomy. World J Hepatol. 2017;9(18):815–22.

64. Slankamenac K, Breitenstein S, Held U, Beck-Schimmer B, Puhan MA, Clavien PA. Development and validation of a prediction score for postoperative acute renal failure following liver resection. Ann Surg. 2009;250:720–8.

65. Tomozawa A, Ishikawa S, Shiota N, Cholvisudhi P, Makita K. Perioperative risk factors for acute kidney injury after liver resection surgery: an historical cohort study. Can J Anaesth. 2015;62:753–61.

66. Ford MK, Beattie SW, Wijeysundera DN. systematic review: prediction of perioperative cardiac complications and mortality by the revised cardiac risk index. Ann Intern Med. 2010;152:26–35.

67. Kambakamba P, Slankamenac K, Tschuor C, et al. Epidural analgesia and perioperative kidney function after major liver resection. Br J Surg. 2015;102:805–12.

68. Kim CS, Oak CY, Kim HY, et al. Incidence, predictive factors, and clinical outcomes of acute kidney injury after gastric surgery for gastric cancer. PLoS ONE. 2013;8:e82289.

69. Sun LY, Wijeysundera DN, Tait GA, Beattie WS. Association of intraoperative hypotension with acute kidney injury after elective noncardiac surgery. Anesthesiology. 2015;123:515–23.

70. de Haan JE, Hoorn EJ, de Geus HRH. Acute kidney injury after liver transplantation: recent insights and future perspectives. Best Pract Res Clin Gastroenterol. 2017;31(2):161–9.

71. Chen J, Singhapricha T, Hu K-Q, et al. Postliver transplant acute renal injury and failure by the RIFLE criteria in patients with normal pretransplant serum creatinine concentrations: a matched study. Transplantation. 2011;91:348–53.

72. Thakar CV, Kharat V, Blanck S, Leonard AC. Acute kidney injury after gastric bypass surgery. Clin J Am Soc Nephrol. 2007;2(3):426–30.

73. Weingarten TN, Gurrieri C, McCaffrey JM, et al. Acute kidney injury following bariatric surgery. Obes Surg. 2013;23(1):64–70.

74. Almac E, Ince C. The impact of storage on red cell function in blood transfusion. Best Pract Res Clin Anaesthesiol. 2007;21(2):195–208.

75. Koch C, Li L, Sessler D, et al. Duration of red-cell storage and complications after cardiac surgery. N Engl J Med. 2008;358(12):1229–39.

76. Karkouti K, Wijeysundera D, Yau TM, et al. Acute kidney injury after cardiac surgery. Focus on modifiable risk factors. Circulation. 2009;119(4):495–502.

77. Ricci Z, Romagnoli S, Ronco C. Perioperative intravascular volume replacement and kidney insufficiency. Best Pract Res Clin Anaesthesiol. 2012;26(4):463–74.

78. Myburgh JA, Finfer S, Bellomo R, et al. Hydroxyethyl starch or saline for fluid resuscitation in intensive care. N Engl J Med. 2012;367:1901–11.

79. Perel P, Roberts I, Ker K. Colloids versus crystalloids for fluid resuscitation in critically ill patients. Cochrane Database Syst Rev. 2013;2:CD000567.

80. Raiman M, Mitchell C, Biccard B, Rodseth R. Comparison of hydroxyethyl starch colloids with crystalloids for surgical patients: a systematic review and meta-analysis. Eur J Anaesthesiol. 2016;33(1):42–8.

81. Zazzeron L, Gattinoni L, Caironi P, et al. Role of albumin, starches and gelatins versus crystalloids in volume resuscitation of critically ill patients. Curr Opin Crit Care. 2016;22(5):428–36.

82. Shaw AD, Kellum JA. The risk of AKI in patients treated with intravenous solutions containing hydroxyethyl starch. Clin J Am Soc Nephrol. 2013;8(3):497–503.

83. Kim SK, Choi SS, Sim JH, et al. Effect of hydroxyethyl starch on acute kidney injury after living donor hepatectomy. Transplant Proc. 2016;48(1):102–6.

84. Vives M, Callejas R, Duque P, et al. Modern hydroxyethyl starch and acute kidney injury after cardiac surgery: a prospective multicentre cohort. Br J Anaesth. 2016;117(4):458–63.

85. Umegaki T, Uba T, Sumi C, et al. Impact of hydroxyethyl starch 70/0.5 on acute kidney injury after gastroenterological surgery. Korean J Anesthesiol. 2016;69(5):460–7.

86. Sear J. Kidney dysfunction in the postoperative period. Br J Anaesth. 2005;95(1):20–32.

87. Carmichael P, Carmichael AR. Acute renal failure in the surgical setting. ANZ J Surg. 2003;73:144–53.

88. Levy EM, Viscoli CM, Horwitz RI. The effect of acute renal failure on mortality. A cohort analysis. JAMA. 1996;275:1489–94.

89. Grams ME, Rabb H. The distant organ effects of acute kidney injury. Kidney Int. 2012;81:942–8.

90. Kerrigan CL, Stotland MA. Ischemia reperfusion injury: a review. Microsurgery. 1993;14:165–75.

91. Welborn MB, Oldenburg HS, Hess PJ, et al. The relationship between visceral ischemia, proinflammatory cytokines, and organ injury in patients undergoing thoracoabdominal aortic aneurysm repair. Crit Care Med. 2000;28:3191–7.

92. Gobe G, Willgoss D, Hogg N, Schoch E, Endre Z. Cell survival or death in renal tubular epithelium after ischemia- reperfusion injury. Kidney Int. 1999;56:1299–304.

93. Neves JB, Jorge S, Lopes JA. Acute kidney injury: epidemiology, diagnosis, prognosis, and future directions. EMJ Nephrol. 2015;3(1):90–6.

94. Chertow GM, Burdick E, Honour M, Bonventre JV, Bates DW. Acute kidney injury, mortality, length of stay, and costs in hospitalized patients. J Am Soc Nephrol. 2005;16:3365–70.

95. Lopes JA, Fernandes P, Jorge S, et al. Acute kidney injury in intensive care unit patients: a comparison between the RIFLE and the Acute Kidney Injury Network classifications. Crit Care. 2008;12(R110):16–31.

96. Ostermann M, Chang RW. Acute kidney injury in the intensive care unit according to RIFLE. Crit Care Med. 2007;35:1837–43.

97. Lai CF, Wu VC, Huang TM, et al. Kidney function decline after a non-dialysis-requiring acute kidney injury is associated with higher long-term mortality in critically ill survivors. Crit Care. 2012;16:R123.

98. Coca SG, Peixoto AJ, Garg AX, Krumholz HM, Parikh CR. The prognostic importance of a small acute decrement in kidney function in hospitalized patients: a systematic review and meta-analysis. Am J Kidney Dis. 2007;50(5):712–20.

99. Li X, Hassoun HT, Santora R, Rabb H. Organ crosstalk: the role of the kidney. Curr Opin Crit Care. 2009;15:481–7.

100. Coca SG, Yusuf B, Shlipak MG, Garg AX, Parikh CR. Long-term risk of mortality and other adverse outcomes after acute kidney injury: a systematic review and meta-analysis. Am J Kidney Dis. 2009;53:961–73.

101. Linder A, Fjell C, Levin A, Walley KR, Russell JA, Boyd JH. Small acute increases in serum creatinine are associated with decreased long-term survival in the critically ill. Am J Respir Crit Care Med. 2014;189(9):1075–81.

102. Ferenbach DA, Bonventre JV. Mechanisms of maladaptive repair after AKI leading to accelerated kidney ageing and CKD. Nat Rev Nephrol. 2015;11(5):264–76.

103. Coca SG, Singanamala S, Parikh CR. Chronic kidney disease after acute kidney injury: a systematic review and meta-analysis. Kidney Int. 2012;81:442–8.

104. Spurgeon-Pechman KR, Donohoe DL, Mattson DL, Lund H, James L, Basile DP. Recovery from acute renal failure predisposes hypertension and secondary renal disease in response to elevated sodium. Am J Physiol Renal Physiol. 2007;293:F269–78.

105. Basile DP. The endothelial cell in ischemic acute kidney injury: implications for acute and chronic function. Kidney Int. 2007;72:151–6.

106. Sarafidis PA, Bakris GL. Microalbuminuria and chronic kidney disease as risk factors for cardiovascular disease. Nephrol Dial Transplant. 2006;21:2366–74.

107. Go AS, Chertow GM, Fan D, McCulloch CE, Hsu CY. Chronic kidney disease and the risks of death, cardiovascular events, and hospitalization. N Engl J Med. 2004;351:1296–305.

108. Gameiro J, Neves JB, Rodrigues N, et al. Acute kidney injury, long-term renal function and mortality in patients undergoing major abdominal surgery: a cohort analysis. Clin Kidney J. 2016;9(2):192–200.

5

The prognostic value of bispectral index and suppression ratio monitoring after out-of-hospital cardiac arrest

Ward Eertmans[1,2]* ⓘ, Cornelia Genbrugge[1,2], Margot Vander Laenen[2], Willem Boer[2], Dieter Mesotten[1,2], Jo Dens[1,3], Frank Jans[1,2] and Cathy De Deyne[1,2]

Abstract

Background: We investigated the ability of bispectral index (BIS) monitoring to predict poor neurological outcome in out-of-hospital cardiac arrest (OHCA) patients fully treated according to guidelines.

Results: In this prospective, observational study, 77 successfully resuscitated OHCA patients were enrolled in whom BIS, suppression ratio (SR) and electromyographic (EMG) values were continuously monitored during the first 36 h after the initiation of targeted temperature management at 33 °C. The Cerebral Performance Category (CPC) scale was used to define patients' outcome at 180 days after OHCA (CPC 1–2: good–CPC 3–5: poor neurological outcome). Using mean BIS and SR values calculated per hour, receiver operator characteristics curves were constructed to determine the optimal time point and threshold to predict poor neurological outcome. At 180 days post-cardiac arrest, 39 patients (51%) had a poor neurological outcome. A mean BIS value ≤ 25 at hour 12 predicted poor neurological outcome with a sensitivity of 49% (95% CI 30–65%), a specificity of 97% (95% CI 85–100%) and false positive rate (FPR) of 6% (95% CI 0–29%) [AUC: 0.722 (0.570–0.875); $p = 0.006$]. A mean SR value ≥ 3 at hour 23 predicted poor neurological with a sensitivity of 74% (95% CI 56–87%), a specificity of 92% (95% CI 78–98%) and FPR of 11% (95% CI 3–29%) [AUC: 0.836 (0.717–0.955); $p < 0.001$]. No relationship was found between mean EMG and BIS < 25 ($R^2 = 0.004$; $p = 0.209$).

Conclusion: This study found that mean BIS ≤ 25 at hour 12 and mean SR ≥ 3 at hour 23 might be used to predict poor neurological outcome in an OHCA population with a presumed cardiac cause. Since no correlation was observed between EMG and BIS < 25, our calculated BIS threshold might assist with poor outcome prognostication following OHCA.

Keywords: Bispectral index, Suppression ratio, Prognostication, Out-of-hospital cardiac arrest, Neuromonitoring, Neurological outcome

Background

Once admitted to the Intensive Care Unit (ICU), post-anoxic brain injury is considered as the predominant cause of death in patients admitted after cardiac arrest (CA) [1, 2]. The implementation of targeted temperature management (TTM) in the post-CA setting improved neurological outcome substantially, but delayed neuro-prognostication until at least 72 h after CA [3–7]. Nevertheless, early and reliable prognostication is most appreciated to inform relatives. Moreover, it could avoid futile and expensive treatment efforts in out-of-hospital cardiac arrest (OHCA) patients with irreversible brain damage.

Current guidelines recommend the use of a neuroprognostication algorithm including four main modalities

*Correspondence: ward.eertmans@uhasselt.be
[1] Department of Medicine and Life Sciences, Hasselt University, Diepenbeek, Belgium
Full list of author information is available at the end of the article

which should be used in conjunction with each other whenever possible, i.e. clinical neurological examination, electrophysiology, biomarkers and brain imaging [5, 7, 8]. Unfortunately, most of the recommended prognostic markers are labour-intensive and above all require trained experts for correct interpretation. In recent years, the potential use of bispectral index (BIS) and to a lesser extent suppression ratio (SR) monitoring has been investigated in the post-CA setting [9–15]. Although these studies demonstrated that BIS and SR values could be used to predict poor neurological outcome, this monitoring option was not yet implemented in the neuroprognostication algorithm proposed by current guidelines [5]. Its use in brain-injured CA patients is namely associated with certain limitations. The BIS monitor was originally designed to monitor intraoperative awareness during anaesthesia, possibly implying that physicians treating post-CA patients are unfamiliar with its use [16]. Additionally, BIS monitoring is exposed to potential confounders of which high electromyographic (EMG) activity is acknowledged as the predominant one within CA research, causing falsely elevated BIS values [17]. In previous BIS studies, neuromuscular blockers (NMB) were administered continuously in all patients to minimize EMG activity interference although its constant use is not in line with current guidelines [18]. Altogether, these limitations question the clear benefit of this user-friendly monitoring option to assist with neuroprognostication. Therefore, this prospective, observational study aimed to assess the ability of BIS monitoring to predict poor neurological outcome in OHCA patients fully treated according to guidelines.

Methods

Study population

A prospective, observational study was performed between March 2011 and May 2015 in a Belgian tertiary care hospital (Ziekenhuis Oost-Limburg, Genk). All adult comatose survivors successfully resuscitated from OHCA with a presumed cardiac cause were admitted to the Coronary Care Unit (CCU) and were considered as eligible for this study. According to the institutional post-CA care protocol, all patients were treated uniformly and BIS monitoring was started immediately after admission to CCU [19]. Approval from the local Committee for Medical Ethics was obtained prior to study onset (11/06) and written informed consent was obtained from patient's next of kin.

Patient management

The institutional post-resuscitation protocol has been described previously [19, 20]. To summarize, TTM at 33 °C was initiated immediately after arrival at the emergency department by administering cold saline intravenously (4 °C—15–30 ml/kg). Urgent coronary angiography was performed followed by a percutaneous coronary intervention when indicated. TTM was further mechanically induced after CCU admission and maintained at 33 °C for 24 h using either endovascular (Icy cathether, CoolGard® 3000, Alsius, Irvine, CA, USA) or surface (ArcticGel™ pads, Arctic Sun® 5000, Medivance, Louisville, Colorado, USA) cooling systems. Subsequently, patients were rewarmed over the following 12 h (0.3 °C/h). Both cooling systems were equipped with a feedback loop system to control target temperature using an oesophageal temperature probe. All patients were intubated, mechanically ventilated and sedated with propofol, midazolam and remifentanil. Within the period of TTM, sedation doses were titrated to obtain values between − 3 and − 5 on the Richmond Agitation-Sedation scale. According to current guidelines, cisatracurium was only administered in case of shivering [18]. After the return to normothermia, sedation was reduced to evaluate patients' neurological status properly. Patients not ready for extubation owing to circulatory or respiratory issues or due to persisting coma were kept sedated under the lowest dose needed to tolerate the endotracheal tube. EEGs were performed on clinical indication, and antiepileptic drugs were given in case of epileptic activity. Every EEG was characterized by a description of the posterior dominant rhythm (or absence thereof) and amplitude as well as the presence of non-dominant rhythms. Lateralization and the presence of artefacts was described where applicable. If present, epileptic activity was described as interictal, ictal or as status epilepticus. A status epilepticus was defined as continuous epileptic activity including rhythmic focal or generalized spikes lasting for more than 5 min and was considered as therapy-refractory in case of persistent epileptic activity in spite of at least two lines of antiepileptic drugs. Once the neurological, hemodynamic and respiratory status had been recovered sufficiently, patients were extubated.

Bispectral index and suppression ratio monitoring

Bilateral BIS monitoring was initiated as soon as possible after CCU admission using the BIS VISTA™ (Aspect Medical Systems, Inc. Norwood, USA). A six-electrode frontotemporal bilateral sensor was applied to the patient's forehead. The BIS monitor is a simplified EEG monitor that uses fast Fourier transformation to convert raw frontal EEG signals into simple and real-time BIS numbers ranging from 0 (iso-electric EEG) to 100 (normal electrical activity in awake subjects). Additionally, a SR is calculated, representing the percentage of each 63-s period that is iso-electric [21]. Finally, EMG activity is another parameter calculated by the BIS monitor describing the electromyographic content of the EEG signal and ranges from 0 (no EMG activity) to 100 (large EMG activity). BIS, SR and EMG values were continuously recorded and stored during the hypothermic and rewarming phase (i.e. 36 h). Although treating physicians (cardiologists) were not blinded to values displayed on the BIS monitor, decisions to withdraw life support were never based on these parameters and the dosage of sedatives was not titrated based on BIS values.

Withdrawal of treatment policy

In patients not regaining consciousness despite complete cessation of sedation, maximal supportive treatment was provided until at least 72 h after normothermia was reached. Together with clinical neurological examination, malignant EEG patterns (i.e. status epilepticus, persisting burst suppression rhythms or long-lasting cerebral inactivity) were considered as the first-line support for the decision to withdraw therapy, and in specific, when seizures remained therapy-refractory or if other EEG rhythms with a poor prognosis remained present on subsequent EEG assessments. In case subsequent EEGs were inconclusive or when patients failed to wake up after the end of active temperature control, SSEPs and/or brain CT were performed. In line with international guidelines, absent corneal and pupillary reflexes, bilateral absence of the N20 component of SSEPs and refractory epileptic activity was considered to support this decision to withdraw therapy [22].

Outcome assessment

The primary endpoint was neurological outcome defined by the Cerebral Performance Category (CPC) at 180 days post-CA. According to the scale classification, CPC1 is indicative for good cerebral performance; CPC2 implies moderate disability with sufficient cerebral functioning for independent daily-life activity; CPC3 indicates severe neurological sequelae; CPC4 implies coma or vegetative state; and CPC5 stands for death [23]. In this study, a CPC1–2 and CPC3–5 was considered as good and poor neurological outcome, respectively.

Statistical analysis

Statistical analysis was performed using SPSS version 22.0 (SPSS Inc, Chicago, USA). Equal distribution was tested with a Kolmogorov–Smirnov test. Depending on normality, categorical data were compared between patients with a good and poor neurological outcomes using Fisher exact or Chi-Square tests, while unpaired t tests or Mann–Whitney U tests were used to compare continuous data. BIS, SR and EMG values were stored per second and left and right values were averaged. Mean BIS, SR and EMG values were then calculated per hour

from initiation of TTM onwards and were used for data analysis. To assess the predictive ability of BIS and SR, receiver operating characteristic (ROC) curves were constructed at each hour using mean BIS and SR values and the Youden index was calculated for each ROC curve (Youden index = sensitivity + specificity − 1). The optimal time point and threshold to predict poor neurological outcome was determined based on the highest Youden index across all ROC curves. Relative risk ratios of poor neurological outcome were computed for the presence of single BIS and SR values between given intervals on the respective optimal time points. In addition, regression curves were fitted (including the calculation of the Pearson correlation coefficient) to describe the relationship between mean EMG and BIS values below and above our calculated (optimal) BIS threshold. Survival analyses were executed using Kaplan–Meier curves and log-rank statistic. p values < 0.05 were considered as significant.

Results

Between March 2011 and May 2015, 121 eligible OHCA patients were consecutively enrolled in this study. Forty-four patients were excluded from further analysis for following reasons: no recording of BIS values ($n = 34$), initiation of BIS monitoring at day 2 ($n = 4$) and incoherence between time stamp and start of BIS monitoring ($n = 6$). In total, 77 successfully resuscitated OHCA survivors were prospectively included. At 180 days post-CA, 38 patients (49%) had a good (CPC1–2), while 39 patients (51%) had a poor neurological outcome (CPC5). There were no patients with a CPC 3 or 4 at 180 days following CA. Baseline characteristics, patient's severity at admission and complications within the post-resuscitation management phase are summarized in Table 1 for both outcome groups. Sedation doses were in general higher in patients with a good neurological outcome. In total, 44 (57%) patients received NMB during the period of TTM, with no difference in the NMB dosage between both outcome groups ($p = 0.804$; Table 2).

In 27 out of the 39 (69%) patients with a poor (neurological) outcome (CPC5), therapy was withdrawn at day 10 (6–20) post-CA and they died due to extensive neurological injury. First, 19 out of these 27 patients had a therapy-refractory status epilepticus. On top of persistent seizure activity, six and four out of these 19 patients had bilateral absent cortical responses on SSEP and diffuse brain oedema on CT, respectively. One patient with therapy-refractory seizures developed a septic shock after TTM at 33 °C ended and died 6 days after CCU admission. Another patient died 2 days after admission due to multi-organ failure in addition to persistent epileptic activity. Despite aggressive antiepileptic therapy, the other seven patients remained in a comatose vegetative

Table 1 Baseline characteristics and post-resuscitation management and complications

Characteristic	Good neurological outcome (N = 38)	Poor neurological outcome (N = 39)	p
Age	67 ± 13	61 ± 13	0.034
Male	31 (82)	31 (80)	0.817
Co-morbidities			
Diabetes	2 (5)	10 (26)	0.025
Chronic kidney insufficiency	2 (5)	6 (15)	0.263
Cerebrovascular disease	2 (5)	2 (5)	1.000
Acute myocardial infarction	6 (16)	5 (13)	0.755
Arterial hypertension	16 (42)	17 (44)	1.000
Hyperlipidemia	15 (39)	16 (41)	1.000
Cardiac arrest variables			
Initial rhythm			0.003
Shockable	33 (87)	20 (56)	
Non-shockable	5 (13)	16 (44)	
Witnessed arrest	34 (92)	33 (87)	0.479
Bystander CPR	18 (47)	20 (51)	0.821
BLS duration (min)	8 (0–14)	10 (0–12)	0.561
ALS duration (min)	12 (8–21)	15 (10–28)	0.348
Number of shocks	2 (1–5)	1 (0–4)	0.111
Time emergency call—ROSC (min)	28 ± 19	32 ± 15	0.388
Post-resuscitation management			
Percutaneous Coronary Intervention	27 (71)	17 (44)	0.015
Cooling, endovascular/surface	20 (53)/18 (47)	15 (38)/24 (62)	0.265
Time to target temperature (min)	140 (73–295)	141 (107–195)	0.652
Intra-aortic balloon pump	11 (29)	6 (15)	0.178
Post-resuscitation complications			
Post-resuscitation shock	16 (42)	21 (54)	0.365
ARDS	4 (11)	7 (18)	0.517
Pneumonia	21 (55)	17 (44)	0.365
Acute kidney injury	9 (24)	12 (31)	0.610
Renal replacement therapy	3 (8)	3 (8)	1.000
Status epilepticus	1 (3)	20 (51)	<0.001
Burst suppression	4 (11)	16 (41)	0.004
Cause of death			
Neurological injury	–	27 (69)	–
Post-cardiac arrest shock	–	10 (26)	–
Other	–	2 (5)	–
CCU days	19 (12–32)	9 (6–17)	<0.001

Data are shown as mean ± SD, median with interquartile range and n (%)

ALS Advanced Life Support, ARDS Acute Respiratory Distress Syndrome, BLS Basic Life Support, CCU Coronary Care Unit, CPR cardiopulmonary resuscitation, ROSC return of spontaneous circulation

Statistical significant values indicate in italics (p < 0.05)

state in whom therapy was withdrawn after 10 (9–32) days. Second, a bilateral absent cortical response (N20) on SSEP was the main reason for withdrawal of life-sustaining treatment in four out of these 27 patients. Third, two patients did not recover neurologically 2–3 weeks following CA, and EEGs persistently showed burst-suppression patterns. Finally, two patients had long-lasting cerebral inactivity based on EEG in whom a brain CT showed diffuse cerebral oedema indicative for extensive cerebral swelling.

Figure 1 displays the evolution of mean BIS and SR values over the first 36 h from the initiation of TTM onwards in patients with good and poor neurological outcomes. After calculating the mean BIS and SR per

Table 2 Sedation doses and neuromuscular blockage

Sedatives	Good neurological outcome	Poor neurological outcome	p value
Propofol (mg/kg/h)	2.54 ± 0.51	1.35 ± 0.05	0.071
Remifentanil (µg/kg/min)	0.15 ± 0.07	0.10 ± 0.01	0.210
Midazolam (µg/kg/min)	1.45 ± 0.34	0.85 ± 0.21	0.156
Cisatracurium (mg/kg/h)[a]	0.13 (0.03–0.17)	0.10 (0.07–0.14)	0.804

Data are presented as mean ± SD and median with interquartile ranges

[a] Cisatracurium was administered in 20 and 24 patients with a good and poor neurological outcome, respectively

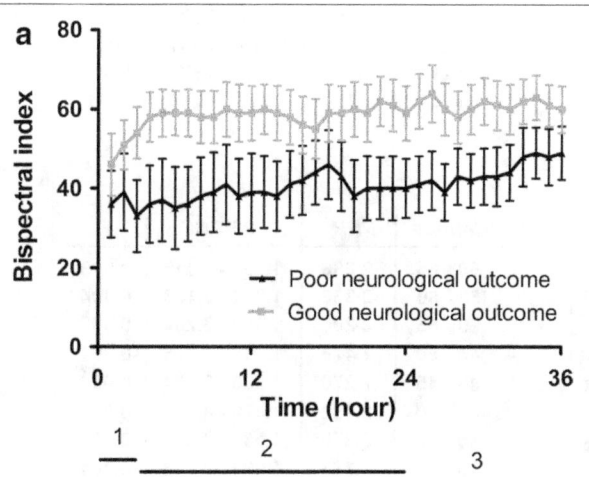

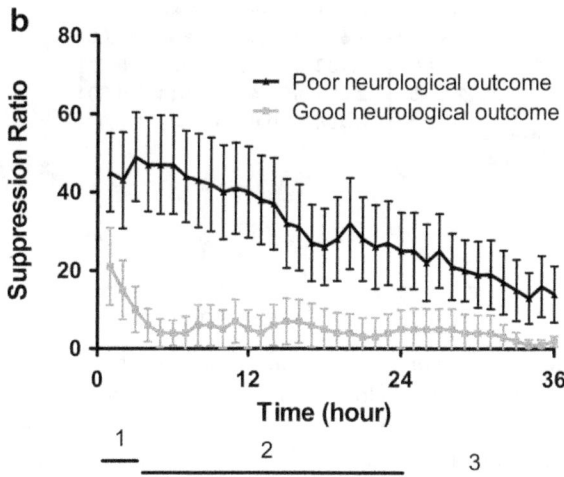

Fig. 1 Evolution of mean BIS and SR during targeted temperature management. Hourly mean BIS (**a**) and SR values (**b**) are shown with their 95% CI in patients with a good and poor neurological outcome. Patients with a poor neurological outcome had significantly higher BIS and lower SR values during (1) the induction phase ($p = 0.002$ and $p < 0.001$, respectively), (2) the hypothermic phase ($p < 0.001$ and $p < 0.001$, respectively) and (3) rewarming phase ($p < 0.001$ and $p < 0.001$, respectively)

hour, the optimal time point which provided the best sensitivity and specificity to predict poor neurological

outcome was determined. A mean BIS value below or equal to 25 at hour 12 predicted poor neurological outcome with a sensitivity of 49% (95% CI 30–65%) and specificity of 97% (95% CI 85–100%) [AUC: 0.722 (0.570–0.875); $p = 0.006$]. Only one patient with a mean BIS ≤ 25 at hour 12 survived with a good neurological outcome. This corresponded to a false positive rate (FPR) of 6% (95% CI 0–29%). A mean SR value above or equal to 3 at hour 23 predicted poor neurological outcome with a sensitivity of 74% (95% CI 56–87%) and specificity of 92% (95% CI 78–98%) [AUC: 0.836 (0.717–0.955); $p < 0.001$]. This corresponded to a FPR of 11% (95% CI 3–29%). Three patients with a mean SR ≥ 3 at hour 23 had a good neurological outcome.

At these optimal time points, relative risk ratios of poor neurological outcome were calculated for the presence of single BIS and SR values per second between given intervals (Fig. 2). Patients experiencing at least one BIS ≤ 25 at hour 12 had a 2.3-fold higher risk of poor neurological outcome (95% CI 1.38–3.85; $p = 0.001$). On the other hand, the presence of at least a single SR ≥ 3 at hour 23 was associated with a 4.4-fold higher risk of poor neurological outcome (95% CI 2.09–9.30; $p < 0.001$).

The overall relationship between mean EMG and BIS was best described by a quadratic regression curve ($Y = 29.64 - 0.228X + 0.007X^2$; $R^2 = 0.671$; $p < 0.001$; Fig. 3). To account for possible EMG interferences on our calculated BIS threshold, regression curves were fitted between mean EMG and BIS values below and above 25. This analysis showed no relationship between mean EMG and BIS values below 25 ($Y = 28.10 + 0.043X$; $R^2 = 0.004$; $p = 0.209$), implying that EMG interference below our calculated BIS threshold is rather negligible. In contrast, a significant relationship was observed between mean EMG and BIS values above 25 ($Y = 30.35 - 0.263X + 0.007X^2$; $R^2 = 0.650$; $p < 0.001$; Fig. 3).

Survival curves are presented in Fig. 4. Patients with a mean BIS ≤ 25 at hour 12 were at high risk of poor neurological outcome (log-rank test $p < 0.001$; Fig. 4a). Patients with a mean SR ≥ 3 at hour 23 had a high risk for poor neurological outcome (log-rank test $p < 0.001$; Fig. 4b). A mean BIS ≤ 25 at hour 12 together with a mean SR ≥ 3 at

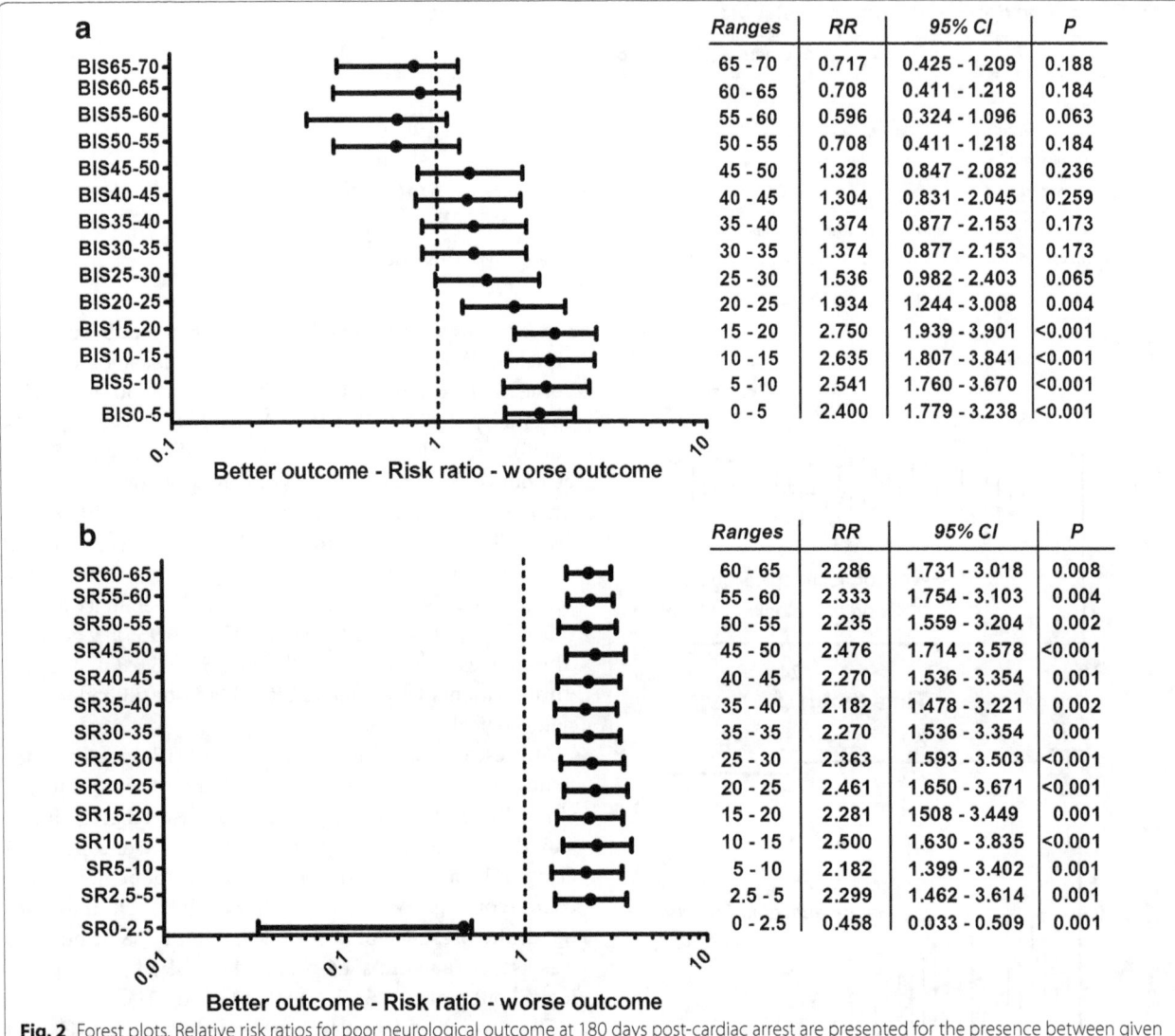

Fig. 2 Forest plots. Relative risk ratios for poor neurological outcome at 180 days post-cardiac arrest are presented for the presence between given BIS (**a**) and SR (**b**) ranges at hour 12 and 23, respectively

hour 23 was associated with poor neurological outcome (log-rank test $p < 0.001$; Fig. 4c).

Discussion

This study shows that BIS monitoring might assist with the prediction of poor neurological outcome in OHCA patients fully treated according to current guidelines. Mean BIS values below or equal to 25 at hour 12 and mean SR values above or equal to 3 at hour 23 were associated with poor neurological outcome in OHCA patients.

Consistent with previous studies, patients with a poor neurological outcome had lower BIS and higher SR values during the entire period of TTM. Up to now, the optimal time point and threshold to predict poor neurological

outcome remain questionable. In the post-CA setting, mean BIS values below 40 or mean SR values above 40 during the first 4 h after cardiopulmonary resuscitation were shown to be early predictors for poor outcome [24]. According to Stammet et al. [14], a mean BIS value of 23 calculated over 12.5 h achieved a specificity and sensitivity of 89 and 86%, respectively. In line with these data, the optimal time point to predict poor neurological outcome in our patient cohort was at hour 12 using a mean BIS value of 25 reaching a specificity of 97%. As such, this is the first study which found a nearly similar BIS threshold to predict poor neurological outcome at a more or less identical time point. Furthermore, we demonstrated that a SR value of 3 at hour 23 had an even higher predictive power for poor outcome and its presence was associated

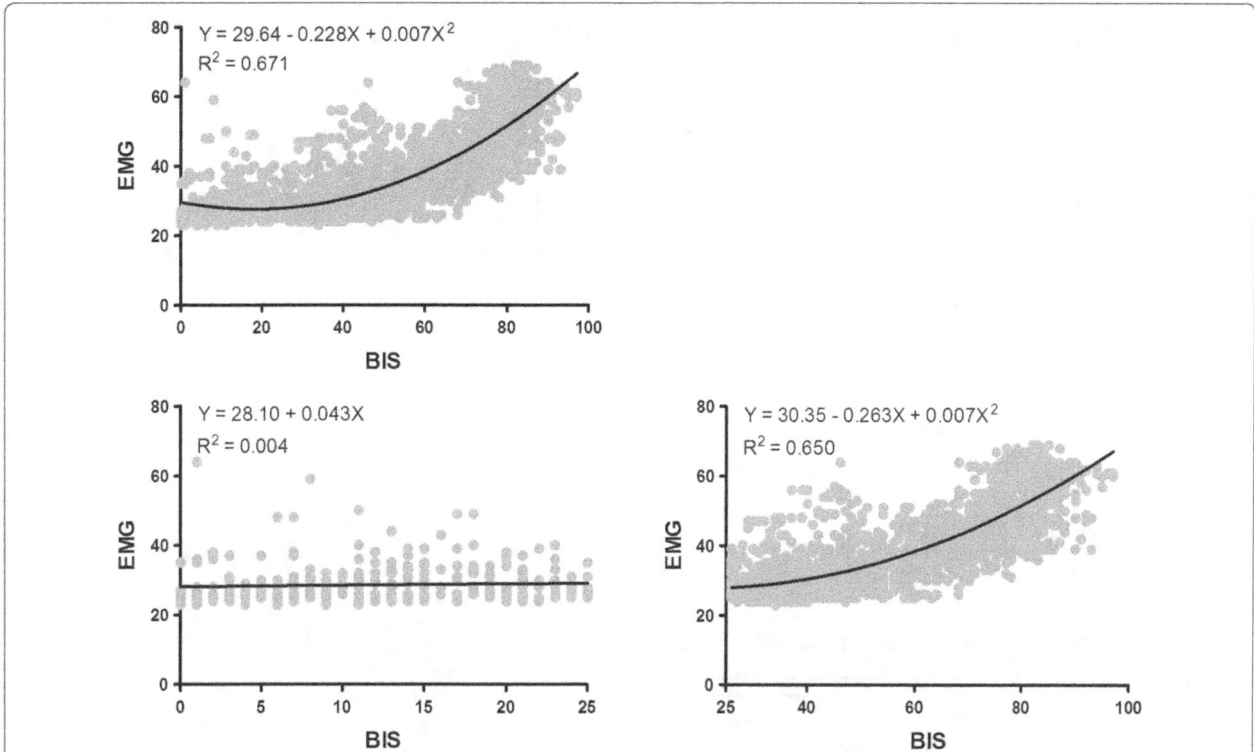

Fig. 3 Correlation between EMG and BIS. The overall relationship between mean EMG and BIS is best described by a quadratic regression curve. No correlation is present between mean EMG and BIS below 25

with a fourfold higher risk to decease. Unfortunately, others did not assess the prognostic performance of SR longitudinally, which prevents us from comparing these results with current literature [10, 24]. For that reason, future studies are warranted to validate the value of SR as early prognostic marker in comparison to BIS.

BIS monitoring is known to be subjected to several confounding factors although this study confirms its potential to assist with early neuroprognostication [10, 11, 14, 15, 24, 25]. One of the predominant confounders is high EMG activity interference which is known to falsely elevate the BIS value [17]. In previous BIS studies, any influence of EMG activity on the BIS value was excluded by the continuous administration of NMB in all study patients although several undesirable effects have been associated with its routine use. Besides an increased risk on pneumonia and ICU-acquired weakness, continuous administration of NMB during TTM delays neurological examination and masks seizures [26–28]. Our patient cohort, however, was treated according to current guidelines, which suggest to limit the use of NMB to patients who experience shivering [18]. This allowed us to assess whether BIS monitoring was still able to predict poor neurological outcome after OHCA even though EMG activity interference was not minimized in all study patients. In fact, no correlation was observed between EMG and BIS values below or equal to our calculated threshold of 25, implying that EMG activity interference below this cut-off value is most likely negligible. Nonetheless, it is plausible to assume that the calculated sensitivity of our BIS threshold would have been higher if NMB were administered continuously.

In general, our results strengthen the hypothesis that BIS monitoring could be used as early prognostic tool after OHCA. Nevertheless, early neuroprognostication has always been challenging. It has become even more complicated within the era of TTM with guidelines currently suggesting to postpone prognostication until at least 72 h after OHCA [29, 30]. Still, it is desirable to identify patients with no prospect of full neurological recovery as early as possible. Therefore, prognostic markers should always achieve a high specificity with narrow confidence intervals. Using mean BIS values at hour 12 and mean SR values at hour 23, we were able to predict poor neurological outcome with a specificity of 97 and 92%, respectively. To compare our results, established neurophysiological tools such as SSEPs and EEGs reach a comparably high specificity [31, 32]. However, prognostic markers cannot be used on its own unless they reach a FPR of 0%. A false classification of patients with a

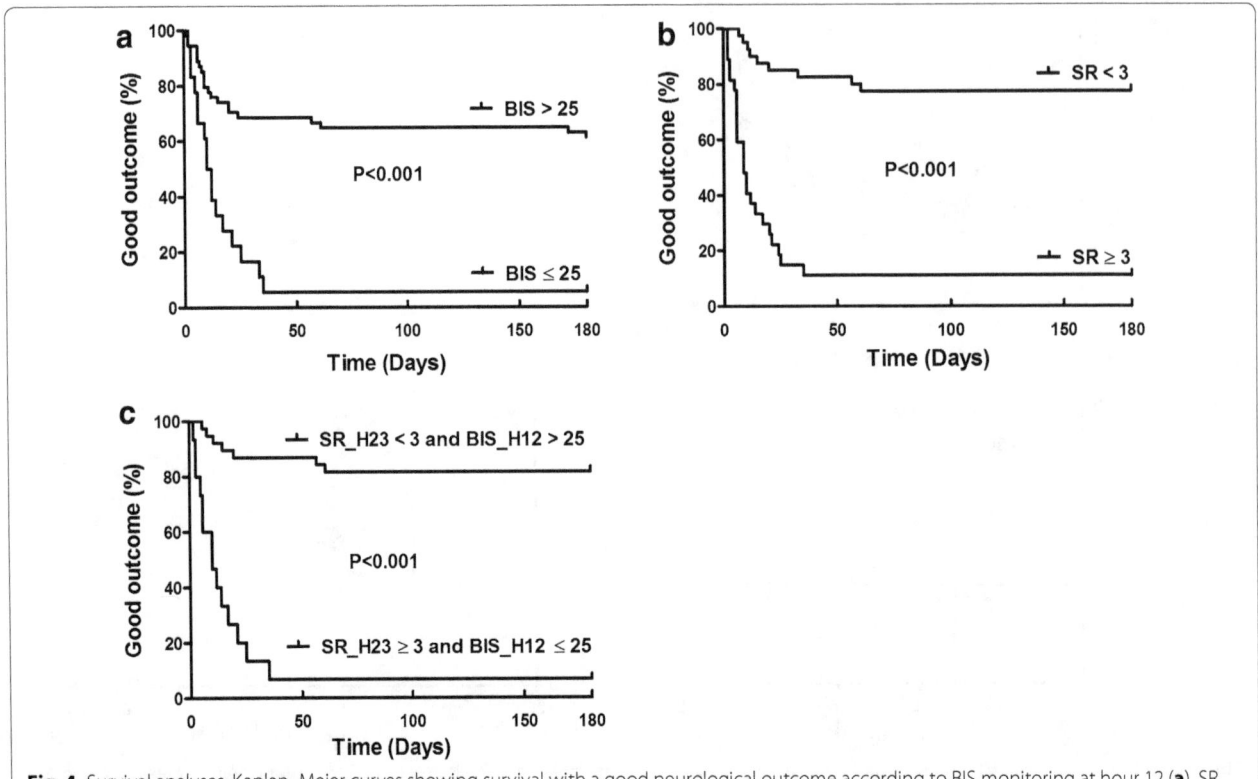

Fig. 4 Survival analyses. Kaplan–Meier curves showing survival with a good neurological outcome according to BIS monitoring at hour 12 (**a**), SR monitoring at hour 23 (**b**) or both (**c**)

favourable prognosis would namely result in an ethically unacceptable decision to withdraw medical treatment. Therefore, our results should be interpreted with caution and we do not advise to use BIS or SR as single parameter for outcome prediction. Currently, the benefit of a multimodal approach using an entire battery of prognostic markers is being investigated [12, 33]. Based on our results, future studies are needed to elucidate whether poor neurological outcome can be predicted with a false positive ratio of 0% by combining BIS and SR values with other highly specific parameters. For now, this study only confirmed the value of BIS and SR as potential early outcome predictors.

Several limitations need to be acknowledged. First, this was a single-centre study with a limited sample size. Second, physicians were not blinded since visual confirmation is required to assess signal quality. Nonetheless, BIS and SR values were not used in the decision of withdrawal of life-sustaining therapy. Third, it has been demonstrated that BIS values decrease under hypothermic conditions [34, 35]. Nevertheless, TTM at 33 °C unlikely influenced our results as all patients were treated uniformly and time to target temperature did not differ between both patient cohorts. Still, the ability of BIS

monitoring to predict poor neurological outcome in patients treated with TTM at 36 °C remains to be elucidated. Finally, mean BIS and SR values were calculated per hour although these are not available in clinical practice. Nevertheless, Stammet et al. [14] demonstrated that a minute-by-minute analysis did not provide additional prognostic information. Therefore, we believe that mean BIS and SR values per hour should be implemented in the current BIS monitor as they might assist with neuroprognostication.

Conclusions

This study shows that mean BIS values below or equal to 25 at hour 12 and mean SR values above or equal to 3 at hour 23 predicted poor neurological outcome in OHCA patients fully treated according to current guidelines. These results underline the possible potential of BIS monitoring to assist with early neuroprognostication in successfully resuscitated OHCA patients treated with TTM at 33 °C. Future studies are now warranted which should focus on the contribution of BIS and SR values to the multimodal neuroprognostication algorithm advised by current guidelines.

Abbreviations
BIS: bispectral index; CA: cardiac arrest; CCU: Coronary Care Unit; CPC: Cerebral Performance Category; EEG: electro-encephalography; EMG: electro-myographic activity; FPR: false positive rate; ICU: Intensive Care Unit; NMB: neuromuscular blockers; OHCA: out-of-hospital cardiac arrest; ROC: receiver operating characteristic; SR: suppression ratio; SSEP: somatosensory evoked potential; TTM: targeted temperature management.

Authors' contributions
WE was responsible for the study execution, data management, data analysis, data interpretation, and manuscript writing. CG was responsible for the study design, study execution, oversight of data management, data interpretation and critically revising the manuscript. MV, WB and FJ were responsible for study design, interpretation of results and manuscript editing. JD and CDD were responsible for the conception, study design, study execution, data interpretation and manuscript editing. All authors read and approved the final manuscript.

Author details
[1] Department of Medicine and Life Sciences, Hasselt University, Diepenbeek, Belgium. [2] Department of Anaesthesiology, Intensive Care, Emergency Medicine and Pain Therapy, Ziekenhuis Oost-Limburg, Schiepse Bos 6, 3600 Genk, Belgium. [3] Department of Cardiology, Ziekenhuis Oost-Limburg, Schiepse Bos 6, 3600 Genk, Belgium.

Acknowledgements
The authors wish to thank the residents, nursing and medical staff of the Coronary Care Unit of Ziekenhuis Oost-Limburg for their cooperation and support in this study.

Competing interests
The research institution of author Ward Eertmans received honoraria from Medtronic for giving a lecture on the CAS Annual Meeting 2017. The remaining authors have declared that they do not have any conflicts of interest.

Funding
This work was supported by the Limburg Clinical Research Program (LCRP) UHasselt-ZOL-Jessa, supported by the foundation Limburg Sterk Merk, Hasselt University, Ziekenhuis Oost-Limburg and Jessa Hospital.

References
1. Lemiale V, Dumas F, Mongardon N, Giovanetti O, Charpentier J, Chiche JD, et al. Intensive care unit mortality after cardiac arrest: the relative contribution of shock and brain injury in a large cohort. Intensive Care Med. 2013;39(11):1972–80.
2. Dragancea I, Rundgren M, Englund E, Friberg H, Cronberg T. The influence of induced hypothermia and delayed prognostication on the mode of death after cardiac arrest. Resuscitation. 2013;84(3):337–42.
3. Hypothermia after Cardiac Arrest Study G. Mild therapeutic hypothermia to improve the neurologic outcome after cardiac arrest. N Engl J Med. 2002;346(8):549–56.
4. Bernard SA, Gray TW, Buist MD, Jones BM, Silvester W, Gutteridge G, et al. Treatment of comatose survivors of out-of-hospital cardiac arrest with induced hypothermia. N Engl J Med. 2002;346(8):557–63.
5. Nolan JP, Soar J, Cariou A, Cronberg T, Moulaert VR, Deakin CD, et al. European Resuscitation Council and European Society of Intensive Care Medicine Guidelines for post-resuscitation care 2015: section 5 of the European Resuscitation Council Guidelines for Resuscitation 2015. Resuscitation. 2015;95:202–22.
6. Nielsen N, Wetterslev J, Cronberg T, Erlinge D, Gasche Y, Hassager C, et al. Targeted temperature management at 33 degrees C versus 36 degrees C after cardiac arrest. N Engl J Med. 2013;369(23):2197–206.
7. Sandroni C, Cariou A, Cavallaro F, Cronberg T, Friberg H, Hoedemaekers C, et al. Prognostication in comatose survivors of cardiac arrest: an advisory statement from the European Resuscitation Council and the European Society of Intensive Care Medicine. Resuscitation. 2014;85(12):1779–89.
8. Rossetti AO, Rabinstein AA, Oddo M. Neurological prognostication of outcome in patients in coma after cardiac arrest. Lancet Neurol. 2016;15(6):597–609.
9. Stammet P, Werer C, Mertens L, Lorang C, Hemmer M. Bispectral index (BIS) helps predicting bad neurological outcome in comatose survivors after cardiac arrest and induced therapeutic hypothermia. Resuscitation. 2009;80(4):437–42.
10. Seder DB, Fraser GL, Robbins T, Libby L, Riker RR. The bispectral index and suppression ratio are very early predictors of neurological outcome during therapeutic hypothermia after cardiac arrest. Intensive Care Med. 2010;36(2):281–8.
11. Leary M, Fried DA, Gaieski DF, Merchant RM, Fuchs BD, Kolansky DM, et al. Neurologic prognostication and bispectral index monitoring after resuscitation from cardiac arrest. Resuscitation. 2010;81(9):1133–7.
12. Stammet P, Wagner DR, Gilson G, Devaux Y. Modeling serum level of s100beta and bispectral index to predict outcome after cardiac arrest. J Am Coll Cardiol. 2013;62(9):851–8.
13. Seder DB, Dziodzio J, Smith KA, Hickey P, Bolduc B, Stone P, et al. Feasibility of bispectral index monitoring to guide early post-resuscitation cardiac arrest triage. Resuscitation. 2014;85(8):1030–6.
14. Stammet P, Collignon O, Werer C, Sertznig C, Devaux Y. Bispectral index to predict neurological outcome early after cardiac arrest. Resuscitation. 2014;85(12):1674–80.
15. Burjek NE, Wagner CE, Hollenbeck RD, Wang L, Yu C, McPherson JA, et al. Early bispectral index and sedation requirements during therapeutic hypothermia predict neurologic recovery following cardiac arrest. Crit Care Med. 2014;42(5):1204–12.
16. Punjasawadwong Y, Phongchiewboon A, Bunchungmongkol N. Bispectral index for improving anaesthetic delivery and postoperative recovery. Cochrane Database Syst Rev. 2014;6:CD003843.
17. Vivien B, Di Maria S, Ouattara A, Langeron O, Coriat P, Riou B. Overestimation of Bispectral Index in sedated intensive care unit patients revealed by administration of muscle relaxant. Anesthesiology. 2003;99(1):9–17.
18. Murray MJ, DeBlock H, Erstad B, Gray A, Jacobi J, Jordan C, et al. Clinical practice guidelines for sustained neuromuscular blockade in the adult critically ill patient. Crit Care Med. 2016;44(11):2079–103.
19. Meex I, Dens J, Jans F, Boer W, Vanhengel K, Vundelinckx G, et al. Cerebral tissue oxygen saturation during therapeutic hypothermia in post-cardiac arrest patients. Resuscitation. 2013;84(6):788–93.
20. Genbrugge C, Eertmans W, Meex I, Van Kerrebroeck M, Daems N, Creemers A, et al. What is the value of regional cerebral saturation in post-cardiac arrest patients? A prospective observational study. Crit Care. 2016;20(1):327.
21. Johansen JW. Update on bispectral index monitoring. Best Pract Res Clin Anaesthesiol. 2006;20(1):81–99.
22. Peberdy MA, Callaway CW, Neumar RW, Geocadin RG, Zimmerman JL, Donnino M, et al. Part 9: post-cardiac arrest care: 2010 American Heart Association Guidelines for Cardiopulmonary Resuscitation and Emergency Cardiovascular Care. Circulation. 2010;122(18 Suppl 3):S768–86.
23. Grenvik A, Safar P. Brain failure and resuscitation. New York: Churchill Livingstone; 1981.
24. Selig C, Riegger C, Dirks B, Pawlik M, Seyfried T, Klingler W. Bispectral index (BIS) and suppression ratio (SR) as an early predictor of unfavourable neurological outcome after cardiac arrest. Resuscitation. 2014;85(2):221–6.
25. Riker RR, Stone PC Jr, May T, McCrum B, Fraser GL, Seder D. Initial bispectral index may identify patients who will awaken during therapeutic hypothermia after cardiac arrest: a retrospective pilot study. Resuscitation. 2013;84(6):794–7.
26. Salciccioli JD, Cocchi MN, Rittenberger JC, Peberdy MA, Ornato JP, Abella BS, et al. Continuous neuromuscular blockade is associated with decreased mortality in post-cardiac arrest patients. Resuscitation. 2013;84(12):1728–33.
27. Lascarrou JB, Le Gouge A, Dimet J, Lacherade JC, Martin-Lefevre L, Fiancette M, et al. Neuromuscular blockade during therapeutic hypothermia after cardiac arrest: observational study of neurological and infectious outcomes. Resuscitation. 2014;85(9):1257–62.
28. Price D, Kenyon NJ, Stollenwerk N. A fresh look at paralytics in the critically ill: real promise and real concern. Ann Intensive Care. 2012;2(1):43.

29. Perman SM, Kirkpatrick JN, Reitsma AM, Gaieski DF, Lau B, Smith TM, et al. Timing of neuroprognostication in postcardiac arrest therapeutic hypothermia*. Crit Care Med. 2012;40(3):719–24.

30. Cronberg T, Horn J, Kuiper MA, Friberg H, Nielsen N. A structured approach to neurologic prognostication in clinical cardiac arrest trials. Scand J Trauma Resusc Emerg Med. 2013;21:45.

31. Kamps MJ, Horn J, Oddo M, Fugate JE, Storm C, Cronberg T, et al. Prognostication of neurologic outcome in cardiac arrest patients after mild therapeutic hypothermia: a meta-analysis of the current literature. Intensive Care Med. 2013;39(10):1671–82.

32. Rossetti AO, Oddo M, Logroscino G, Kaplan PW. Prognostication after cardiac arrest and hypothermia: a prospective study. Ann Neurol. 2010;67(3):301–7.

33. Taccone F, Cronberg T, Friberg H, Greer D, Horn J, Oddo M, et al. How to assess prognosis after cardiac arrest and therapeutic hypothermia. Crit Care. 2014;18(1):202.

34. Mathew JP, Weatherwax KJ, East CJ, White WD, Reves JG. Bispectral analysis during cardiopulmonary bypass: the effect of hypothermia on the hypnotic state. J Clin Anesth. 2001;13(4):301–5.

35. Honan D, Doherty D, Frizelle H. A comparison of the effects on bispectral index of mild vs. moderate hypothermia during cardiopulmonary bypass. Eur J Anaesthesiol. 2006;23(5):385–90.

6

Does metformin exposure before ICU stay have any impact on patients' outcome?

Sebastien Jochmans[1]*[ID], Jean-Emmanuel Alphonsine[2], Jonathan Chelly[1], Ly Van Phach Vong[3], Oumar Sy[3], Nathalie Rolin[3], Olivier Ellrodt[3], Mehran Monchi[1] and Christophe Vinsonneau[4]

Abstract

Background: Impact of metformin exposure before ICU stay remains controversial. Metformin is thought to induce lactic acidosis and haemodynamic instability but may reduce ICU mortality. We evaluated its influence on outcome in diabetic patients admitted in the ICU and then compared two different populations based on the presence of septic shock.

Methods: We conducted a retrospective cohort study in a 24-bed French ICU between October 2010 and December 2013, including all ICU-admitted diabetic patients.

Results: Among 635 diabetic patients admitted during the study period, 131 (21%) were admitted with septic shock. Multivariate analysis showed no difference in hospital mortality in all metformin users (OR 0.75 [95% CI 0.44–1.28]; $p = 0.29$), except in the septic shock subgroup (OR 0.61; 95% CI [0.37–0.99]; $p = 0.04$) despite higher vasopressor dosages in the first hours after shock onset. Blood lactate level was higher in metformin users than in non-metformin users in all patients ($p < 0.001$), in septic shock patients ($p < 0.001$) and in patients without kidney injury ($p < 0.001$). Metformin users did not have more septic shock from unknown aetiology ($p = 0.65$) or unknown pathogen ($p = 0.99$).

Conclusions: Metformin use before admission to ICU did not affect in-hospital mortality. However, for patients with septic shock, mortality was lower, despite worse clinical presentation on admission. Blood lactate levels were always higher with or without septic shock and indifferent of kidney function.

Keywords: Metformin, Septic shock, Diabetes, Lactic acidosis, ICU

Background

Metformin is increasingly used as an oral antidiabetic (OAD) agent, especially in patients with type 2 diabetes mellitus. Metformin inhibits hepatic glucose production, reduces intestinal glucose absorption and improves glucose metabolism [1].

Its use is associated with a reduction in cardiovascular morbidity and mortality, in comparison with insulin, other OADs or diet alone, in non-acutely ill patients [2, 3]. It is thought to induce or worsen lactic acidosis, especially in acute renal or liver dysfunction [4]. But in a recent meta-analysis pooling 347 trials involving long-run metformin use, the authors found no case of metformin-associated lactic acidosis (MALA), as well as no difference in blood lactate level related to metformin use [5]. These results were confirmed in a large cohort of diabetic patients treated with metformin despite various metformin contraindications, in which no MALA has been described by the authors [2].

In the ICU, MALA has been described in renal, liver, pulmonary or cardiovascular chronic failure [6], and several case reports described fatal or non-fatal MALA in acute conditions. In contrast, a recent retrospective

*Correspondence: sebastien.jochmans@gmail.com
[1] Département de Médecine Intensive et Unité de Recherche Clinique, Groupe Hospitalier Sud Ile-de-France, Hôpital de Melun, 77000 Melun, France
Full list of author information is available at the end of the article

study in 17 Danish ICUs found that prior to admission metformin use was associated with a reduction in 30-day mortality [3].

Our main objective in this study was to evaluate the influence of pre-admission metformin use on outcome in diabetic ICU patients and in a subgroup experiencing septic shock (an acute condition known to induce lactic acidosis [7, 8]). Secondary objectives were to assess MALA incidence and blood lactate levels in ICU patients with diabetes, treated or not by metformin, with or without septic shock.

Methods

We performed a retrospective cohort study in our Intensive Care Medicine Department between October 2010 and December 2013. The study protocol was approved by the French Intensive Care Society (FICS)—Société de Réanimation de Langue Française (SRLF)—ethical review board.

Patients

Inclusion and exclusion criteria

All patients admitted within the study period with a history of diabetes treated by insulin or oral antidiabetics were included. So-called diabetic patients treated only with diet were considered as unconfirmed diabetes and were excluded. The other exclusion criteria were as follows:

Unknown chronic antidiabetic treatment, modifications of antidiabetic treatment during the month before ICU admission and unavailable arterial blood gas sample within 4 h after ICU admission.

Data collection

Collected clinical features were as follows: age, sex, height, weight, Simplified Acute Physiology Score II (SAPS II), main admission cause, metformin contraindication ('Definitions' paragraph below), ICU admission biomarkers (leucocytes, platelets, haemoglobin, creatinine, C-reactive protein, bilirubin and/or INR if available), arterial blood gas samples at day 1, all bacteriological tests, vasopressor dosages (close to the initiation even outside the ICU), urinary output and amount of intravascular input during the first 24 h, the use of invasive ventilation and renal replacement therapy, the presence of acute respiratory distress syndrome (ARDS), ICU and hospital length of stay and vital status.

Definitions

Usual metformin contraindications (adapted from the instructions for the use of the medicinal product) were defined as:

1. Chronic respiratory failure (previous pulmonary function tests, history of acute respiratory decompensation, oxygen or non-invasive ventilation at home, sleep apnoea) and/or
2. Chronic cardiac failure (history of pulmonary oedema, left ventricular ejection fraction < 45%) and/or
3. Chronic renal disease (calculated creatinine clearance with Modification of Diet in Renal Disease [MDRD] < 60 mL/min/1.73 m^2) and/or
4. Chronic liver disease (history of cirrhosis, previous INR > 1.2) and/or
5. Myocardial infarction during the previous month

Septic shock was defined according to the Surviving Sepsis Campaign definition [9]. Acute kidney injury was defined using Kidney Disease Improving Global Outcome (KDIGO) classification [10] and was considered for any stage of the classification.

Statistical analysis

Continuous variables were expressed as median [25th–75th interquartile range] or mean ± standard deviation [95% confidence interval] (after Shapiro–Wilks test) and compared using nonparametric Mann–Whitney (or Student's t test) and linear regression tests. Categorical variables were expressed as n (%) and compared using Chi-square or Fisher's exact tests. All tests were two-tailed assuming alpha risk = 0.05. All collected data were analysed in univariate analysis regarding ICU and hospital survivals. We included in forward and backward stepwise multivariate regression models as covariates all data with $p < 0.1$ in univariate analysis, with stratification by metformin use. We applied these models in ICU patients and in the subgroups of septic shock and metformin users with usual contraindication. We performed a post hoc validity assessment of the regression models by receiver operating characteristic (ROC) curves, and we selected as the result the model with the best area under the curve. Results of multivariate regression test were expressed by odds ratio (95% confidence interval). Prognostic value of blood lactate level on mortality was tested with ROC curves (results expressed by area under the curve [AUC] % (95% confidence interval)), sensitivity and sensibility.

Statistical analysis and graphic representations were performed with SPSS Statistics V20 software (IBM®, New York, NY, USA) and Prism 6 software (GraphPad Software Inc.®, San Diego, CA, USA).

Results

Among the 3871 patients admitted in our ICU during the study period, 635 (16.4%) were finally included (study flowchart is available in Additional file 1: Figure S1), including 131 (20.6%) patients with septic shock at day 1 after ICU admission.

Metformin use before admission was found in 240 patients (37.8%) and was similar regarding occurrence or non-occurrence of septic shock ($p = 0.69$). Ratio of metformin use in patients with one or more usual contraindications was high (119 (49.6%)) with a similar rate in septic shock patients ($p = 0.54$).

ICU admission and hospital stay

The main characteristics of ICU diabetics at admission and during ICU or hospital stays are specified in Table 1 and Additional file 1: Table S1. In our study cohort, 588 (92.6%) patients were admitted for a medical cause, mainly for acute respiratory failure (266 (41.9%)). There was no difference between metformin users (MET) and non-metformin users (NO-MET) in the reason for admission. MET were younger with less chronic respiratory and renal failures. They had higher blood lactate level ($p < 0.001$), lower bicarbonate ($p < 0.01$) and also lower serum creatinine ($p < 0.001$) with less acute kidney injury ($p < 0.001$). Severity score (SAPS II) and need in organ support (i.e. invasive mechanical ventilation, vasopressor, renal replacement therapy) were similar. Among MET, there was no difference in lactate level between patients with or without usual contraindication ($p = 0.86$) (Additional file 1: Table S2).

The main characteristics for diabetics with septic shock at admission and during ICU or hospital stays are specified in Table 2 and Additional file 1: Tables S3 and S4. Aetiologies of shock are specified in Additional file 1: Table S3. There was no difference between MET and NO-MET regarding unknown aetiology ($p = 0.65$) and unknown pathogen ($p = 0.99$) (Additional file 1: Table S4). MET with septic shock had higher blood lactate than NO-MET at admission ($p < 0.001$) and during the first 12 h (Fig. 1). Bicarbonate was lower ($p < 0.01$). They also received more renal replacement therapy ($p = 0.02$), while they had less chronic renal failure and there was no significant difference in serum creatinine, pH, day 1 urinary output or acute kidney injury occurrence. In MET, there was a linear correlation between blood lactate and serum creatinine ($\rho = 0.36$; $p < 0.01$) in contrast to NO-MET ($\rho = 0.09$; $p = 0.41$) (Additional file 1: Figures S2 and S3). However, lactate was even higher in MET ($p < 0.001$) with normal kidney function (MDRD creatinine clearance > 60 mL/min/1.73 m^2).

Septic shock severity can also be evaluated by the amount of vascular filling and the dose of vasopressors. There was no difference in the number of patients with intensive vascular filling (i.e. more than 50 mL/kg/day) between MET and NO-MET, but there was a statistical trend for higher maximal dose of noradrenaline in MET

Table 1 Cohort of ICU diabetics: main characteristics at ICU admission, during ICU stay and ICU/hospital outcome

	ICU diabetics	No metformin	Metformin
N	635	395 (62.2)	240 (37.8)
Age (y)	71 [61–79]	73 [62.5–80]	68 [60–78]*
Men	408 (64.3)	255 (64.6)	153 (63.8)
SAPS II	39 [31–52]	40 [32–52]	38 [29–51]
Usual metformin contraindication	387 (60.9)	268 (67.9)	119 (49.6)*
Chronic respiratory insufficiency	190 (29.9)	132 (33.4)	58 (24.2)*
Chronic cardiac insufficiency	138 (21.7)	92 (23.3)	46 (19.2)
Chronic liver disease	75 (11.8)	49 (12.4)	26 (10.8)
Chronic kidney failure	144 (22.7)	128 (32.4)	16 (6.7)*
Recent myocardial infarction	8 (1.3)	5 (1.3)	3 (1.3)
pH	7.36 [7.28–7.42]	7.36 [7.29–7.43]	7.36 [7.27–7.42]
PaCO$_2$ (mmHg)	36 [29–43]	37 [30–44]	36 [28–43]
HCO$_3$ (mmHg)	21.3 [17–25.2]	21.9 [17.5–26]	20.4 [15.3–24]*
Lactate (mmol/L)	1.4 [0.9–2.4]	1.2 [0.8–2.1]	1.8 [1.1–3.9]*
INR	1.25 [1.06–1.71]	1.26 [1.06–1.65]	1.24 [1.07–1.77]
Bilirubin (µmol/L)	10 [7–16]	10 [7–16]	10 [7–16]
C-reactive protein (mg/L)	34 [8–115]	35 [8–115]	32 [8–115]
Haemoglobin (g/dL)	11.2 [9.6–13]	11.1 [9.6–12.7]	11.7 [9.7–13.4]
Leucocytes (G/L)	11.2 [8.1–15.3]	10.8 [7.5–14.6]	11.7 [8.4–16.3]
Platelets (G/L)	213 [155–277]	207 [155–271]	219 [157–293]
Creatinine (µmol/L)	131 [85–238]	153 [90–285]	108 [80–174]*
Acute kidney injury	392 (61.7)	268 (67.8)	124 (51.7)*
Renal replacement therapy	113 (17.8)	72 (18.2)	41 (17.1)
Vasopressors	229 (36.1)	136 (34.4)	93 (38.8)
Invasive ventilation	230 (36.2)	139 (35.2)	91 (37.9)
ICU length of stay (d)	6 [3–10]	6 [3.5–10]	6 [3–9]
ICU death	117 (18.4)	75 (19)	42 (17.5)
Hospital length of stay (d)	12 [6–23]	12 [6–23]	13 [7–23]
Hospital death	140 (22)	92 (23.3)	48 (20)

Values are *n* (%) or median [IQR 25th–75th]

* $p < 0.05$ between metformin and no metformin

($p = 0.09$). Vasopressor dose was significantly higher in MET the first hours after reaching criteria for septic shock (Fig. 2).

Mortality and length of stay

ICU or hospital lengths of stay as well as ICU death showed no statistically significant difference between MET and NO-MET in the cohort of diabetics and in the

Table 2 Subgroup of ICU diabetics with septic shock: main characteristics at ICU admission, during ICU stay and ICU/hospital outcome

	Septic shocks	No metformin	Metformin
N	131	79 (60.3)	52 (39.7)
Age (y)	70 [63–78]	71 [64–78]	66 [61–78]
Men	89 (67.9)	56 (70.9)	33 (63.5)
SAPS II	52 [42–69]	48 [40–68]	57 [46–68]
Usual metformin contraindication	79 (60.3)	56 (70.9)	23 (44.2)*
Chronic respiratory failure	30 (22.9)	21 (26.6)	9 (17.3)
Chronic cardiac failure	27 (20.6)	20 (25.3)	7 (13.5)
Chronic liver disease	26 (19.8)	18 (22.8)	8 (15.4)
Chronic renal failure	19 (14.5)	16 (20.3)	3 (5.8)*
Recent myocardial infarction	1 (0.8)	1 (1.3)	0
pH	7.32 [7.2–7.38]	7.32 [7.23–7.39]	7.26 [7.17–7.38]
PaCO$_2$ (mmHg)	34 [27–42]	35 [29–43]	34 [24–42]
HCO$_3$ (mmHg)	18.2 [13.3–22.2]	19.7 [14.7–24.1]	15.5 [10.1–19.9]*
Lactate (mmol/L)	2.2 [1.1–5]	1.4 [1–2.8]	4.5 [2.1–8.7]*
INR	1.5 [1.2–2.3]	1.6 [1.3–2.9]	1.4 [1.1–1.9]
Bilirubin (μmol/L)	12 [8–24]	13 [8–26]	10 [8–19]
C-reactive protein (mg/L)	95 [24–224]	98 [30–225]	85 [14–212]
Haemoglobin (g/dL)	10.6 [9.1–12.4]	10.7 [9.3–12.4]	10.5 [9.1–12.4]
Leucocytes (G/L)	12.1 [8.3–19.6]	11.9 [8.5–19]	12.9 [8.4–21.6]
Platelets (G/L)	185 [119–265]	199 [120–273]	173 [118–252]
Creatinine (μmol/L)	167 [113–326]	163 [108–276]	176 [123–364]
Urinary output day 1 (mL)	1200 [553–2200]	1200 [558–1925]	1425 [443–2400]
Number of patients with vascular filling > 50 mL/kg ≥ 1 day	76 (60.3)	42 (58.4)	34 (69.4)
Maximum dose of noradrenaline			
(mg/h)	2 [1–4.3]	2 [1–3.5]	3.5 [1.3–5]*
(μg/kg/min)	0.43 [0.22–0.95]	0.4 [0.21–0.76]	0.61 [0.23–1.16]
Maximum dose of adrenaline			
(mg/h)	2.5 [1.5–6]	3 [1.5–6.3]	2.5 [1.4–6]
(μg/kg/min)	0.61 [0.25–1.22]	0.52 [0.22–1.3]	0.66 [0.27–0.98]
Noradrenaline duration (h)	39 [18–64]	48 [19–71]	36 [15–59]
Adrenaline duration (h)	36 [9–90]	36 [14–90]	30 [6–102]
Vasopressor duration (h)	48 [24–96]	48 [24–97]	36 [23–72]
Acute kidney injury	104 (79.4)	62 (78.5)	42 (80.8)
ARDS	48 (36.6)	27 (34.2)	21 (40.4)
Renal replacement therapy	51 (38.9)	24 (30.4)	27 (51.9)*
Invasive ventilation	96 (73.3)	56 (70.9)	40 (76.9)
ICU length of stay (d)	9 [5–16]	9 [6–19]	7 [4–13]
Hospital length of stay (d)	15 [7–29]	15 [8–29]	16 [4–26]
ICU death	51 (38.9)	31 (39.2)	20 (38.5)
Hospital death	53 (40.5)	33 (41.8)	20 (38.5)

Values are n (%) or median [IQR 25th–75th]

* p < 0.05 between metformin and no metformin

subgroup of septic shock patients. Hospital death was not significantly different in multivariate regression model analysis (OR 0.75 [0.44–1.28]; $p = 0.29$) (Additional file 1: Table S5). In the subgroup of septic shock patients, metformin was associated with a lower mortality after multivariate analysis with odds ratio 0.61 [95% CI 0.36–0.99]; $p = 0.049$ (Table 3).

Blood lactate levels showed a prognostic value in MET (AUC 67.3% (95% CI 58.3–76.4); $p = 0.001$) and NO-MET (AUC 68.6% (61.5–75.8); $p < 0.001$) of the cohort

Does metformin exposure before ICU stay have any impact on patients'...

53

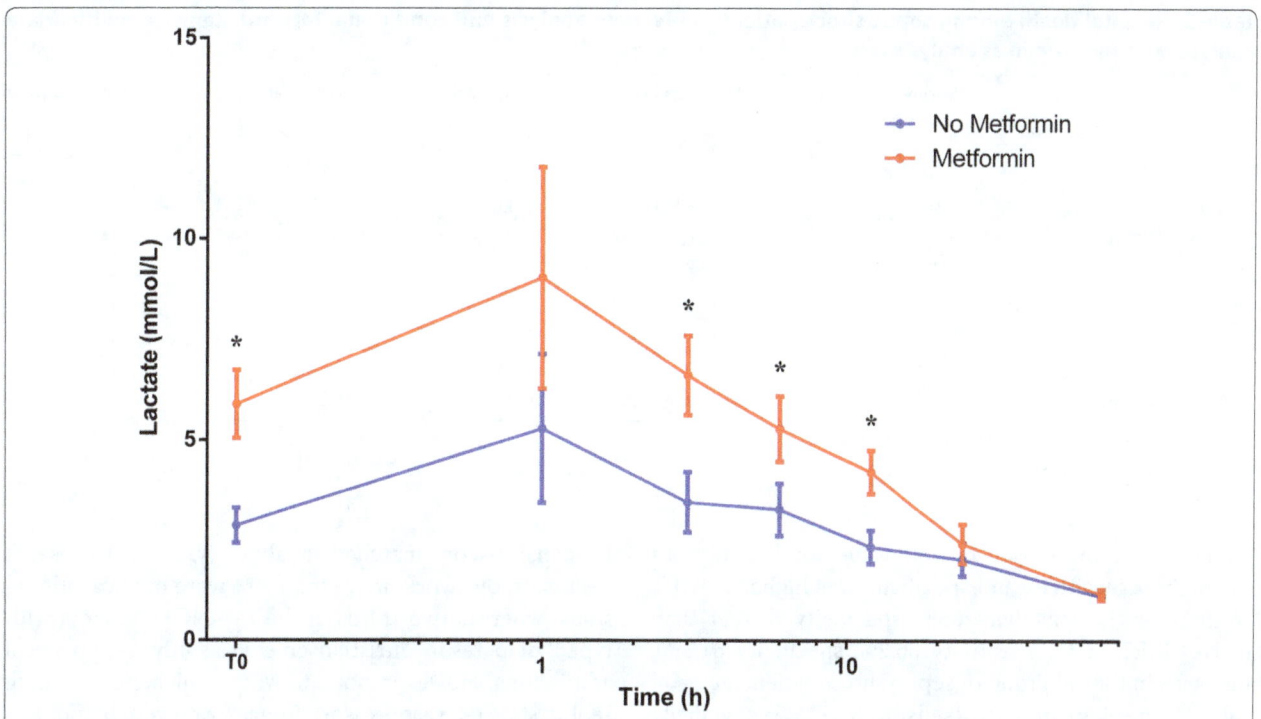

Fig. 1 Initial evolution of lactate level in ICU diabetics sustaining septic shock with or without pre-admission metformin treatment. T0: time of septic shock diagnosis. Abscissa axis is log 10 scale. *$p < 0.05$

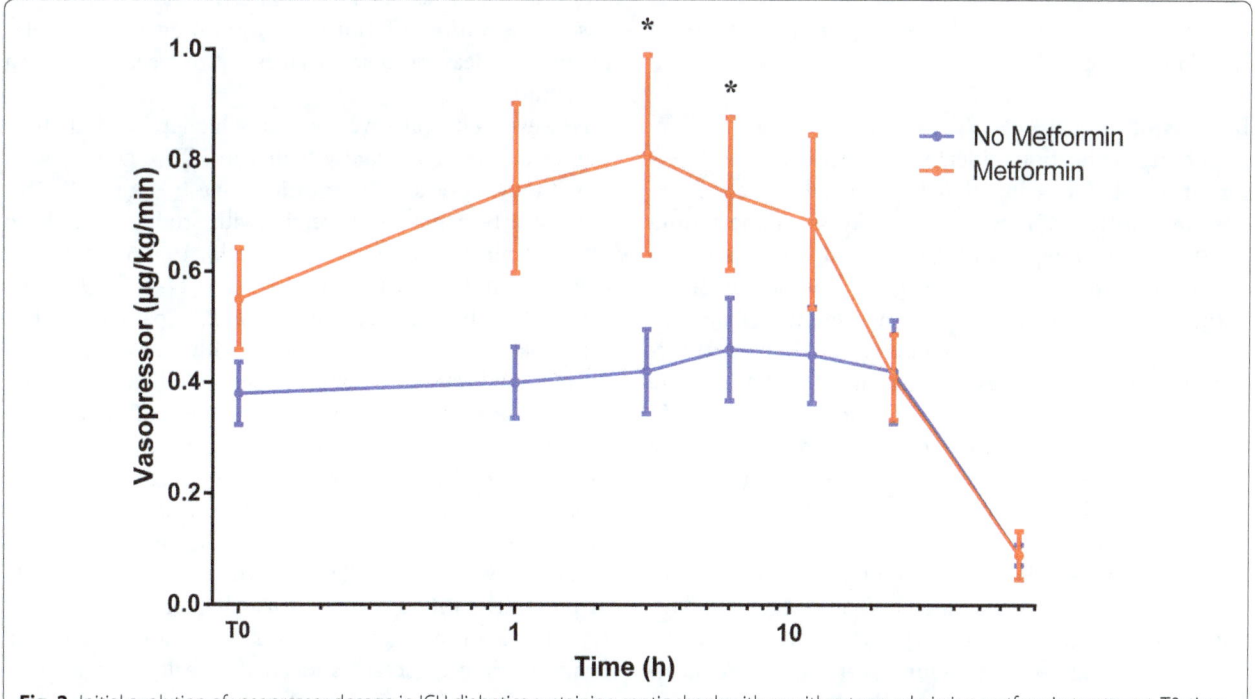

Fig. 2 Initial evolution of vasopressor dosage in ICU diabetics sustaining septic shock with or without pre-admission metformin treatment. T0: time of septic shock diagnosis. Abscissa axis is log 10 scale. *$p < 0.05$

and also in MET (AUC 66.7% (51.5–81.9); $p = 0.05$) and   NO-MET (AUC 65.5% (53–78.1); $p = 0.02$) of shocked

Table 3 Hospital death among septic shock patients: univariate analysis and conditional forward stepwise multivariate analysis with metformin as analysis factor

	Survivor	Non-survivor	P-univariate	Odds ratio	P-multivariate
N	80 (61.1)	51 (38.9)	–	–	–
Men	49 (61.3)	40 (78.4)	0.055	NS	NS
SAPS II	49 [40–61]	65 [46–80]	0.001	1.05 (1.04–1.07)	< 0.001
Metformin (n)	32 (40)	20 (39.2)	1	0.61 (0.37–0.99)	0.049
Lactate (mmol/L)	1.7 [1–3.9]	3.2 [1.4–7.1]	0.003	1.21 (1.1–1.34)	< 0.001
ARDS (n)	23 (28.8)	25 (49)	0.03	NS	NS
RRT (n)	24 (30)	27 (52.9)	0.011	NS	NS
Invasive ventilation (n)	48 (60)	48 (94.1)	< 0.001	NS	NS
Urinary output day 1 (mL)	1400 [675–2400]	1030 [65–1900]	0.03	NS	NS

$a = 0.05$. Area under the curve of the multivariate model = 0.786

RRT renal replacement therapy, *NS* not significant

patients. But prognostic cut-off value for lactate with the highest sensitivity and specificity was higher in MET (2.15 mmol/L, sensitivity 65%, specificity 61.6%) than in NO-MET (1.35, sensitivity 66.2%, specificity 61.3%). Likewise in the subgroup of septic shock patients, cut-off values were 4.45 mmol/L (sensitivity 57.9%, specificity 56.7%) versus 1.45 mmol/L (sensitivity 58.1%, specificity 56.2%), respectively.

Among MET, there was no significant difference in hospital death between patients with or without usual contraindication (OR 1.24 [0.48–3.2]; $p = 0.66$) (Additional file 1: Table S6).

Discussion

In our large cohort on critically ill diabetic patients, metformin use before admission to ICU did not affect in-hospital mortality; however, pre-admission metformin treatment was independently associated with a decrease in hospital mortality in the group of septic shock patients, even with an initial clinical presentation appearing more severe. Indeed, independent of kidney function, vasopressor dosages and serum lactate levels were higher during the first hours after shock onset in MET. Nevertheless, metformin did not seem to induce shock per se because there was no more septic shock from unknown aetiology or unknown pathogens in MET than in NO-MET.

A beneficial association between metformin and mortality has been already described both in selected patients with chronic heart failure [11], liver disease [12, 13], mild-to-moderate kidney failure [14] which are usual contraindications, and in ICU patients [3]. In this latter study, based on retrospective analysis of Northern Denmark database, 30-day mortality was lower in metformin users than in non-metformin users with adjusted hazard ratio = 0.8 (95% confidence interval 0.71–0.95).

Propensity-score-matched analyses yielded the same results. In our work, more than 90% were medical admissions, whereas two-thirds of the 7404 ICU patients with type 2 diabetes in Christiansen et al.'s study were surgical admissions. However, no data were available concerning septic shocks, vasopressor dosages or even blood lactate levels. Mechanisms of this beneficial effect remain unclear: in ICU patients, metformin may supply higher amounts of lactate serving as an energetic carbon source and therefore is available for ischaemic tissues with glucose preservation. Metformin may also decrease cellular hypoxia of less perfused tissues by decreasing oxygen consumption.

However, clinical severity seems higher in MET. Lactate levels are significantly higher in ICU diabetics with or without septic shock (Additional file 1: Figure S4). This issue still remains controversial with studies finding no effect of metformin on lactate rate [5, 15, 16] or, on the contrary, finding an increased lactate [17–27]. One reason for this discrepancy may be that ICU patients, unlike other patients, suffer acute stress with endogenous catecholamine release leading to increased lactate levels through adrenergic receptor stimulation. Physiological studies showed that metformin enhances lactate production and decreases oxygen consumption [23–25] by inhibiting mitochondrial chain complexes [19, 22–24, 27]. Therefore, in our study, prognostic cut-off values are higher in MET, especially when there is a septic shock, as previously found [28]. It is usually admitted that lactic acidosis in metformin users is due to a reduced renal drug clearance. Lactate and creatinine levels (and creatinine clearance) are linearly correlated in our study as previously shown [17, 18, 21, 26, 29–31]. But lactate levels remain higher in patients without kidney injury with metformin than without. This last issue was only previously described in case reports and one cohort study [26], although another study failed to find hyper-lactatemia when kidney function was normal [29]. MET probably received more haemodialysis for the purpose of either correcting deeper hypobasemia or eliminating plasma metformin.

- Vasopressor dosages are higher in septic shock diabetics with pre-admission metformin. This increase in catecholamines need, which has not been previously described, is not due to acidosis per se because pH values are similar with or without metformin. Recent data suggest that metformin decreases adenylate cyclase activity and therefore cyclic AMP concentration [32]. The effects of vasopressors are mediated by adrenergic receptors, G protein and adenylate cyclase stimulations leading to an increase in cyclic AMP concentration. It is assumed that it is necessary to increase vasopressor dosages in order to obtain the same haemodynamic effect and compensate decreased adenylate cyclase activity induced by metformin. Indeed, metformin does not seem to produce sepsis-like shock because there is as much septic shock of unknown aetiology or germ in MET than in NO-MET. However, metformin actually seems to worsen the criteria usually used to assess the severity of septic shocks.

Finally, in our study, patients treated with metformin despite the presence of the usual contraindications do not have higher lactate levels. The mortality rate is not increased either. These contraindications have been challenged for several years so that metformin seems deleterious only in terminal kidney disease [33]. Our collected data did not allow us to evaluate outcome according to the intensity of each organ failure. It is possible that our patients had mainly mild-to-moderate lung, liver, heart or kidney injury that would be insufficient to worsen outcome or lactate level.

Our study is subject to certain limitations. First, it is a retrospective study, avoiding observation bias, but with selection bias due to non-inclusion of patients with missing data. Thus, we cannot determine whether metformin users are more likely to be admitted to ICU than other antidiabetics' takers, and also whether the presence of a contraindication for its use is linked to a higher rate of hospitalization. The lack of randomization of metformin therapy does not indicate whether the improvement in observed survival is due to metformin itself or whether the clinical presentation and biological characteristics of patients taking metformin appear to be 'falsely' more severe. We have included in our logis-

tic regression model certain parameters such as lactate and bicarbonate levels, which are both influenced by the presence of metformin and most likely do not have the same prognostic value in patients previously untreated by metformin. Similarly, elevated doses of vasopressors, which are used as a criterion for poor outcome for example in the SOFA score, may not carry the same prognostic significance. Metformin blood dosage has never been performed. However, it seems linearly correlated to lactate concentration [18, 21, 31]. Lastly, comparison between MET treated or non-treated by renal replacement therapy was unfeasible because analysis would lack power and be statistically unreliable. If current scientific opinion suggests its use in metformin overdose, there is no strong proof. There is indeed a contradiction between studies finding a beneficial association between sepsis and metformin and in contrast the desire to eliminate metformin by haemodialysis. Therefore, we suggest that future studies should seek to answer two questions: Is there a benefit in giving metformin during the first hours of septic shock in diabetic patients previously untreated by metformin? Is there really a benefit in the early elimination of metformin by haemodialysis in diabetic patients with septic shock and without acute kidney injury?

Conclusions

Metformin use before admission to ICU is associated with a decrease in mortality in septic shock patients despite a worse clinical presentation on admission. Metformin users have higher lactate levels independent of kidney function and need higher vasopressor dosages during the first hours of septic shock. Metformin does not seem to induce shock per se. The presence or absence of one of the usual contraindications to taking metformin does not alter lactate levels or hospital mortality.

Abbreviations

AMP: adenosine monophosphate; ARDS: acute respiratory distress syndrome; AUC: area under the curve; ICU: intensive care unit; KDIGO: Kidney Disease Improving Global Outcome; MALA: metformin-associated lactic acidosis; MDRD: Modification of Diet in Renal Disease; MET: metformin users; NO-MET: non-metformin users; OAD: oral antidiabetic; ROC: receiver operating characteristic; RRT: renal replacement therapy; SAPS II: Simplified Acute Physiology Score II; SOFA: Sepsis-Related Organ Failure Assessment score.

Authors' contributions

SJ, JEA, CV and MM had the original idea; SJ dealt with the administrative files and authorizations; SJ, JEA, JC, LVPV, OE, OS and NR collected data; SJ and MM performed the statistical analysis; and SJ, JC and CV wrote the manuscript. All authors read and approved the final manuscript.

Authors' information
First results of this study have been presented by JEA during the 44th Annual Congress of the French Intensive Care Society in Paris 2016.

Author details
[1] Département de Médecine Intensive et Unité de Recherche Clinique, Groupe Hospitalier Sud Ile-de-France, Hôpital de Melun, 77000 Melun, France. [2] Service de Réanimation Médicale, AP-HP, Hôpital Bicêtre, 94270 Le Kremlin-Bicêtre, France. [3] Département de Médecine Intensive, Groupe Hospitalier Sud Ile-de-France, Hôpital de Melun, 77000 Melun, France. [4] Service de Réanimation Polyvalente, Hôpital de Bethune, 62408 Bethune, France.

Acknowledgements
We are indebted to Charles Timoney and Sean A. Freeman for manuscript corrections.

Competing interests
SJ received fees from ResMed. JC received fees from Hamilton Medical. CV received fees from Astute Medical. The remaining authors have disclosed that they do not have any competing interest. None of these competing interests are related to the present manuscript.

Funding
No external source of funding.

References
1. Gong L, Goswami S, Giacomini KM, Altman RB, Klein TE. Metformin pathways: pharmacokinetics and pharmacodynamics. Pharmacogenet Genomics. 2012;22(11):820–7.
2. Eurich DT, Weir DL, Majumdar SR, Tsuyuki RT, Johnson JA, Tjosvold L, et al. Comparative safety and effectiveness of metformin in patients with diabetes mellitus and heart failure: systematic review of observational studies involving 34,000 patients. Circ Heart Fail. 2013;6(3):395–402.
3. Christiansen CF, Johansen MB, Christensen S, O Brien JM, Tønnesen E, Sørensen HT. Preadmission metformin use and mortality among intensive care patients with diabetes: a cohort study. Crit Care. 2013;17(5):R192.
4. Arroyo D, Melero R, Panizo N, Goicoechea M, Rodríguez-Benítez P, Vinuesa SG, et al. Metformin-associated acute kidney injury and lactic acidosis. Int J Nephrol. 2011;2011:749653.
5. Salpeter SR, Greyber E, Pasternak GA, Salpeter EE. Risk of fatal and nonfatal lactic acidosis with metformin use in type 2 diabetes mellitus. Cochrane Database Syst Rev. 2010;4:CD002967.
6. Cicero AFG, Tartagni E, Ertek S. Metformin and its clinical use: new insights for an old drug in clinical practice. Arch Med Sci. 2012;8(5):907–17.
7. Kjelland CB, Djogovic D. The role of serum lactate in the acute care setting. J Intensive Care Med. 2010;25(5):286–300.
8. Rishu AH, Khan R, Al-Dorzi HM, Tamim HM, Al-Qahtani S, Al-Ghamdi G, et al. Even mild hyperlactatemia is associated with increased mortality in critically ill patients. Crit Care. 2013;17(5):R197.
9. Dellinger RP, Levy MM, Rhodes A, Annane D, Gerlach H, Opal SM, et al. Surviving sepsis campaign: international guidelines for management of severe sepsis and septic shock, 2012. Intensive Care Med. 2013;39(2):165–228.
10. Kidney Disease: Improving Global Outcomes (KDIGO) Acute Kidney Injury Work Group. KDIGO clinical practice guideline for acute kidney injury. Kidney Int Suppl. 2012;2:1–138.
11. Romero SP, Andrey JL, Garcia-Egido A, Escobar MA, Perez V, Corzo R, et al. Metformin therapy and prognosis of patients with heart failure and new-onset diabetes mellitus. A propensity-matched study in the community. Int J Cardiol. 2013;166(2):404–12.
12. Zhang X, Harmsen WS, Mettler TA, Kim WR, Roberts RO, Therneau TM, et al. Continuation of metformin use after a diagnosis of cirrhosis significantly improves survival of patients with diabetes. Hepatology. 2014;60(6):2008–16.
13. Harris K, Smith L. Safety and efficacy of metformin in patients with type 2 diabetes mellitus and chronic hepatitis C. Ann Pharmacother. 2013;47(10):1348–52.
14. Inzucchi SE, Lipska KJ, Mayo H, Bailey CJ, McGuire DK. Metformin in patients with type 2 diabetes and kidney disease: a systematic review. JAMA. 2014;312(24):2668–75.
15. Chang C-H, Sakaguchi M, Dolin P. Epidemiology of lactic acidosis in type 2 diabetes patients with metformin in Japan. Pharmacoepidemiol Drug Saf. 2016;25(10):1196–203.
16. Kamber N, Davis WA, Bruce DG, Davis TME. Metformin and lactic acidosis in an Australian community setting: the Fremantle Diabetes Study. Med J Aust. 2008;188(8):446–9.
17. Sipahi S, Solak Y, Acikgoz SB, Genc AB, Yildirim M, Yilmaz U, et al. Retrospective analysis of lactic acidosis-related parameters upon and after metformin discontinuation in patients with diabetes and chronic kidney disease. Int Urol Nephrol. 2016;48(8):1305–12.
18. Cucchiari D, Podestà MA, Merizzoli E, Calvetta A, Morenghi E, Angelini C, et al. Dose-related effects of metformin on acid-base balance and renal function in patients with diabetes who develop acute renal failure: a cross-sectional study. Acta Diabetol. 2016;53(4):551–8.
19. DeFronzo R, Fleming GA, Chen K, Bicsak TA. Metformin-associated lactic acidosis: current perspectives on causes and risk. Metabolism. 2016;65(2):20–9.
20. Hitchings AW, Archer JRH, Srivastava SA, Baker EH. Safety of metformin in patients with chronic obstructive pulmonary disease and type 2 diabetes mellitus. COPD. 2015;12(2):126–31.
21. Adam WR, O'Brien RC. A justification for less restrictive guidelines on the use of metformin in stable chronic renal failure. Diabet Med J Br Diabet Assoc. 2014;31(9):1032–8.
22. Piel S, Ehinger JK, Elmér E, Hansson MJ. Metformin induces lactate production in peripheral blood mononuclear cells and platelets through specific mitochondrial complex I inhibition. Acta Physiol Oxf Engl. 2015;213(1):171–80.
23. Protti A, Lecchi A, Fortunato F, Artoni A, Greppi N, Vecchio S, et al. Metformin overdose causes platelet mitochondrial dysfunction in humans. Crit Care. 2012;16(5):R180.
24. Protti A, Fortunato F, Monti M, Vecchio S, Gatti S, Comi GP, et al. Metformin overdose, but not lactic acidosis per se, inhibits oxygen consumption in pigs. Crit Care. 2012;16(3):R75.
25. Protti A, Russo R, Tagliabue P, Vecchio S, Singer M, Rudiger A, et al. Oxygen consumption is depressed in patients with lactic acidosis due to biguanide intoxication. Crit Care. 2010;14(1):R22.
26. Liu F, Lu J, Tang J, Li L, Lu H, Hou X, et al. Relationship of plasma creatinine and lactic acid in type 2 diabetic patients without renal dysfunction. Chin Med J (Engl). 2009;122(21):2547–53.
27. Dykens JA, Jamieson J, Marroquin L, Nadanaciva S, Billis PA, Will Y. Biguanide-induced mitochondrial dysfunction yields increased lactate production and cytotoxicity of aerobically-poised HepG2 cells and human hepatocytes in vitro. Toxicol Appl Pharmacol. 2008;233(2):203–10.
28. Filho RR, Rocha LL, Corrêa TD, Pessoa CMS, Colombo G, Assuncao MSC. Blood lactate levels cutoff and mortality prediction in sepsis-time for a reappraisal? A retrospective cohort study. Shock. 2016;46(5):480–5.
29. Lepelley M, Giai J, Yahiaoui N, Chanoine S, Villier C. Lactic acidosis in diabetic population: is metformin implicated? Results of a matched case-control study performed on the type 2 diabetes population of Grenoble Hospital University. J Diabetes Res. 2016;2016:3545914.

30. Eppenga WL, Lalmohamed A, Geerts AF, Derijks HJ, Wensing M, Egberts A, et al. Risk of lactic acidosis or elevated lactate concentrations in metformin users with renal impairment: a population-based cohort study. Diabetes Care. 2014;37(8):2218–24.

31. Duong JK, Furlong TJ, Roberts DM, Graham GG, Greenfield JR, Williams KM, et al. The role of metformin in metformin-associated lactic acidosis (MALA): case series and formulation of a model of pathogenesis. Drug Saf. 2013;36(9):733–46.

32. Miller RA, Chu Q, Xie J, Foretz M, Viollet B, Birnbaum MJ. Biguanides suppress hepatic glucagon signaling by decreasing production of cyclic AMP. Nature. 2013;494(7436):256–60.

33. Hung S-C, Chang Y-K, Liu J-S, Kuo K-L, Chen Y-H, Hsu C-C, et al. Metformin use and mortality in patients with advanced chronic kidney disease: national, retrospective, observational, cohort study. Lancet Diabetes Endocrinol. 2015;3(8):605–14.

7

The prognostic impact of abdominal surgery in cancer patients with neutropenic enterocolitis: a systematic review and meta-analysis, on behalf the Groupe de Recherche en Réanimation Respiratoire du patient d'Onco-Hématologie (GRRR-OH)

Colombe Saillard[1*], Lara Zafrani[2], Michael Darmon[3,4], Magali Bisbal[4,5], Laurent Chow-Chine[5], Antoine Sannini[5], Jean-Paul Brun[5], Jacques Ewald[6], Olivier Turrini[6], Marion Faucher[5], Elie Azoulay[2,4,7] and Djamel Mokart[4,5]

Abstract

Neutropenic enterocolitis (NE) is a diagnostic and therapeutic challenge associated with high mortality rates, with controversial opinions on its optimal management. Physicians are usually reluctant to select surgery as the first-choice treatment, concerns being raised regarding the potential risks associated with abdominal surgery during neutropenia. Nevertheless, no published studies comforted this idea, literature is scarce and surgery has never been compared to medical treatment. This review and meta-analysis aimed to determine the prognostic impact of abdominal surgery on outcome of neutropenic cancer patients presenting with NE, versus medical conservative treatment. This meta-analysis included studies analyzing cancer patients presenting with NE, treated with surgical or medical treatment, searched by PubMed and Cochrane databases (1983–2016), according to PRISMA recommendations. The endpoint was hospital mortality. Fixed-effects models were used. The meta-analysis included 20 studies (385 patients). Overall estimated mortality was 42.2% (95% CI = 40.2–44.2). Abdominal surgery was associated with a favorable outcome with an OR of 0.41 (95% CI = 0.23–0.74; $p = 0.003$). Pre-defined subgroups analysis showed that neither period of admission, underlying malignancy nor neutropenia during the surgical procedure, influenced this result. Surgery was not associated with an excess risk of mortality compared to medical treatment. Defining the optimal indications of surgical treatment is needed.

Keywords: Neutropenic enterocolitis, Typhlitis, Cancer patients, Abdominal surgery, Meta-analysis

Background

Neutropenic enterocolitis (NE) or typhlitis is a serious complication of neutropenia characterized by segmental ulceration and inflammation with necrosis of ileum, cecum and ascending colon [1]. NE was initially described in an autopsy study of children with acute leukemia [2] and evolved to an entity encountered in neutropenic patients [3–8]. The pathogenesis of NE is poorly understood and probably multifactorial. Immunosuppression induced by neutropenia, combined with chemotherapy toxicity, tumoral infiltration, intramural hemorrhage and inflammatory reaction lead to direct mucosal injury, up to necrotizing damages and microbial

*Correspondence: saillardc@ipc.unicancer.fr
[1] Haematology Department, Institut Paoli Calmettes, 232 Boulevard Sainte Marguerite, 13009 Marseille Cedex 09, France
Full list of author information is available at the end of the article

translocation. Patients typically present with gastrointestinal (GI) symptoms, in a context of neutropenia, usually following chemotherapy, with bowel wall thickening and positive microbiological samples. Recently, revised diagnostic criteria have been proposed [9]. NE incidence is unknown, reports ranging from 0.8 to 26% [8]. NE carries a poor prognosis, with mortality rates up to 80%, due to complications such as bowel perforation, ischemia, necrosis and septic shock evolution [5, 9, 10].

NE optimal management is controversial, with some advising abdominal surgery [4, 11–16], and others advocating medical conservative treatment including broad-spectrum antibiotherapy, bowel rest and general supportive care [8, 17, 18]. Physicians are often reluctant to surgery, because of neutropenia and thrombopenia. When surgery is indicated, the question of delaying it until neutropenia resolution arises.

Major advances have been made in the last decade in onco-hematology patients, particularly in the management of septic shock [19, 20], critically ill onco-hematology patients admitted to the intensive care unit (ICU) [21], neutropenic cancer patients [12, 22] and organ failures including acute respiratory failure [23–27]. Surprisingly, no major improvements have been reported in neutropenic cancer patients presenting with surgical acute abdominal syndrome [28]. Surgical treatment has never been evaluated neither compared to medical treatment, NE being rare, literature scarce and mainly based on small observational reports, case series or case reports. Surgeons and onco-hematologists are usually reluctant to select surgery as the first-choice treatment, concerns being raised regarding the potential risks associated with abdominal surgery during neutropenia, which is furthermore frequently associated with thrombopenia. Nevertheless, no published studies comforted this idea. Moreover, neutropenia is not considered anymore as an unfavorable prognostic factor in critically ill cancer patients, as recently published in a large meta-analysis [22]. Surgery even appeared to be associated with a good prognosis in a recent publication in neutropenic cancer patients with acute abdominal pain [12].

To determine the prognostic impact of abdominal surgery, compared to medical conservative treatment, on short-term mortality of neutropenic cancer patients presenting with NE, we conducted a systematic review and meta-analysis. Secondary objectives were to assess the influence of surgery on outcome in pre-specified subgroups, according to underlying malignancy, period of admission and the presence of neutropenia during the surgery procedure.

Methods

Review

These systematic review and meta-analysis were reported following criteria set by the PRISMA (Preferred Reporting Items for Systematic reviews and Meta-Analyses) statement and the MOOSE (Meta-analysis Of Observational Studies in Epidemiology) group [29–34]. This study was registered on the international register for prospective reviews PROSPERO (number CRD42016048952).

Study outcome

The aim of this meta-analysis was to determine the prognostic impact of abdominal surgery, compared to medical treatment, on short-term outcome of neutropenic cancer patients presenting with NE. The selected endpoint was overall hospital mortality.

Search strategy and eligibility assessment

First, public-domain databases including PubMed and the Cochrane database were searched by using exploded Medical Subject Headings and the appropriate corresponding keywords: "NEUTROPENIC ENTEROCOLITIS" OR "TYPHLITIS." The research was restricted to English-written abstracts with full-text articles available concerning humans from January 1983 to 2016. References cited in the articles of interest and published reviews were manually searched to find any additional reports. The search was rerun immediately prior to analysis to ensure that the most current information was presented. Abstracts were carefully checked and studies focusing on children or patients aged lower than 18 years old, case reports and studies failing to focus on neutropenic patients were excluded. There were no restrictions in terms of underlying malignancy or study type. In case series, a minimum of three patients were needed with at least one patient in each treatment arm to be analyzed.

All remaining references were then downloaded for consolidation, elimination of duplicates and further analysis. Four authors (CS, LZ, MD, DM) independently determined the eligibility of all studies identified in the initial research. Any disagreements were resolved by discussion. The flowchart of publications selection is presented in Fig. 1.

Data extraction and quality assessment

The authors carried out data extraction working in pairs. Disagreements were resolved by discussion among authors and in case of persistent disagreement by adjudication of a third evaluator.

For each included trial, information was extracted on the following: study design, follow-up period, studied

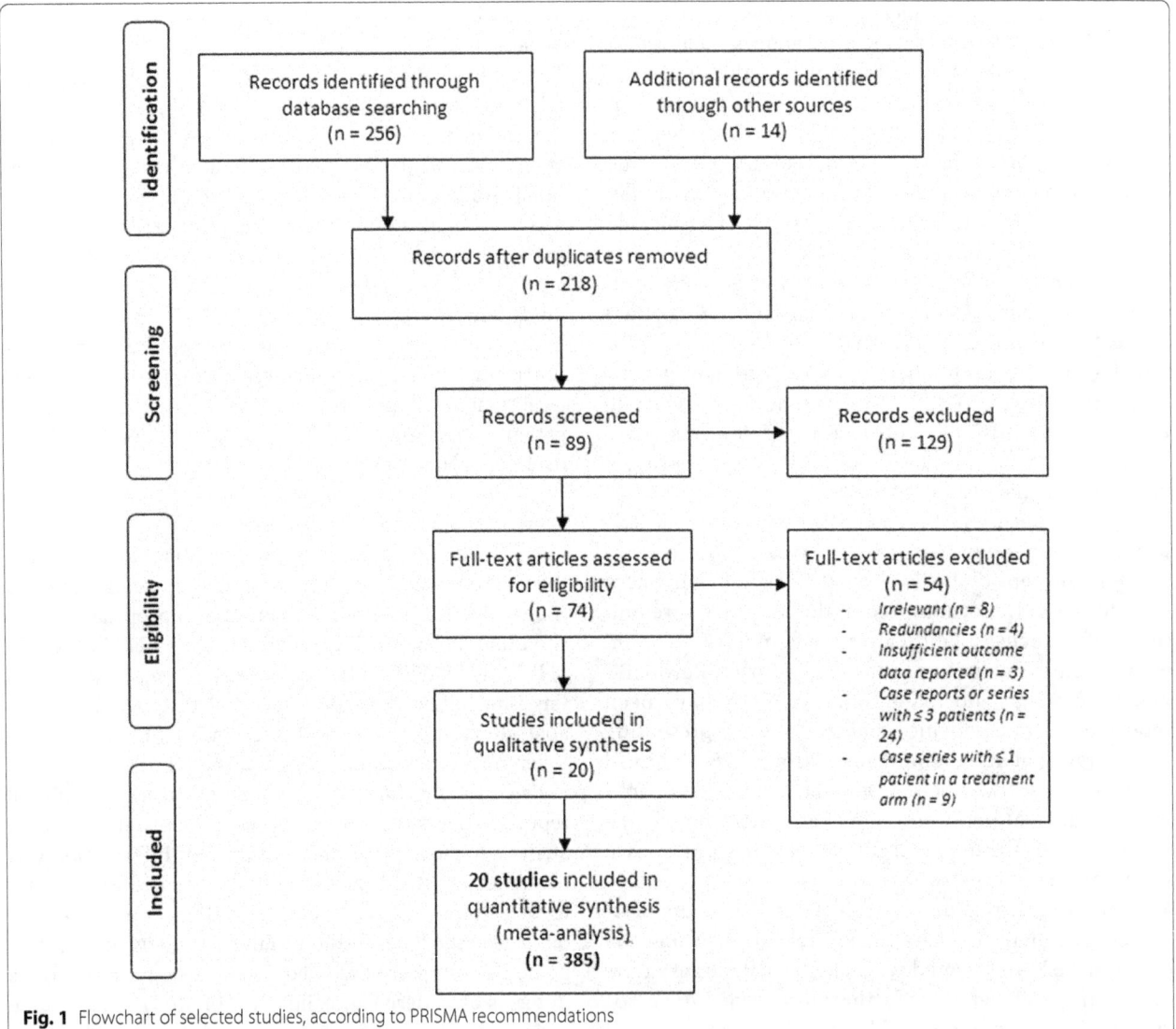

Fig. 1 Flowchart of selected studies, according to PRISMA recommendations

population, number of patients included, period of inclusion, median age, underlying malignancy, rate of allogeneic hematopoietic stem cell transplantation recipients, neutropenia duration, number of patients undergoing surgery during the neutropenic phase, outcome (overall hospital mortality) of patients with and without abdominal surgery, type of surgery, pathological findings and microbiological documentation.

Risk of bias was assessed using the Cochrane's Tool to Assess Risk of Bias in Cohort Studies (http://methods. cochrane.org/bias/reporting-biases). However, all the studies were homogenous in terms of methodology, all of them being retrospective, single-center with small-sample size cohorts including many case series and case reports, making standard scale or checklists difficult to apply.

Statistical analysis

Results were analyzed using Review Manager 5.1 (Cochrane Collaboration, Oxford, UK). Overall hospital mortality of included patients and mortality in included studies are reported as median (interquartiles). The summary estimates of odd ratios (OR) were calculated using the fixed-effects model and presented as forest plots after pooling. All estimates are presented as proportion with two-sided 95% confidence interval (95% CI). The pooled OR, symbolized by a solid diamond at the bottom of the forest plot (the width of which represents the 95% CI), is the best estimate of the pooled outcome. Publication bias was assessed by visually inspecting the funnel plot.

Three subgroups analyzes were preplanned, in order to evaluate the impact of abdominal surgery on outcome according to underlying malignancy (solid tumor, hematological malignancy or both), median ICU admission period (before or after 2003) and neutropenia the day of surgery defined by a neutrophil count < 0.5 G/L (when neutropenia status during surgery procedure was not specified, patients were not analyzed in this subgroup analysis).

A p value of less than 0.05 was considered statistically significant. Cochrane's χ^2 test and I^2 test for heterogeneity were used to assess interstudy heterogeneity. The χ^2 test assessed whether observed differences in results were compatible with chance alone, and the I^2 described the percentage of the variability in effect estimates resulting from heterogeneity rather than from sampling error. An I^2 test for heterogeneity above 0.25 was considered as moderate heterogeneity. Statistically significant heterogeneity was considered present at χ^2 $p < 0.10$ and $I^2 > 50\%$. We used the fixed-effects model as heterogeneity was low in our analyses.

Results

The initial search yielded 270 citations, of which 52 were excluded for duplication. Among these records, 129 were excluded as irrelevant to the scope of this review. For the 89 remaining records, abstracts were carefully checked, and 74 full-text articles focusing on NE cancer patients' management were selected for further evaluation. Articles considered as irrelevant, redundant, with insufficient outcome data reported or less than three patients (including at least one in each treatment arm), or including patients under 18 were excluded. Finally, 20 studies, with a total of 385 patients fulfilled our eligibility criteria and were included (Fig. 1) [9–11, 35–50].

Characteristics of included studies

Included studies were published from 1983 to 2015. All were retrospective and single-center, except one which included eight academic institutions [9]. Study designs consisted of small-size observational studies, case reports (including ≥ 3 patients) and cases series. The sample size of included patients ranged from 3 to 88 patients. Study populations varied across studies, including ten studies focusing on hematology patients ($n=229$) [36–38, 40, 41, 43, 45, 47, 50], one on patients with solid malignancies ($n=4$) [49] and the nine others on onco-hematology patients with no further details [9–11, 35, 39, 42, 44, 46, 48]. Allogenic hematopoietic stem cell recipients represented 93 patients (24%). The outcome variable was overall hospital mortality in all studies. On the total of 385 patients, 76 underwent abdominal surgery, versus 309 benefiting from medical conservative treatment. The detail of surgery procedures, pathological findings and microbial documentation is reported in Tables 1 and 2.

Outcome

Overall estimated mortality rate was 42.2% (95% CI = 40.2–44.2). Overall estimated mortality rates of patients undergoing surgical or medical treatment were 26.6% (95% CI = 19.7–33.4%) and 43.7% (95% CI = 40.1–47.3%), respectively. Funnel plot analysis failed to identify publication bias (Fig. 2). Overall, abdominal surgery was not deleterious and was associated with a favorable outcome, compared to medical conservative treatment, with an OR of 0.41 (95% CI = 0.23–0.74; $p = 0.003$) (Fig. 3). Heterogeneity was low ($I^2 = 15\%$).

Association of abdominal surgery with outcome in the pre-defined subgroups

- Influence of inclusion period (before or after 2003)

Mortality according to the inclusion period is displayed in Fig. 4. Inclusion period did not modify the results of abdominal surgery in neutropenic cancer patients with NE. Before 2003, patients undergoing surgery had a better prognosis compared to patients receiving medical treatment, with an OR of 0.44 (95% CI = 0.23–0.85; $p = 0.01$). After 2003, the association of surgery with outcome tended to decrease over time, with an OR of 0.32 (95% CI = 0.09–1.23; $p = 0.1$).

- Influence of underlying malignancy

In hematology patients, who usually undergo deeper and longer periods of neutropenia, surgery remains associated with a favorable outcome, suggesting that underlying malignancy did not influence outcome (Fig. 5). In studies with pooled oncology and hematology patients, patients undergoing surgery tended to have a better prognosis compared to patients receiving medical treatment, with an OR of 0.48 (95% CI = 0.2–1.16; $p = 0.1$). In studies focusing on patients with heamatological malignancies, the results of surgery were once again favorable with an OR of 0.35 (95% CI = 0.16–0.79; $p = 0.01$). The comparison between surgical and medical treatment could not be performed in oncology patients specifically, as only one publication focused on patients with solid tumors.

- Influence of neutropenia during the surgical procedure

Mortality according to the presence of neutropenia during the surgical procedure is displayed in Fig. 6. It assessed immediate surgery versus surgical procedures delayed after neutropenia resolution. The presence of neutropenia during surgical procedure, compared to patients medically treated, was not deleterious on outcome with an overall OR of 0.87 (95% CI = 0.26–2.89, $p = 0.8$).

Table 1 Surgical procedures in patients undergoing abdominal surgery and pathological findings

Study and year of publication	n/n'	Surgical procedures	Pathological findings	Surgery indication	Mortality after surgery
Mulholland 1983	3/4	Right hemicolectomy with ileostomy (n = 1), Subtotal colectomy with ileostomy (n = 1), No resection (n = 1)	Extensive mucosal and submucosal necrosis. No perforation. The submucosa was edematous	Cecal perforation (2), Colic perforation (1)	2/3
Mower 1986	8/13	Laparotomy without resection (n = 3), Right hemicolectomy (n = 4), Terminal ileal resection (n = 1)	Isolated ileocecal inflammation, edema or pneumatosis without evidence of necrosis or infarction	Perforation (5), Exploratory laparotomy (3)	1/8, 5/8 dead at 4 months
Moir 1986	6/16	Right hemicolectomy, ileostomy, and mucous fistula (n = 3), Divided ileostomy (n = 1), Local resection, ileostomy, abscess drainage (n = 2)	In all, cecal ulceration and mucosal thickening with intense submucosal and mucosal edema. The more severe cases showed hemorrhagic infarction	Severe systemic sepsis, Persistent tenderness, rebound, Pneumatosis, Bowel instruction, Paracolic abcesses, Right flank myonecrosis	2/6
Starnes 1986	5/23	/	/	Cholecystitis, Right lower quadrant typhlitis, Splenic infarction, Diverticular perforation, Large bowel obstruction	0/5
Villar 1987	18/19	Exploratory laparotomy (n = 4), Colectomy (n = 3), Drainage of hepatic abscesses (n = 3), Enterolysis (n = 3), Simoid resection (n = 1), Cholecystectomy (n = 1), Appendicectomy (n = 1), Ligation of esophageal varices and splenectomy (n = 1), Meckel's resection (n = 1)	/	Enterocolitis (4), Sepsis (3), Hepatic abscesses (3), Bowel obstruction (3), Cholecystitis (1), Appendicitis (1)	3/18
Wade 1992	6/22	Appendectomy (n = 2), No bowel resection (n = 1), Right hemicolectomy (n = 1), Diverting colostomy (n = 1), Cholecystectomy (n = 1)	/	Appendicitis (2), Digestive hemorrhage (1), Cecum perforation (1), Prevention of perineal excoriation (1), Cholecystitis (1)	3/6
Abbasoglu 1993	2/3	Appendectomy and cecum exteriorization (n = 1), Laparotomy and sigmoid exteriorization (n = 1)	Ulceration, thrombosed vessels and necrotic areas in the mucosa and submucosa. Necrosis involving all layers, sigmoid perforation	Appendix perforation, Colon perforation	1/2
Buyukasik 1997	3/20	Bowel resection and enterostomy (n = 3)	Ischemic and hemorrhagic mucosal and submucosal necroses extending focally to serosal surface, microvascular thromboses, submucosal edema, bacterial infiltrates with the absence of inflammatory response and necrotic mucosal pseudo-membranes	/	0/3
Gomez 1998	1/18	Exploratory laparotomy (n = 1)	Edematous and thickened cecum and ascending colon	/	/

Table 1 continued

Study and year of publication	n/n'	Surgical procedures	Pathological findings	Surgery indication	Mortality after surgery
Song 1998	2/14	End jejunostomy and fistula (n=1) No bowel resection (n=1)	Ischemia of the entire small bowel, and right colon most severely involving the distal ileum with focal areas of transmural necrosis. Thickened inflamed cecum	Medical treatment failure (1) Peritoneal signs (1)	1/2
Ibrahim 2000	3/6	Right hemicolectomy (n=1) Left hemicolectomy (n=1) Left hemicolectomy (n=1)	Necrotic bowel. Multiple ulcerations of the sigmoid colonic wall and acute and chronic inflammation, acute serositis and perforation. Histologically, extensive ischemic damage was evident, as well as vascular changes, including thrombosis and revascularization associated with mucosal regeneration. Perforation of the descending sigmoid colon. Transmural necrosis associated with perforation was histologically evident	Pneumoperitoneum (2) Severe abdominal pain (1)	1/3
Cartoni 2001	1/88	Left hemicolectomy (n=1)	Ulceration and hemorrhagic necrosis of the intestinal mucosa in all cases, together with a mild-to-moderate mononuclear inflammatory infiltrate	/	0/1
Gorschluter 2002	5/13	Cholecystectomy (n=2) Left-sided colostomy (n=1) Laparotomy (n=1) Appendectomy (n=1)	Diffuse serous inflammation	/	0/5
Kirkpatrick 2003	1/11	Total colectomy (n=1)	Digestive perforation	/	/
Hsu 2004	2/9	Laparotomy (n=2)	Bowel necrosis and peritonitis	/	/
Batlle 2007	6/7	Ileocolic resection (n=1) Right hemicolectomy with ileostomy (n=5)	Typhlitis confirmed. Ulcerated mucosa. Massive edema	/	/
Badgwell 2008	3/17	Right colectomy (n=2) Left colectomy (n=1)	/	/	0/3
Gondal 2010	4/16	/	/	/	/

Table 1 continued

Study and year of publication	n/n'	Surgical procedures	Pathological findings	Surgery indication	Mortality after surgery
Mokart 2017	58/58	/	/	No cause (1) Primary peritonitis (2) Tumoral infiltration (12) Digestive graft versus host disease (2) NE (3) Invasive digestive aspergillosis (3) Digestive bleeding (5) Appendicitis (2) Cholecystitis (3) Sigmoiditis (8) Gastrointestinal obstruction (8) Mesenteric ischemia (2) Others (7)	18/58
Sachak 2015	15/19	Segmental resection (n = 15)	Gross mucosal abnormalities with a patchy distribution. Histologic abnormalities always involved the cecum and/or right colon with other bowel segments variably involved. NE lesions were not seen in the appendix or rectum. Pathologic features included necrosis and hemorrhage. Many cases were characterized by infiltrating organisms in an inflammatory depleted background	/	4/19

n patients undergoing surgery, *n'* total number of patients. *NE* neutropenic enterocolitis

Table 2 Microbial documentation reported in the selected studies

Type of samples	Pathogens identified
Blood cultures	Bacteria
	Klebsiella pneumonia ($n=2$)
	Pseudomonas aeruginosa ($n=1$)
	Escherichia coli ($n=14$)
	Enterococcus faecium ($n=6$)
	Enterobacter aerogenes ($n=1$)
	Clostridium septicum ($n=1$)
	Aeromonas hydrophilia ($n=1$)
	Clostridium perfringens ($n=1$)
	Bacteroides fragilis ($n=1$)
	Gram-negative bacilli (non-specified) ($n=39$)
	Stenotrophomonas maltophilia ($n=1$)
	Staphylococcus aureus ($n=1$)
	Staphylococcus epidermidis ($n=2$)
	Alpha-hemolytic streptococcus ($n=1$)
	Viridans streptococcus ($n=1$)
	Gram-positive Cocci (non-specified) ($n=8$)
	Bacteria (non-specified) ($n=13$)
	Fungi
	Candida krusei ($n=1$)
	Candida glabrata ($n=1$)
	Fungemia ($n=4$)
	Candida (non-specified) ($n=1$)
	Virus
	Cytomegalovirus ($n=1$)
Peroperative digestive samples	Bacteria
	Pseudomonas aeruginosa ($n=4$)
	Escherichia coli ($n=1$)
	Klebsiella pneumonia ($n=1$)
	Diphteroides ($n=1$)
	Acinetobacter anitratus ($n=1$)
	Clostridium difficile ($n=2$)
	Bacteroides fragilis ($n=1$)
	Enterobacter aerogenes ($n=1$)
	Gram-negative bacilli (non-specified) ($n=21$)
	Gram-positive bacilli (non-specified) ($n=2$)
	Fungi
	Aspergillus fumigatus ($n=1$)
	Candida glabrata ($n=2$)
	Candida krusei ($n=1$)
	Candida (non-specified) ($n=7$)
	Virus
	Cytomegalovirus ($n=1$)

Table 2 continued

Type of samples	Pathogens identified
Autopsy samples	*Candida albicans* ($n=3$)
	Candida glabrata ($n=1$)
	Aspergillus fumigatus ($n=1$)
	Aspergillosis pneumonia ($n=5$)
	Fungal pneumonia ($n=3$)
	Kidney and thyroid candida abscess ($n=1$)
Stool samples	*Clostridium difficile* ($n=8$)
	Pseudomonas aeruginosa ($n=1$)
	Escherichia coli ($n=1$)
	Candida glabrata ($n=2$)
	Yeasts (non-specified) ($n=3$)
	Adenovirus ($n=1$)

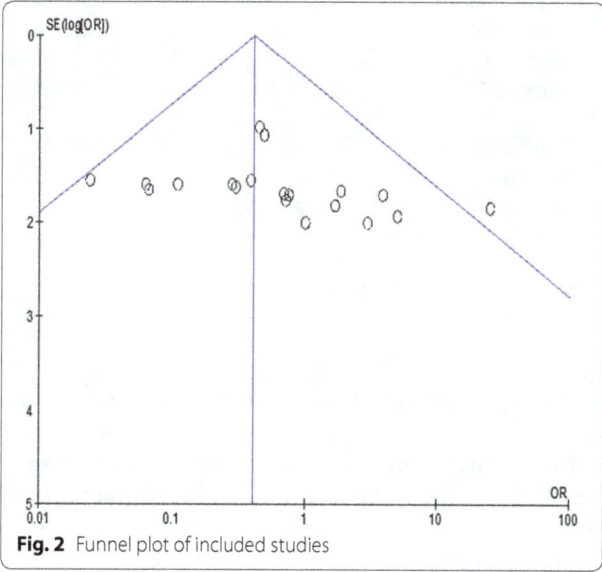

Fig. 2 Funnel plot of included studies

Discussion

This systematic review and meta-analysis, including 385 patients, assessed the prognostic association of abdominal surgery on outcome in neutropenic cancer patients presenting with NE compared to medical conservative treatment. It suggested that surgery was not associated with an increased mortality. According to our results, surgery was not deleterious, regardless of underlying malignancy, time period and the presence of neutropenia at the time of surgery. Interestingly, NE overall mortality was 42.2% (95% IC$=$40.2–44.2), which is particularly encouraging compared to the literature from the 1980s. Moreover, recent data supported the good prognosis associated with NE in a large prospective study of

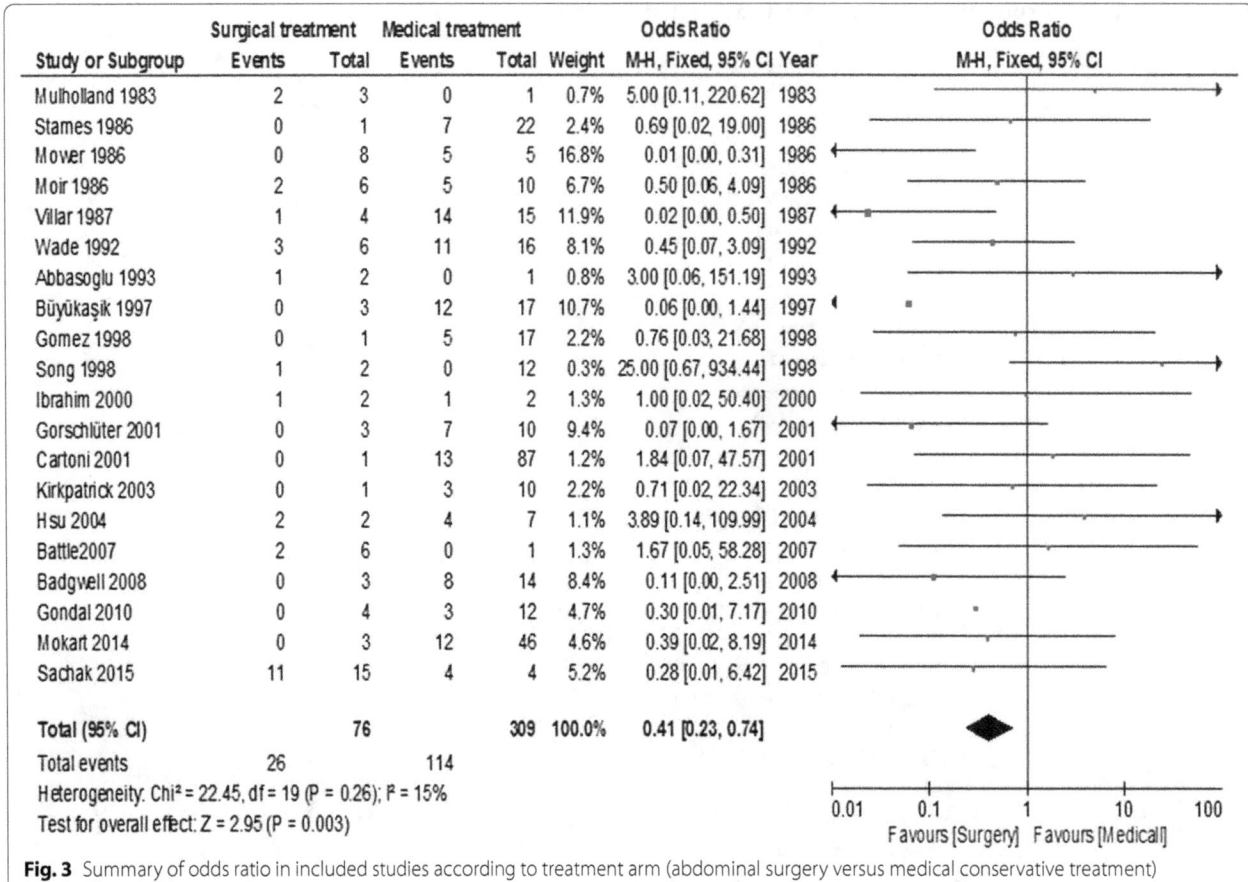

Study or Subgroup	Surgical treatment		Medical treatment			Odds Ratio		Odds Ratio
	Events	Total	Events	Total	Weight	M-H, Fixed, 95% CI	Year	M-H, Fixed, 95% CI
Mulholland 1983	2	3	0	1	0.7%	5.00 [0.11, 220.62]	1983	
Starnes 1986	0	1	7	22	2.4%	0.69 [0.02, 19.00]	1986	
Mower 1986	0	8	5	5	16.8%	0.01 [0.00, 0.31]	1986	
Moir 1986	2	6	5	10	6.7%	0.50 [0.06, 4.09]	1986	
Villar 1987	1	4	14	15	11.9%	0.02 [0.00, 0.50]	1987	
Wade 1992	3	6	11	16	8.1%	0.45 [0.07, 3.09]	1992	
Abbasoglu 1993	1	2	0	1	0.8%	3.00 [0.06, 151.19]	1993	
Büyükaşik 1997	0	3	12	17	10.7%	0.06 [0.00, 1.44]	1997	
Gomez 1998	0	1	5	17	2.2%	0.76 [0.03, 21.68]	1998	
Song 1998	1	2	0	12	0.3%	25.00 [0.67, 934.44]	1998	
Ibrahim 2000	1	2	1	2	1.3%	1.00 [0.02, 50.40]	2000	
Gorschlüter 2001	0	3	7	10	9.4%	0.07 [0.00, 1.67]	2001	
Cartoni 2001	0	1	13	87	1.2%	1.84 [0.07, 47.57]	2001	
Kirkpatrick 2003	0	1	3	10	2.2%	0.71 [0.02, 22.34]	2003	
Hsu 2004	2	2	4	7	1.1%	3.89 [0.14, 109.99]	2004	
Battle 2007	2	6	0	1	1.3%	1.67 [0.05, 58.28]	2007	
Badgwell 2008	0	3	8	14	8.4%	0.11 [0.00, 2.51]	2008	
Gondal 2010	0	4	3	12	4.7%	0.30 [0.01, 7.17]	2010	
Mokart 2014	0	3	12	46	4.6%	0.39 [0.02, 8.19]	2014	
Sachak 2015	11	15	4	4	5.2%	0.28 [0.01, 6.42]	2015	
Total (95% CI)		76		309	100.0%	0.41 [0.23, 0.74]		
Total events	26		114					

Heterogeneity: Chi² = 22.45, df = 19 (P = 0.26); I² = 15%
Test for overall effect: Z = 2.95 (P = 0.003)

Fig. 3 Summary of odds ratio in included studies according to treatment arm (abdominal surgery versus medical conservative treatment)

critically ill neutropenic cancer patients admitted to the ICU [12].

The optimal management of NE has been a matter of debate [1, 8, 11, 51]. Physicians are frequently reluctant to select surgery as the first-choice treatment in neutropenic patients, based on a potential risk of higher infectious and hemorrhagic complications, although no publications support this idea. Interestingly, an appropriately early indication for appendectomy or cholecystectomy in neutropenic hematology patients was not associated with problematic postoperative course [52, 53]. Similarly, in 85 hematology patients who underwent surgery for acute abdominal complication, neutropenia and thrombopenia were not associated with outcome [54]. Moreover, data obtained in non-cancer patients with thrombocytopenia suggest that even high-risk hemorrhage surgical intervention such as splenectomy carried a low risk of morbidity and mortality [55].

Due to improvements in general supportive care, recent studies reported the success of conservative non-surgical management in most patients diagnosed with NE. It includes immediate broad-spectrum antimicrobial therapy adapted to local microbiological ecology

and patients' colonization [56–59], general supportive care (intravenous fluid support, parenteral nutrition and nasogastric suction if necessary, platelet transfusions in patients with severe thrombocytopenia, antalgic treatment) and bowel rest [8]. We could not analyze the impact of granulocyte colony stimulating factor (G-CSF) due to insufficient data. Its routine use remains of uncertain benefit and cannot be recommended [60]. Patients should be carefully monitored using repeated imaging to assess bowel wall thickness in addition to clinical response, as relapses can occur [61]. We found that the protective association of abdominal surgery with outcome tended to decrease over time compared to conservative treatment, probably because major advances have been made in the last decade in the medical management of severe sepsis and septic shock [19, 20], management of onco-hematology patients including in the ICU setting [21, 62] and including neutropenic patients [12, 22] and organ failures management [24–27]. Interestingly, surgery did not become deleterious, whereas medical management improved. Surgical interventions are generally reserved for selected cases of NE based on criteria first proposed by Shamberger et al., including: (a)

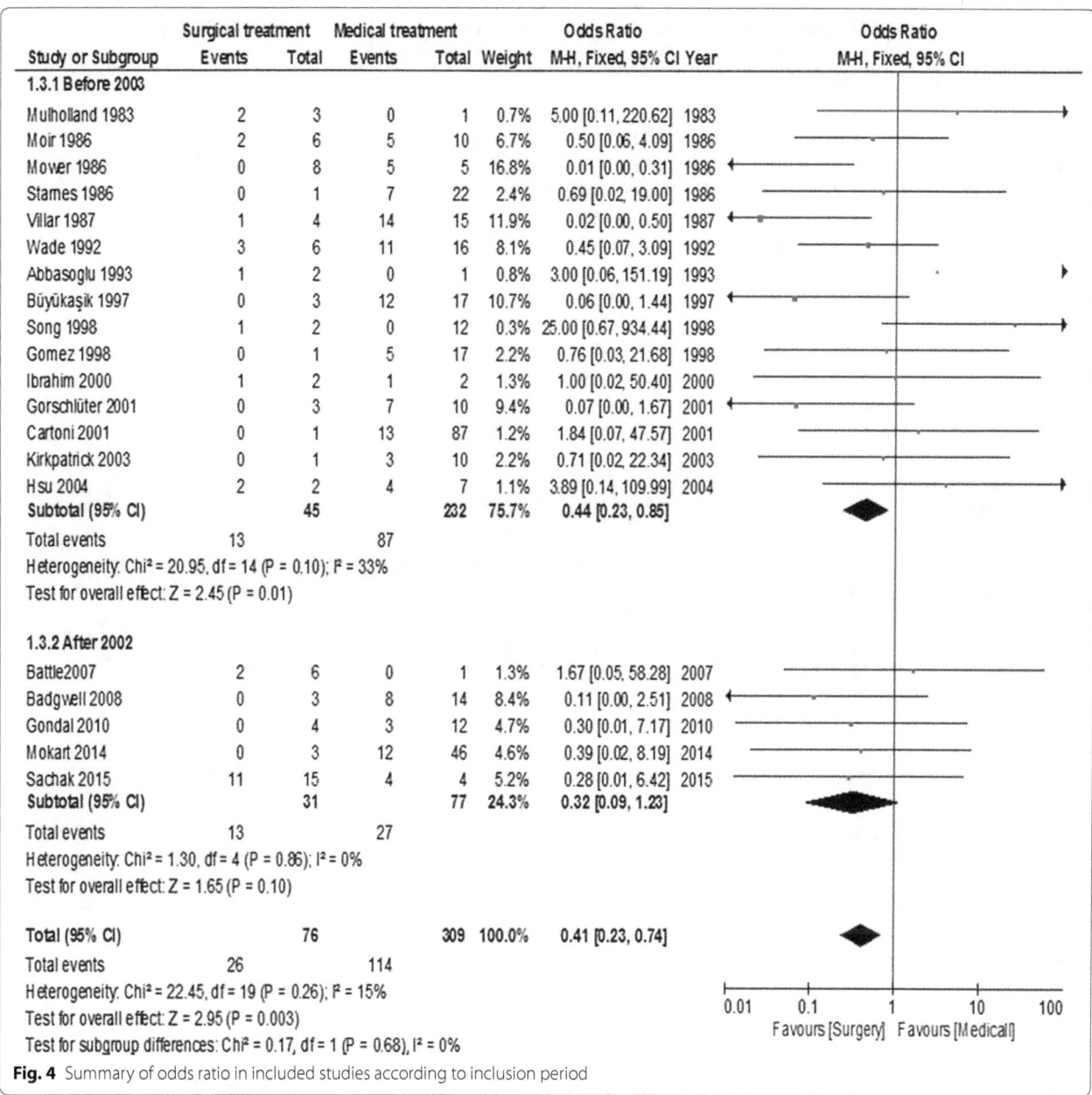

Study or Subgroup	Surgical treatment		Medical treatment		Weight	Odds Ratio M-H, Fixed, 95% CI	Year	Odds Ratio M-H, Fixed, 95% CI
	Events	Total	Events	Total				
1.3.1 Before 2003								
Mulholland 1983	2	3	0	1	0.7%	5.00 [0.11, 220.62]	1983	
Moir 1986	2	6	5	10	6.7%	0.50 [0.06, 4.09]	1986	
Mower 1986	0	8	5	5	16.8%	0.01 [0.00, 0.31]	1986	
Starnes 1986	0	1	7	22	2.4%	0.69 [0.02, 19.00]	1986	
Villar 1987	1	4	14	15	11.9%	0.02 [0.00, 0.50]	1987	
Wade 1992	3	6	11	16	8.1%	0.45 [0.07, 3.09]	1992	
Abbasoglu 1993	1	2	0	1	0.8%	3.00 [0.06, 151.19]	1993	
Büyükaşik 1997	0	3	12	17	10.7%	0.06 [0.00, 1.44]	1997	
Song 1998	1	2	0	12	0.3%	25.00 [0.67, 934.44]	1998	
Gomez 1998	0	1	5	17	2.2%	0.76 [0.03, 21.68]	1998	
Ibrahim 2000	1	2	1	2	1.3%	1.00 [0.02, 50.40]	2000	
Gorschlüter 2001	0	3	7	10	9.4%	0.07 [0.00, 1.67]	2001	
Cartoni 2001	0	1	13	87	1.2%	1.84 [0.07, 47.57]	2001	
Kirkpatrick 2003	0	1	3	10	2.2%	0.71 [0.02, 22.34]	2003	
Hsu 2004	2	2	4	7	1.1%	3.89 [0.14, 109.99]	2004	
Subtotal (95% CI)		45		232	75.7%	0.44 [0.23, 0.85]		
Total events	13		87					
Heterogeneity: Chi² = 20.95, df = 14 (P = 0.10); I² = 33%								
Test for overall effect: Z = 2.45 (P = 0.01)								
1.3.2 After 2002								
Battle 2007	2	6	0	1	1.3%	1.67 [0.05, 58.28]	2007	
Badgwell 2008	0	3	8	14	8.4%	0.11 [0.00, 2.51]	2008	
Gondal 2010	0	4	3	12	4.7%	0.30 [0.01, 7.17]	2010	
Mokart 2014	0	3	12	46	4.6%	0.39 [0.02, 8.19]	2014	
Sachak 2015	11	15	4	4	5.2%	0.28 [0.01, 6.42]	2015	
Subtotal (95% CI)		31		77	24.3%	0.32 [0.09, 1.23]		
Total events	13		27					
Heterogeneity: Chi² = 1.30, df = 4 (P = 0.86); I² = 0%								
Test for overall effect: Z = 1.65 (P = 0.10)								
Total (95% CI)		76		309	100.0%	0.41 [0.23, 0.74]		
Total events	26		114					
Heterogeneity: Chi² = 22.45, df = 19 (P = 0.26); I² = 15%								
Test for overall effect: Z = 2.95 (P = 0.003)								
Test for subgroup differences: Chi² = 0.17, df = 1 (P = 0.68); I² = 0%								

Favours [Surgery]   Favours [Medical]

Fig. 4 Summary of odds ratio in included studies according to inclusion period

the persistence of gastrointestinal bleeding despite correction of coagulopathy, thrombocytopenia and neutropenia; (b) free air in the intraperitoneal cavity indicative of bowel perforation; (c) clinical deterioration despite optimal medical management; and (d) the development of other indications for surgery such as appendicitis [63]. However, these criteria have never been evaluated. Another indication should be evaluated, concerning patients with bowel wall thickness greater than 10 mm, who carry a high mortality rate, because they may benefit from a surgical management [38].

Even when the surgery indication is clear, the optimal timing of surgery is debated. For symptomatic septic neutropenic patients, neutropenia recovery represents a high-risk period in which the clinical status is likely to worsen [64]. Waiting for neutropenia resolution remains debated because this approach might expose patients to a septic degradation toward septic shock. Interestingly, Badgwell recently suggested to delay surgery until neutropenia recovery, although he demonstrated in the same publication that surgery was independently associated with a good outcome, regardless of the duration of neutropenia, which appears as a conflicting message

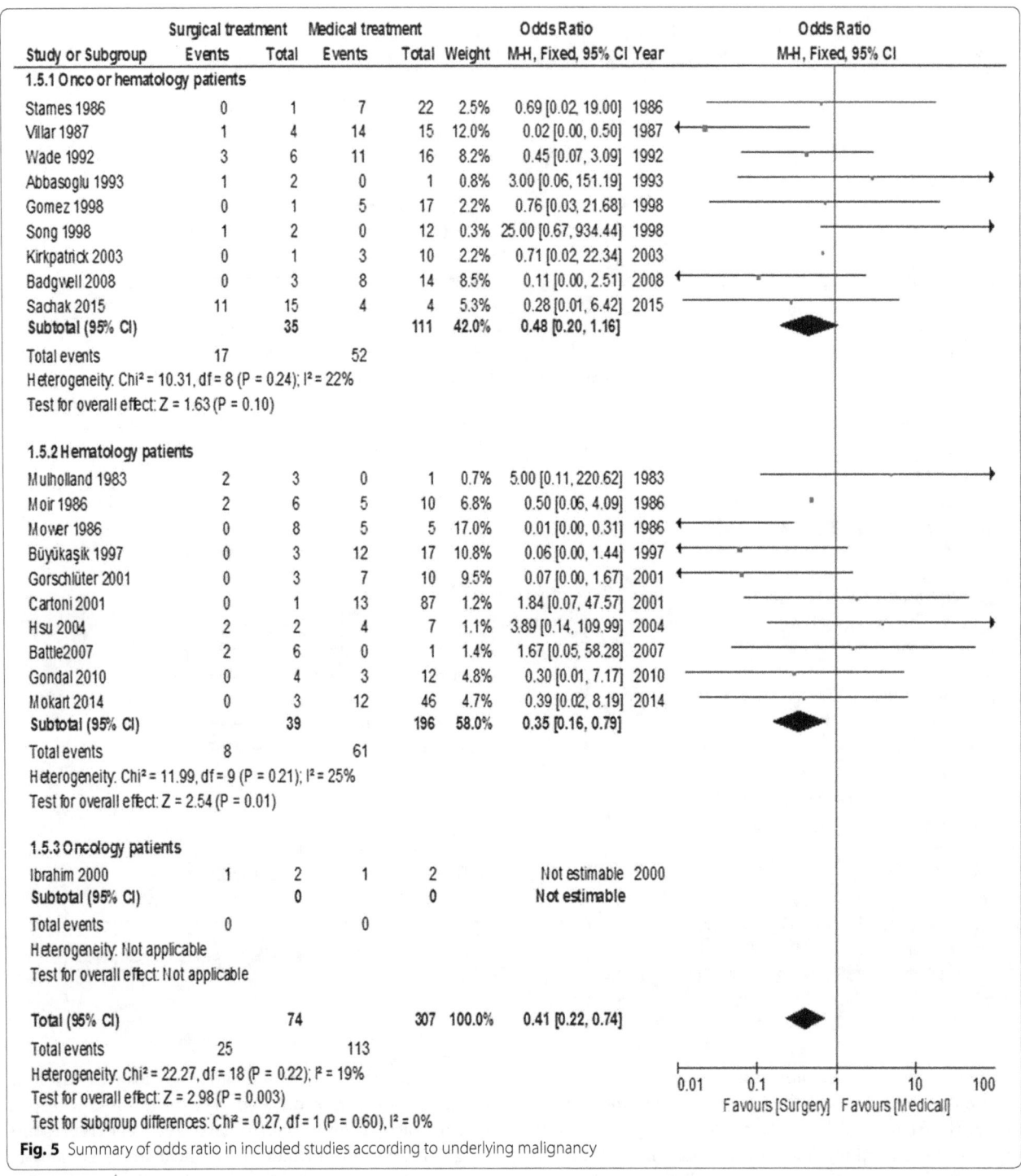

Fig. 5 Summary of odds ratio in included studies according to underlying malignancy

[11]. An expert panel from the French Intensive Care Society stated that neutropenia and thrombocytopenia should not modify the timing of surgery in patients with suspicion of digestive tract perforation [16], without any robust publication to rely on. Recent data demonstrated that preoperative septic shock and renal replacement

therapy were independently associated with an increased mortality in hematology patients who underwent surgery for an acute abdominal complication [54]. We showed that surgery during the neutropenic period did not modify the prognosis, suggesting that surgery should probably not be delayed. It is important to note that some

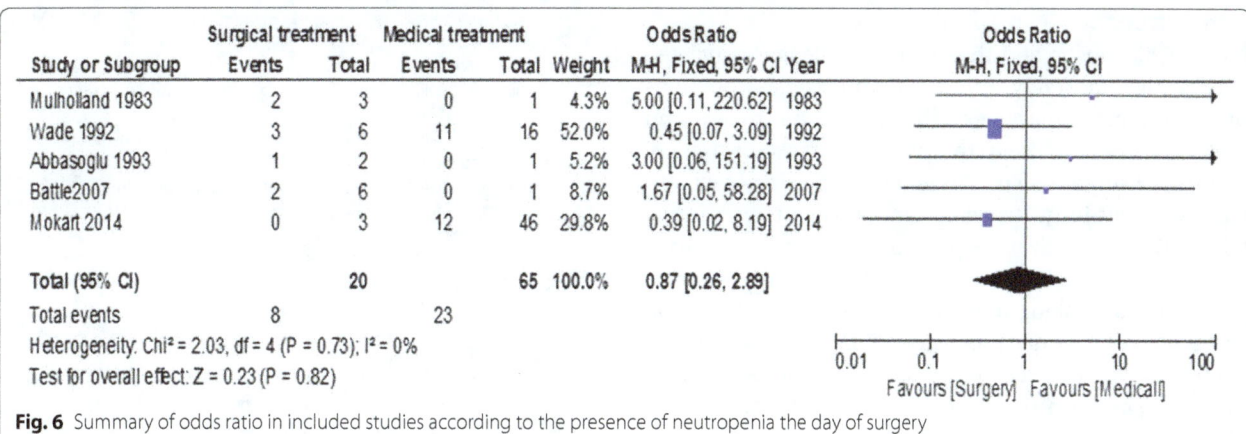

Fig. 6 Summary of odds ratio in included studies according to the presence of neutropenia the day of surgery

patients included in the meta-analysis underwent surgery lately at the stage of septic shock and multi-organ failures. Despite these severe situations, abdominal surgery was not associated with an increased mortality, suggesting that the prognostic impact of surgical management may be underestimated. We could not analyze early versus delayed surgical procedures. The influence of an early surgical strategy on outcome deserves to be evaluated, as we know that an early management is associated with a better prognosis [65, 66].

Our results indicated that surgery was not deleterious. Considering that inadequately treated typhlitis carries a high risk of death [6] and that the lack of surgical management was found to be a significant adverse prognostic factor [9, 11], larger indications of abdominal surgery should probably be evaluated. In tricky situations, exploratory laparotomy could probably be performed, as it seems not to be associated with an increased mortality, and represents an effective way to treat NE, perform microbiological samples and remove infectious inoculum. Pathological reports revealed that white laparotomy was uncommon. Infectious documentation is crucial in these patients, as the absence of diagnosis is a well-known adverse prognostic factor [27]. In the absence of microbial diagnosis, the place of empirical antifungal treatment is questionable, at the light of reported microbiological data.

We acknowledge several limitations. The main one is the strength of evidence in the literature concerning NE therapy, which is extremely poor. Available data are limited to low-quality studies, which are all retrospective, single-center, small-sample cohorts, case reports or case series. Moreover, there is a wide heterogeneity in patients, underlying malignancy, neutropenia duration and immunosuppression. There is also a bias in treatment allocation arm according to centers experience and case-volume, surgical indications differing among the studies. The wide admission period did not reflect all recent improvements and results can therefore be influenced. Moreover, study inclusion period was estimated using median inclusion period. This surrogate is, however, imperfect, a few studies being performed over large period. Lastly, several concerns existed with respect to the terminology of NE, because definition criteria evolved over time. It has been shown that clinical impressions are frequently inaccurate, initial clinical diagnosis being correct in only 53% of cases after autopsy or surgery confirmation [10]. Lastly, this study included various types of abdominal surgery, ranging from cholecystectomy to bowel necrosis with peritonitis, with different ranges of severity (no organ dysfunctions to multi-organ failure) prior to surgery, which can represent important cofounder factors.

However, in the absence of prospective studies or large retrospective cohorts, this meta-analysis may represent the best evidence supporting the absence of increased mortality associated with abdominal surgery in neutropenic cancer patients with NE. We do not know whether surgery is superior or comparable to medical treatment, but it did not appear as deleterious. However, surgical therapy can be useful. Delaying surgical therapy due to neutropenia, thrombocytopenia, or other chemotherapy or malignancies associated reasons is not recommended.

These data strengthen the indications of surgical management in the cases of GI or septic complications and question the place of surgery in other cases. These results may lead to conduct future clinical trials, including homogeneous cohorts of patients in terms of abdominal surgery and organ failure severity, in order to determine optimal surgery indications and evaluate the place of early surgical management in this context.

Conclusions

NE is a diagnostic and therapeutic challenge associated with a high mortality rate, with controversial opinions on its optimal management. This systematic review and meta-analysis suggested the absence of excess risk of abdominal surgery on outcome versus conservative medical treatment in neutropenic cancer patients presenting with NE. Major advances have been made in the management of sepsis and supportive care in onco-hematology patients, making medical treatment essential in all cases. However, surgery appeared to be associated with a favorable outcome when indicated. Additional studies are needed to confirm these results and investigate the best indications of surgical treatment.

Abbreviations

CI: confidence interval; GI: gastro-intestinal; ICU: intensive care unit; MOOSE: meta-analysis of observational studies in epidemiology; NE: neutropenic enterocolitis; OR: odds ratio; PRISMA: preferred reporting items for systematic reviews and meta-analyses.

Authors' contributions

All the authors fulfill all three authorship criteria: conception and design or analysis and interpretation of data, drafting the article and revising it critically for important intellectual content and the final approval of the version to be published. All the authors read and approved the final manuscript.

Author details

[1] Haematology Department, Institut Paoli Calmettes, 232 Boulevard Sainte Marguerite, 13009 Marseille Cedex 09, France. [2] Medical Intensive Care Unit, Saint-Louis University Hospital, AP-HP, Paris, France. [3] Medical-Surgical Intensive Care Unit, Hôpital Nord, Université Jean Monnet, Saint Etienne, France. [4] GRRR-OH (Groupe de Recherche en Réanimation Respiratoire du patient d'Onco-Hématologie), Paris, France. [5] Polyvalent Intensive Care Unit, Department of Anesthesiology and Critical Care, Institut Paoli Calmettes, Marseille, France. [6] Surgery Department, Institut Paoli Calmettes, Marseille, France. [7] Faculté de Médecine, Université Paris Diderot, Sorbonne-Paris-Cité, Paris, France.

Competing interests

The authors declare that they have no competing interests.

References

1. Gorschluter M, Mey U, Strehl J, Ziske C, Schepke M, Schmidt-Wolf IG, et al. Neutropenic enterocolitis in adults: systematic analysis of evidence quality. Eur J Haematol. 2005;75(1):1–13.
2. Moir DH, Bale PM. Necropsy findings in childhood leukaemia, emphasizing neutropenic enterocolitis and cerebral calcification. Pathology. 1976;8(3):247–58.
3. Amromin GD, Solomon RD. Necrotizing enteropathy: a complication of treated leukemia or lymphoma patients. JAMA. 1962;182:23–9.
4. Cunningham SC, Fakhry K, Bass BL, Napolitano LM. Neutropenic enterocolitis in adults: case series and review of the literature. Dig Dis Sci. 2005;50(2):215–20.
5. Katz JA, Wagner ML, Gresik MV, Mahoney DH Jr, Fernbach DJ. Typhlitis. An 18-year experience and postmortem review. Cancer. 1990;65(4):1041–7.
6. Machado NO. Neutropenic enterocolitis: a continuing medical and surgical challenge. N Am J Med Sci. 2010;2(7):293–300.
7. Moir CR, Scudamore CH, Benny WB. Typhlitis: selective surgical management. Am J Surg. 1986;151(5):563–6.
8. Nesher L, Rolston KV. Neutropenic enterocolitis, a growing concern in the era of widespread use of aggressive chemotherapy. Clin Infect Dis. 2013;56(5):711–7.
9. Sachak T, Arnold MA, Naini BV, Graham RP, Shah SS, Cruise M, et al. Neutropenic enterocolitis: new insights into a deadly entity. Am J Surg Pathol. 2015;39(12):1635–42.
10. Wade DS, Nava HR, Douglass HO Jr. Neutropenic enterocolitis. Clinical diagnosis and treatment. Cancer. 1992;69(1):17–23.
11. Badgwell BD, Cormier JN, Wray CJ, Borthakur G, Qiao W, Rolston KV, et al. Challenges in surgical management of abdominal pain in the neutropenic cancer patient. Ann Surg. 2008;248(1):104–9.
12. Mokart D, Darmon M, Resche-Rigon M, Lemiale V, Pene F, Mayaux J, et al. Prognosis of neutropenic patients admitted to the intensive care unit. Intensive Care Med. 2015;41(2):296–303.
13. Koea JB, Shaw JH. Surgical management of neutropenic enterocolitis. Br J Surg. 1989;76(8):821–4.
14. Kunkel JM, Rosenthal D. Management of the ileocecal syndrome. Neutropenic enterocolitis. Dis Colon Rectum. 1986;29(3):196–9.
15. Skibber JM, Matter GJ, Pizzo PA, Lotze MT. Right lower quadrant pain in young patients with leukemia. A surgical perspective. Ann Surg. 1987;206(6):711–6.
16. Schnell D, Azoulay E, Benoit D, Clouzeau B, Demaret P, Ducassou S, et al. Management of neutropenic patients in the intensive care unit (NEWBORNS EXCLUDED) recommendations from an expert panel from the French Intensive Care Society (SRLF) with the French Group for Pediatric Intensive Care Emergencies (GFRUP), the French Society of Anesthesia and Intensive Care (SFAR), the French Society of Hematology (SFH), the French Society for Hospital Hygiene (SF2H), and the French Infectious Diseases Society (SPILF). Ann Intensive Care. 2016;6(1):90.
17. O'Brien S, Kantarjian HM, Anaissie E, Dodd G, Bodey GP. Successful medical management of neutropenic enterocolitis in adults with acute leukemia. South Med J. 1987;80(10):1233–5.
18. Sloas MM, Flynn PM, Kaste SC, Patrick CC. Typhlitis in children with cancer: a 30-year experience. Clin Infect Dis. 1993;17(3):484–90.
19. Dellinger RP, Levy MM, Rhodes A, Annane D, Gerlach H, Opal SM, et al. Surviving Sepsis Campaign: international guidelines for management of severe sepsis and septic shock, 2012. Intensive Care Med. 2013;39(2):165–228.
20. Rivers E, Nguyen B, Havstad S, Ressler J, Muzzin A, Knoblich B, et al. Early goal-directed therapy in the treatment of severe sepsis and septic shock. N Engl J Med. 2001;345(19):1368–77.
21. Azoulay E, Mokart D, Pene F, Lambert J, Kouatchet A, Mayaux J, et al. Outcomes of critically ill patients with hematologic malignancies: prospective multicenter data from France and Belgium—a groupe de recherche respiratoire en reanimation onco-hematologique study. J Clin Oncol. 2013;31(22):2810–8.
22. Bouteloup M, Perinel S, Bourmaud A, Azoulay E, Mokart D, Darmon M. Outcomes in adult critically ill cancer patients with and without neutropenia: a systematic review and meta-analysis of the Groupe de Recherche en Reanimation Respiratoire du patient d'Onco-Hematologie (GRRR-OH). Oncotarget. 2016;8:1860.
23. Azoulay E, Afessa B. The intensive care support of patients with malignancy: do everything that can be done. Intensive Care Med. 2006;32(1):3–5.
24. Azoulay E, Schlemmer B. Diagnostic strategy in cancer patients with acute respiratory failure. Intensive Care Med. 2006;32(6):808–22.
25. Azoulay E, Mokart D, Rabbat A, Pene F, Kouatchet A, Bruneel F, et al. Diagnostic bronchoscopy in hematology and oncology patients with acute respiratory failure: prospective multicenter data. Crit Care Med. 2008;36(1):100–7.
26. Azoulay E, Lemiale V, Mokart D, Pene F, Kouatchet A, Perez P, et al. Acute respiratory distress syndrome in patients with malignancies. Intensive Care Med. 2014;40(8):1106–14.
27. Azoulay E, Pene F, Darmon M, Lengline E, Benoit D, Soares M, et al. Managing critically ill hematology patients: time to think differently. Blood Rev. 2015;29(6):359–67.
28. Hohenberger P, Buchheidt D. Surgical interventions in patients with hematologic malignancies. Crit Rev Oncol Hematol. 2005;55(2):83–91.
29. Beller EM, Glasziou PP, Altman DG, Hopewell S, Bastian H, Chalmers I, et al. PRISMA for Abstracts: reporting systematic reviews in journal and conference abstracts. PLoS Med. 2013;10(4):e1001419.
30. Stroup DF, Berlin JA, Morton SC, Olkin I, Williamson GD, Rennie D, et al.

Meta-analysis of observational studies in epidemiology: a proposal for reporting. Meta-analysis Of Observational Studies in Epidemiology (MOOSE) group. JAMA. 2000;283(15):2008–12.

31. Liberati A, Altman DG, Tetzlaff J, Mulrow C, Gotzsche PC, Ioannidis JP, et al. The PRISMA statement for reporting systematic reviews and meta-analyses of studies that evaluate health care interventions: explanation and elaboration. PLoS Med. 2009;6(7):e1000100.

32. Mahid SS, Hornung CA, Minor KS, Turina M, Galandiuk S. Systematic reviews and meta-analysis for the surgeon scientist. Br J Surg. 2006;93(11):1315–24.

33. Moher D, Liberati A, Tetzlaff J, Altman DG. Preferred reporting items for systematic reviews and meta-analyses: the PRISMA statement. PLoS Med. 2009;6(7):e1000097.

34. Shamseer L, Moher D, Clarke M, Ghersi D, Liberati A, Petticrew M, et al. Preferred reporting items for systematic review and meta-analysis protocols (PRISMA-P) 2015: elaboration and explanation. BMJ. 2015;349:g7647.

35. Abbasoglu O, Cakmakci M. Neutropenic enterocolitis in patients without leukemia. Surgery. 1993;113(1):113–6.

36. Batlle M, Vall-Llovera F, Bechini J, Camps I, Marcos P, Vives S, et al. Neutropenic enterocolitis in adult patients with acute leukemia or stem cell transplant recipients: study of 7 cases. Med Clin (Barc). 2007;129(17):660–3.

37. Buyukasik Y, Ozcebe OI, Haznedaroglu IC, Sayinalp N, Soylu AR, Ozdemir O, et al. Neutropenic enterocolitis in adult leukemias. Int J Hematol. 1997;66(1):47–55.

38. Cartoni C, Dragoni F, Micozzi A, Pescarmona E, Mecarocci S, Chirletti P, et al. Neutropenic enterocolitis in patients with acute leukemia: prognostic significance of bowel wall thickening detected by ultrasonography. J Clin Oncol. 2001;19(3):756–61.

39. Gomez L, Martino R, Rolston KV. Neutropenic enterocolitis: spectrum of the disease and comparison of definite and possible cases. Clin Infect Dis. 1998;27(4):695–9.

40. Gondal G, Johnson E, Paulsen V, Hasan B. Treatment of neutropenic enterocolitis. Tidsskr Nor Laegeforen. 2010;130(2):143–5.

41. Hsu TF, Huang HH, Yen DH, Kao WF, Chen JD, Wang LM, et al. ED presentation of neutropenic enterocolitis in adult patients with acute leukemia. Am J Emerg Med. 2004;22(4):276–9.

42. Kirkpatrick ID, Greenberg HM. Gastrointestinal complications in the neutropenic patient: characterization and differentiation with abdominal CT. Radiology. 2003;226(3):668–74.

43. Mower WJ, Hawkins JA, Nelson EW. Neutropenic enterocolitis in adults with acute leukemia. Arch Surg. 1986;121(5):571–4.

44. Song HK, Kreisel D, Canter R, Krupnick AS, Stadtmauer EA, Buzby G. Changing presentation and management of neutropenic enterocolitis. Arch Surg. 1998;133(9):979–82.

45. Mulholland MW, Delaney JP. Neutropenic colitis and aplastic anemia: a new association. Ann Surg. 1983;197(1):84–90.

46. Starnes HF Jr, Moore FD Jr, Mentzer S, Osteen RT, Steele GD Jr, Wilson RE. Abdominal pain in neutropenic cancer patients. Cancer. 1986;57(3):616–21.

47. Moir CR, Scudamore CH, Benny WB. Typhlitis: selective surgical management. Am J Surg. 1986;151(5):563–6.

48. Villar HV, Warneke JA, Peck MD, Durie B, Bjelland JC, Hunter TB. Role of surgical treatment in the management of complications of the gastrointestinal tract in patients with leukemia. Surg Gynecol Obstet. 1987;165(3):217–22.

49. Ibrahim NK, Sahin AA, Dubrow RA, Lynch PM, Boehnke-Michaud L, Valero V, et al. Colitis associated with docetaxel-based chemotherapy in patients with metastatic breast cancer. Lancet. 2000;355(9200):281–3.

50. Gorschluter M, Glasmacher A, Hahn C, Leutner C, Marklein G, Remig J, et al. Severe abdominal infections in neutropenic patients. Cancer Invest. 2001;19(7):669–77.

51. Chirletti P, Barillari P, Sammartino P, Cardi M, Caronna R, Arcese W, et al. The surgical choice in neutropenic patients with hematological disorders and acute abdominal complications. Leuk Lymphoma. 1993;9(3):237–41.

52. D'Souza S, Lindberg M. Typhlitis as a presenting manifestation of acute myelogenous leukemia. South Med J. 2000;93(2):218–20.

53. Kim KU, Kim JK, Won JH, Hong DS, Park HS. Acute appendicitis in patients with acute leukemia. Korean J Intern Med. 1993;8(1):40–5.

54. Mokart D, Penalver M, Chow-Chine L, Ewald J, Sannini A, Brun JP, et al. Surgical treatment of acute abdominal complications in hematology patients: outcomes and prognostic factors. Leuk Lymphoma. 2017;58:1–8.

55. Kojouri K, Vesely SK, Terrell DR, George JN. Splenectomy for adult patients with idiopathic thrombocytopenic purpura: a systematic review to assess long-term platelet count responses, prediction of response, and surgical complications. Blood. 2004;104(9):2623–34.

56. Freifeld AG, Bow EJ, Sepkowitz KA, Boeckh MJ, Ito JI, Mullen CA, et al. Clinical practice guideline for the use of antimicrobial agents in neutropenic patients with cancer: 2010 Update by the Infectious Diseases Society of America. Clin Infect Dis. 2011;52(4):427–31.

57. Mokart D, Saillard C, Sannini A, Chow-Chine L, Brun JP, Faucher M, et al. Neutropenic cancer patients with severe sepsis: need for antibiotics in the first hour. Intensive Care Med. 2014;40(1):1173–4.

58. Saillard C, Sannini A, Chow-Chine L, Blache JL, Brun JP, Mokart D. Febrile neutropenia in onco-hematology patients hospitalized in Intensive Care Unit. Bull Cancer. 2015;102(4):349–59.

59. Solomkin JS. Evaluating evidence and grading recommendations: the SIS/IDSA guidelines for the treatment of complicated intra-abdominal infections. Surg Infect (Larchmt). 2010;11(3):269–74.

60. Smith TJ, Khatcheressian J, Lyman GH, Ozer H, Armitage JO, Balducci L, et al. 2006 update of recommendations for the use of white blood cell growth factors: an evidence-based clinical practice guideline. J Clin Oncol. 2006;24(19):3187–205.

61. Rolston KV. Neutropenic enterocolitis associated with docetaxel therapy in a patient with breast cancer. Clin Adv Hematol Oncol. 2009;7(8):527–8.

62. Mokart D, Pastores SM, Darmon M. Has survival increased in cancer patients admitted to the ICU? Yes. Intensive Care Med. 2014;40(10):1570–2.

63. Shamberger RC, Weinstein HJ, Delorey MJ, Levey RH. The medical and surgical management of typhlitis in children with acute nonlymphocytic (myelogenous) leukemia. Cancer. 1986;57(3):603–9.

64. Azoulay E, Darmon M. Acute respiratory distress syndrome during neutropenia recovery. Crit Care. 2010;14(1):114.

65. Mokart D, Lambert J, Schnell D, Fouche L, Rabbat A, Kouatchet A, et al. Delayed intensive care unit admission is associated with increased mortality in patients with cancer with acute respiratory failure. Leuk Lymphoma. 2013;54(8):1724–9.

66. Song JU, Suh GY, Park HY, Lim SY, Han SG, Kang YR, et al. Early intervention on the outcomes in critically ill cancer patients admitted to intensive care units. Intensive Care Med. 2012;38(9):1505–13.

Acute kidney injury epidemiology, risk factors, and outcomes in critically ill patients 16–25 years of age treated in an adult intensive care unit

Dana Y. Fuhrman[1]*[ID], Sandra Kane-Gill[2], Stuart L. Goldstein[3], Priyanka Priyanka[4] and John A. Kellum[4]

Abstract

Background: Most studies of acute kidney injury (AKI) have focused on older adults, and little is known about AKI in young adults (16–25 years) that are cared for in an adult intensive care unit (ICU). We analyzed data from a large single-center ICU database and defined AKI using the Kidney Disease Improving Global Outcomes criteria. We stratified patients 16–55 years of age into four age groups for comparison and used multivariable logistic regression to identify associations of potential susceptibilities and exposures with AKI and mortality.

Results: AKI developed in 52.6% ($n = 8270$) of the entire cohort and in 39.8% of the young adult age group (16–25 years). The AUCs for the age categories were similar at 0.754, 0.769, 0.772, and 0.770 for the 16–25-, 26–35-, 36–45-, and 45–55-year age groups, respectively. For the youngest age group, diabetes (OR 1.89; 95% CI 1.09–3.29), surgical reason for admission (OR 1.79; 95% CI 1.44–2.23), severity of illness (OR 1.02; 95% CI 1.02–1.03), hypotension (OR 1.13; 95% CI 1.04–1.24), and certain medications (vancomycin and calcineurin inhibitors) were all independently associated with AKI. AKI was a significant predictor for longer length of stay, ICU mortality, and mortality after discharge.

Conclusions: AKI is a common event for young adults admitted to an adult tertiary care center ICU with an associated increased length of stay and risk of mortality. Potentially modifiable risk factors for AKI including medications were identified for all stratified age groups.

Keywords: Young adult, Acute kidney injury (AKI), Critically ill

Background

An association of acute kidney injury (AKI) and adverse outcomes including length of hospital stay, progression to chronic kidney disease (CKD), and mortality is consistently shown in multiple patient populations [1–6]. In critically ill patients the rates of AKI vary based on the population studied and definition of AKI used, with reported rates of 8–89% for children [7–11] and 7–25% for adults [12–15]. Recently, investigators in the Assessment of Worldwide Acute Kidney Injury, Renal Angina, and Epidemiology (AWARE) study explored the association of AKI with morbidity and mortality in patients 3 months to 25 years of age admitted to a pediatric intensive care unit (ICU) [5]. However, no prior study has investigated specifically the incidence and implications of AKI in the young adult critically ill patient population treated in an adult ICU, a patient group that is growing in adult critical care practices [16].

Given the complexity and diversity of the critical care patient population, it can be challenging to identify and address the numerous risk factors for AKI encountered in the ICU. Since we continue to have no direct pharmacologic therapies for AKI, prevention is of paramount importance. An understanding of the potentially modifiable risk factors that may be unique to different patient groups within the ICU is critical to the prevention of

*Correspondence: dana.fuhrman@chp.edu
[1] Children's Hospital of Pittsburgh, 4401 Penn Avenue, Children's Hospital Drive, Faculty Pavilion Suite 2000, Pittsburgh, PA 15224, USA
Full list of author information is available at the end of the article

AKI. As a result of an increasing number of individuals with childhood chronic illnesses surviving into adulthood [17], there is a need to understand the potentially unique modifiable risk factors for AKI in the 16–25-year-old or young adult ICU population. Little is known about the potential comorbid conditions that may exist in this age group, possibly impacting their AKI incidence and outcomes. As a result of certain comorbid conditions prior to entering the ICU, patients may have a greater exposure to nephrotoxic pharmacologic agents thereby potentially increasing their risk of AKI. Hui-Stickle et al. [18] demonstrated that nephrotoxic medications were the most common cause of acute renal failure for older children and adolescents, while ischemia was the most common etiology in patients 5 years of age or less. There have been no previous studies to date exploring the susceptibilities, exposures, and outcomes of AKI specifically in young adult ICU patients cared for outside of a children's hospital. Thus, we sought to determine if the incidence, risks, and associated outcomes for AKI varied by age across a population of 16–55-year-old ICU patients treated in an adult hospital ICU.

Methods
Study population
After obtaining institutional review board approval, data were obtained from the High-Density Intensive Care (HiDenIC) database, which includes clinical variables on all patients admitted to the University of Pittsburgh,

a tertiary care academic medical center, from July 2000–September 2008. The HiDenIC database includes data on adult patients admitted to one of eight ICUs (medical, cardiac, transplant, surgical, neurological, and trauma). Exclusion criteria were applied including: (1) history of hemodialysis or renal transplant, (2) baseline creatinine > 3.5 mg/dl, (3) liver transplant during the index hospitalization, (4) insufficient information to determine AKI status, and (5) unknown age (Fig. 1). We defined the young adult population as those individuals 16–25 years of age. The remaining cohort was stratified into 10-year age increments including: 26–35 years, 36–45 years, and 46–55 years.

Clinical variables
The risk factors included the analysis are significant predictors of AKI in previous studies [19, 20]. The potential risk factors include sex, race, reference creatinine, estimated glomerular filtration rate (eGFR) derived from the reference creatinine [21], comorbid conditions defined by ICD-9 codes (cardiac disease, CKD, diabetes, fluid overload, history of hypertension, malignancies), admission type (medical or surgical), and moderate anemia (defined by The World Health Organization [22]). Fluid balance was calculated by subtracting total intake from output divided by the admission weight (kg) $\times$ 100 in the first 24 h of ICU admission [23]. We defined fluid overload as a fluid balance > 5%. Severity of illness was evaluated with the Acute Physiology and Chronic Healthy

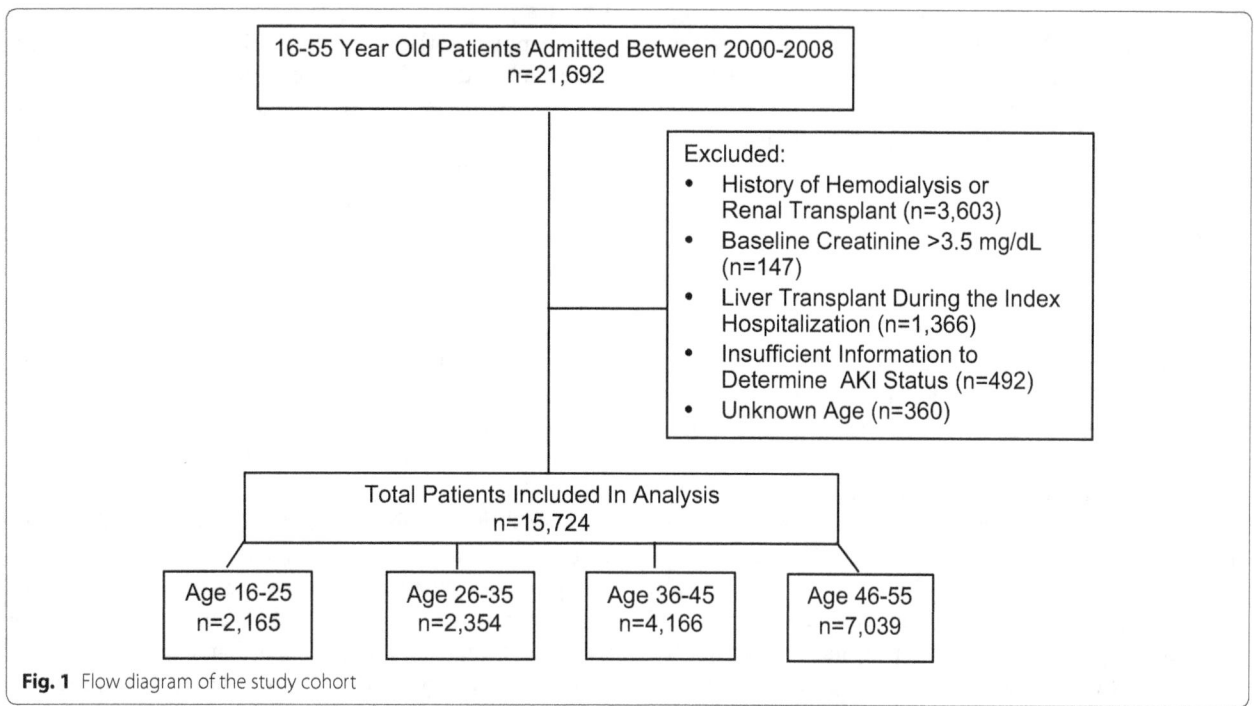

Fig. 1 Flow diagram of the study cohort

Evaluation (APACHE) III score [24]. In the first 24 h of ICU admission, the need for vasopressors, mechanical ventilation as well as concern for sepsis (the ordering of blood cultures and antibiotics within 24 h of each other) was also included. Additionally, we evaluated exposure to potentially nephrotoxic medications within the first 24 h of ICU admission, including angiotensin-converting enzyme inhibitors, angiotensin II receptor blockers, vancomycin, aminoglycosides, antibiotics other than vancomycin or aminoglycosides (including piperacillin/tazobactam, cephalosporins, quinolones, macrolides, sulfonamides, and carbapenems), calcineurin inhibitors, nonsteroidal anti-inflammatory drug (NSAID) medications, acyclovir, mannitol, and phenytoin.

Outcomes

We defined AKI according to the Kidney Disease Improving Global Outcomes (KDIGO) criteria [4]. Any patient meeting the criteria for KDIGO stage 1 or more based on either serum creatinine or urine output during their ICU stay was deemed to have AKI. We defined the reference creatinine as the baseline creatinine when available (lowest value between the most recent hospital creatinine value up to 1 year prior the index hospital admission and the creatinine recorded in the first 24 h of hospital admission) or the lowest value between the creatinine recorded in the first 24 h of hospital admission, first 24 h of ICU admission, and (for patients without a history of CKD) the creatinine derived from the Modification of Diet in Renal Disease (MDRD) equation for creatinine using an eGFR of 75 ml/min/1.73 m² [25, 26]. The reference creatinine was used to determine creatinine changes for defining AKI. We evaluated for each age strata rates of AKI, need for renal replacement therapy (RRT), recovery from RRT, ICU length of stay, hospital length of stay, ICU mortality, hospital mortality, 90-day mortality, and 1-year mortality.

Statistical analysis

Categorical variables were summarized as number and percentage, and continuous variables were summarized as median with interquartile range. Given the large number of patients in the study, statistical differences alone are unlikely to be meaningful. Therefore, we set 10% as a clinically meaningful difference between age groups. Age per 5 years was included as a risk factor for each age group to account for differences within the age groups. To determine the susceptibilities and exposures associated with AKI, multivariable logistic regression was performed whereby: (1) the cohort was stratified by age group (each of 10 years, starting from age 16–25) and (2) with age group as a main effect and accounting for interactions between age group and all other risk factors.

Age-stratified models were built using the following steps: (1) adding each risk factor to age as a continuous variable and using the Wald statistic to determine their significance, (2) the individual size of all variables in step 1 was tested with the Wald statistic as they were added to a multivariable logistic regression model, (3) variables with $p \geq 0.05$ were taken out of the model and a reduced model was fit, and (4) lastly to compare nested models in steps 2 and 3 the likelihood ratio test was used to determine a final model. For the interaction models, in order to find a main effects model, age group was used as a main effect and steps 1 through 4 were repeated. With age retained in the models regardless of significance level, all possible interactions were added one at a time and their significance was determined with the Wald statistic. STATA's "roctab" function was used to assess the area under the receiver operating characteristic curve (AUC) for each age-stratified model. In addition, the "rocreg" function that uses bootstrap (1000 replications) for inference was also used to assess nonparametric ROC estimation under the presence of covariates. Model selection for ICU mortality, hospital mortality, mortality at 90 days after ICU admission, and mortality 1 year after ICU admission across age groups was done using the stepwise selection methodology described above to identify the best model for mortality prediction. Goodness of fit was assessed using Hosmer–Lemeshow [27]. Statistical analyses were performed using STATA software (version SE 14.0, StataCorp LP) and SAS 9.4 with statistical significance set at $p < 0.05$.

Results

After applying the exclusion criteria, 15,724 patients were included in the analysis. The reference creatinine was determined from a documented baseline creatinine in 5543 patients and estimated in 10,181 patients. AKI occurred in 8270 (52.6%) patients. The characteristics of individuals that developed AKI are shown in Table 1. In the 16–25-year-old age group, 39.8% of the patients developed AKI. In all age groups stage I AKI occurred with the greatest frequency. Although stage 3 AKI occurred with the lowest frequency in the 16–25-year-old age group, it occurred in 15% of patients. Only a few variables met our criteria of 10% as a clinically meaningful difference between age groups. Cardiac disease, hypertension, multiple comorbidities, vasopressor use and NSAID use were more common in older adults (Table 1). The distributions for the remainder of the variables were similar between groups.

Sepsis and vancomycin use were found to be highly associated with AKI in the overall cohort as well as for each individual age group. Given that sepsis was defined as the ordering of blood cultures and antibiotics within

Table 1 Patient characteristics by age group (years) with acute kidney injury

Characteristic	16–25 N = 862	26–35 N = 1098	36–45 N = 2189	46–55 N = 4121	All N = 8270
% of age group with AKI	39.8	46.6	52.5	58.5	52.6
Age (years), Median (Q1–Q3)	22 (19–24)	31 (28–33)	41 (39–44)	51 (48–53)	45 (36–51)
Males N (%)	573 (66.5)	670 (61.2)	1304 (60)	2500 (61)	5047 (61)
Race N (%)					
White	597 (69)	790 (72)	1654 (76)	3127 (76)	6168 (76)
Black	132 (15)	131 (12)	226 (10)	409 (10)	898 (11)
Other	133 (15)	177 (16)	309 (14)	585 (14)	1204 (15)
Reference creatinine (mg/dl), median (Q1–Q3)	0.9 (0.7–1.1)	0.9 (0.7–1.1)	0.9 (0.7–1.1)	0.9 (0.7–1.1)	0.9 (0.7–1.1)
eGFR (ml/min/1.73 m^2), median (Q1–Q3)	121.2 (92.8–133)	111.4 (81.9–123.1)	95.7 (79.4–113.9)	86.2 (76.9–104.8)	96.5 (78.6–113.2)
Fluid balance > 5%	111 (12.9)	161 (14.7)	285 (13.1)	485 (11.8)	1042 (12.6)
Cardiac disease N (%)	41 (5)	95 (9)	225 (10)	666 (16)	1027 (12)
Chronic kidney disease N (%)	16 (2)	26 (2)	135 (6)	218 (5)	395 (5)
Diabetes N (%)	50 (6)	102 (9)	227 (10)	741 (18)	1120 (14)
History of hypertension N (%)	59 (7)	135 (12)	459 (21)	1274 (31)	1927 (23)
Malignancy N (%)	7 (0.8)	15 (1)	62 (2.8)	156 (3.8)	240 (3)
Multiple comorbidities N (%)	142 (17)	290 (26)	803 (37)	1889 (46)	3124 (38)
Mechanical ventilation N (%)	580 (67)	684 (62)	1340 (61)	2413 (59)	5017 (61)
Surgical admission N (%)	504 (65)	601 (60)	1128 (57)	2216 (59)	4449 (59)
Suspected sepsis N (%)	122 (14)	198 (18)	395 (18)	698 (17)	1413 (17)
APACHE III score, median (Q1–Q3)	54 (36–72)	53 (34–73)	52 (35–74)	57 (38–80)	55 (37–76)
Vasopressor use N (%)	149 (17)	224 (20)	521 (24)	1125 (27)	2019 (24)
Moderate anemia N (%)	227 (26)	315 (29)	577 (26)	1259 (31)	2378 (29)
Maximum KDIGO N (%)					
Stage 1	400 (46)	444 (41)	738 (34)	1241 (30)	2823 (34)
Stage 2	335 (39)	433 (39)	906 (41)	1783 (43)	3457 (42)
Stage 3	127 (15)	221 (20)	545 (25)	1097 (27)	1990 (24)
Medication exposure N (%)					
ACE inhibitor/ARB	21(2)	27 (2)	93 (4)	269 (7)	410 (5)
Vancomycin	124 (14)	203 (18)	373 (17)	669 (16)	1369 (17)
Aminoglycoside	31 (3.6)	44 (4)	87 (4)	157 (4)	319 (4)
Other Antibiotics	62 (7)	82 (7)	137 (6)	258 (6)	539 (6)
Calcineurin inhibitor	58 (7)	94 (9)	153 (7)	264 (6)	569 (7)
NSAID	40 (5)	90 (8)	269 (12)	716 (17)	1115 (14)
Acyclovir	18 (2)	29 (2.6)	462 (2.1)	67 (1.6)	160 (2)
Mannitol	28 (3)	26 (2)	32 (1.5)	30 (0.7)	116 (1)
Phenytoin	32 (3.7)	24 (2)	47 (2)	82 (2)	185 (2)

AKI acute kidney injury, *eGFR* estimated glomerular filtration rate, *APACHE* Acute Physiology and Chronic Healthy Evaluation, *KDIGO* Kidney Disease Improving Global Outcomes, *ACE* angiotensin-converting enzyme, *ARB* angiotensin II receptor blocker, *NSAID* nonsteroidal anti-inflammatory drug

24 h of each other and vancomycin was the most common antibiotic prescribed, not surprisingly sepsis was highly colinear with vancomycin. Therefore, sepsis was not included in the final individual logistic regression models built for each age group (Table 2). The area under the curve (AUC) for each of the four age groups was similar indicating a comparable ability to predict AKI across the different age strata at 0.754, 0.769, 0.772, and 0.770 for the 16–25-, 26–35-, 36–45-, and 46–55-year-old age groups, respectively. In order to gain more precise estimates, the AUC was re-fitted using bootstrapping and similar AUC values were also determined across the four age strata. Diabetes, APACHE III score, and vancomycin were significantly positively associated with AKI across all age groups. Specifically, for the young adults (ages 16–25), age, race, diabetes, surgical admission, APACHE III score, hypotensive index, vancomycin, calcineurin inhibitor, NSAID, and other nephrotoxic medication

Table 2 Multivariable logistic regression of risk factors for individuals with acute kidney injury compared to those without acute kidney injury by age categories (years)

Characteristic	16–25 OR (95% CI p value)	26–35 OR (95% CI p value)	36–45 OR (95% CI p value)	46–55 OR (95% CI p value)
Age per 5 years	1.39 (1.14–1.69, < 0.01)	1.21 (1.02–1.43, 0.02)	–	–
Black	1.41 (1.04–1.91, 0.02)	–	–	–
Other race	–	–	–	–
Diabetes	1.89 (1.09–3.29, 0.02)	1.86 (1.20–2.89, < 0.01)	1.52 (1.14–2.02, 0.01)	1.55 (1.28–1.85, 0.01)
Fluid balance > 5%	–	–	–	–
Malignancy	–	–	–	–
Hypertension	–	–	–	–
Cardiac disease	–	3.75 (2.23–6.29, < 0.01)	2.00 (1.47–2.72, < 0.01)	1.36 (1.12–1.64, 0.01)
Chronic kidney disease	–	–	–	–
Surgical admission	1.79 (1.44–2.23, < 0.01)	1.39 (1.14–1.71, < 0.01)	1.23 (1.05–1.72, < 0.01)	–
Vasopressor use	–	1.48 (1.04–2.12, 0.03)	1.34 (1.05–1.65, 0.01)	1.41 (1.19–1.69, < 0.01)
Mechanical ventilation	–	1.39 (1.09–2.12, < 0.01)	1.38 (1.16–1.31, < 0.01)	1.53 (1.33–1.73, < 0.01)
Moderate anemia	–	–	–	–
APACHE III score	1.02 (1.02–1.03, < 0.01)	1.02 (1.02–1.26, < 0.01)	1.03 (1.02–1.04, < 0.01)	1.03 (1.03–1.03, < 0.01)
eGFR	–	–	0.98 (0.98–0.99, < 0.01)	0.98 (0.98–0.99, < 0.01)
Hypotensive Index	1.13 (1.04–1.24, < 0.01)	–	–	1.04 (1.01–1.07, 0.01)
ACE inhibitor/ARB	–	–	–	–
Vancomycin	1.46 (1.00–2.13, 0.04)	1.56 (1.13–1.39, < 0.01)	1.39 (1.08–1.77, 0.01)	1.45 (1.18–1.77, < 0.01)
Other antibiotics	–	–	–	–
Calcineurin inhibitor	2.72 (1.45–5.12, < 0.01)	–	2.45 (1.59–3.75, < 0.01)	–
NSAID	0.51 (0.32–0.82, < 0.01)	0.68 (0.49–0.80, 0.02)	0.78 (0.63–0.96, 0.01)	0.92 (0.80–1.07, 0.03)
Other nephrotoxic medications	1.60 (1.03–2.49, 0.03)	–	–	–
AUC (Q1–Q3)	0.754 (0.732–0.776)	0.769 (0.749–0.789)	0.772 (0.757–0.787)	0.770 (0.758–0.781)

OR odds ratio, *CI* confidence interval, *APACHE* Acute Physiology and Chronic Healthy Evaluation, *eGFR* estimated glomerular filtration rate, *ACE* angiotensin-converting enzyme, *ARB* angiotensin II receptor blocker, *NSAID* nonsteroidal anti-inflammatory drug, *ROC* receiver operator curve

use were all significantly associated with AKI (Table 2). Included in the category of other nephrotoxic medications were acyclovir, mannitol, and phenytoin. However, when each of these drugs was included individually in the model, there was no significant association with AKI.

Statistically significant interactions between age groups and the potential risk factors were determined (Table 3). Despite a similar ability to predict AKI across the four age strata, certain risk factors were significantly different with respect to age group. The risk factors that had significant interactions with age were cardiac disease, surgical admission, eGFR, calcineurin inhibitor, NSAID, and other nephrotoxic medication use.

Table 4 shows outcomes of the patients with AKI in each of the four age strata. In the young adult patients, even though only a small number of patients received RRT (*n* = 46), 47.8% of patients that received RRT while hospitalized had no recovery from RRT at 90 days. In the 640 patients in the overall patient cohort that received RRT, 59.4% had no recovery from RRT at 90 days. The ICU and hospital length of stay were similar between age groups. Hospital, ICU, 90-day, and 1-year mortality were

greater in the older adult groups. AKI was a significant predictor of hospital mortality, ICU mortality, mortality at 90 days and mortality at 1 year in the young adult patients (Table 5). Tables 6 and 7 show the significant role that AKI contributed toward predicting hospital and 1 year post-discharge mortality in the 16–25-year-old age group. Patients with AKI had an increased risk of 1 year post-discharge mortality in all age groups (Fig. 2). Among the variables included in the multivariable logistic regression, it was the APACHE III score, a diagnosis of malignancy, and a diagnosis of AKI during the time of ICU admission only that significantly contributed toward predicting mortality 1 year after discharge (Table 7).

Discussion

Even in young adult patients, AKI occurred in 39.8%. Similar to the AWARE study, a strength of this investigation is that we defined AKI using both the KDIGO serum creatinine and urine output criteria, given that defining AKI using serum creatinine has been shown to decrease the sensitivity for AKI detection [5]. Our rate of AKI in the young adult patient cohort falls between the

Table 3 Multivariable logistic regression of interactions between age groups and risk factors associated with AKI

Interaction of age group with	χ^2 (df)	p value*
Race	5.19 (6)	0.52
Diabetes	4.31 (3)	0.22
Cardiac disease	17.55 (3)	< 0.01
Chronic kidney disease	4.67 (3)	0.19
Surgical admission	18.42 (3)	< 0.01
Vasopressor use	1.73 (3)	0.62
Mechanical ventilation	4.57 (3)	0.20
Moderate anemia	2.02 (3)	0.56
APACHE III score	7.07 (3)	0.06
eGFR	16.5 (3)	< 0.01
Hypotensive Index	2.25 (3)	0.52
Vancomycin	1.06 (3)	0.78
Calcineurin inhibitor	12.84 (3)	< 0.01
NSAID	3.30 (3)	< 0.01
Other nephrotoxic medications	8.08 (3)	0.04

AKI acute kidney injury, *APACHE* Acute Physiology and Chronic Healthy Evaluation, *eGFR* estimated glomerular filtration rate, *NSAID* nonsteroidal anti-inflammatory drug

*Each p value comes from a different multivariable logistic regression with age group, 15 risk factors and one interaction

rates reported by AWARE (26.9%) and the Acute Kidney Injury-Epidemiologic Prospective Investigation (AKI-EPI) published in 2015 (57.3%) [5, 28].

Importantly, we show AKI to be a significant predictor of hospital and ICU mortality as well as mortality after discharge in young adult critically ill patients, treated in an adult ICU. Similarly, including both ICU and non-ICU patients less than 18 years of age, Sutherland et al. show a significant association of AKI (defined using the KDIGO criteria) with ICU mortality and hospital length of stay. However, in contrast to our findings, they describe no significant association of AKI with mortality outside of the ICU [6]. Along with differences in patient age, the inclusion of patients with non-ICU AKI in their study may explain the discrepant results when compared to ours, which show AKI to be a significant predictor of hospital and 1 year post-discharge mortality in the 16–25-year-old age group.

Given the poor outcomes associated with AKI in this study as well as prior studies, it is imperative that those caring for critically ill patients identify and address the risk factors that are unique to specific patient groups. The results of this analysis suggest that there are potentially modifiable risk factors for AKI in critically ill young adults. The use of medications such as vancomycin and calcineurin inhibitors was found to be significantly associated with AKI in patients 16–25 years of age. When grouped together, mannitol, acyclovir, and phenytoin were uniquely associated with AKI in the 16–25-year-old cohort. Due to the low rate of use of these medications in our overall patient cohort, we cannot make any determination about AKI risk of each medication individually.

Table 4 Outcomes of patients with acute kidney injury for each of the four age categories (years)

Outcome	Age 16–25	Age 26–35	Age 36–45	Age 46–55	All
Need for RRT N (%)	46 (5.3)	77 (7)	172 (7.9)	345 (8.4)	640 (7.7)
No recovery from RRT at 90 Days N (%)	22 (47.8)	37 (48.1)	92 (53.5)	229 (66.4)	380 (59.4)
ICU length of stay (days), mean (SD)	9.6 (10.7)	10.3 (15.1)	8.7 (11.6)	8.8 (12.9)	9 (12.7)
Hospital length of stay (days), mean (SD)	20.1 (22.2)	21.7 (25.4)	19.5 (24.1)	19.5 (24.2)	19.9 (24.1)
ICU mortality N (%)	51 (5.9)	80 (7.3)	245 (11.2)	486 (11.8)	862 (10.4)
Hospital mortality N (%)	64 (7.4)	107 (9.7)	319 (14.6)	674 (16.4)	1164 (14.1)
90-Day mortality N (%)	67 (7.8)	123 (11.2)	390 (17.8)	860 (20.9)	1440 (17.4)
1-Year mortality N (%)	90 (10.4)	180 (16.4)	498 (22.8)	1145 (27.8)	1913 (23.1)

RRT renal replacement therapy, *ICU* intensive care unit, *SD* standard deviation

Table 5 Multivariable logistic regression of outcomes related to acute kidney injury by age categories (years)

Outcome	Age 16–25 OR (95% CI p value)	Age 26–35 OR (95% CI p value)	Age 36–45 OR (95% CI p value)	Age 46–55 OR (95% CI p value)	All OR (95% CI p value)
Hospital mortality	2.48 (1.25–4.90, < 0.01)	8.63 (1.04–71.70, 0.04)	21.73 (4.02–117.44, < 0.01)	4.88 (2.55–9.34, < 0.01)	2.03 (1.69–2.43, < 0.01)
ICU mortality	2.78 (1.30–5.94, < 0.01)	1.024 (0.58–1.82, 0.934)	1.67 (1.11–2.51, 0.01)	1.48 (1.12–1.97, 0.07)	3.74 (2.09–6.68, < 0.01
Mortality at 90 days	2.04 (1.09–3.82, 0.03)	1.313 (0.84–2.06, 0.233)	2.31 (1.70–3.14, < 0.01)	1.63 (1.34–1.98, < 0.01)	1.78 (1.53–2.07, < 0.01)
Mortality at 1 year	2.25 (1.14–4.45, 0.02)	2.50 (1.50–4.15, < 0.01)	1.98 (1.45–2.70, < 0.01)	1.90 (1.54–2.36, < 0.01)	2.03 (1.74–2.39, < 0.01)

OR odds ratio, *CI* confidence interval, *ICU* Intensive Care Unit

Table 6 Multivariable logistic regression of risk factors for hospital mortality by age categories (years)

Outcome	Age 16–25 OR (95% CI p value)	Age 26–35 OR (95% CI p value)	Age 36–45 OR (95% CI p value)	Age 46–55 OR (95% CI p value)	All OR (95% CI p value)
Age per 5 years	0.73 (0.43–1.23, 0.23)	1.26 (0.88–1.80, 0.20)	1.51 (1.19–1.93, < 0.01)	1.23 (1.04–1.44, 0.01)	1.14 (1.09–1.18, < 0.01)
AKI	2.48 (1.25–4.90, < 0.01)	1.65 (0.98–2.79, 0.05)	2.06 (1.44–2.95, < 0.01)	2.00 (1.56–2.56, < 0.01)	2.03 (1.69–2.43, < 0.01)
APACHE III score	1.03 (1.01–1.03, < 0.01)	1.03 (1.02–1.03, < 0.01)	1.03 (1.02–1.03, < 0.01)	1.03 (1.02–1.03, < 0.01)	1.03 (1.03–1.04, < 0.01)
Hypotensive Index	1.01 (1.01–1.02, < 0.01)	1.00 (0.99–1.01, 0.12)	1.00 (1.00–1.01, < 0.01)	1.00 (1.00–1.00, < 0.01)	1.01 (1.01–1.01, < 0.01)
Vasopressors	3.28 (1.60–6.75, < 0.01)	3.98 (2.46–6.43, < 0.01)	2.46 (1.79–3.38, < 0.01)	1.97 (1.61–2.42, < 0.01)	2.30 (2.0–2.7, < 0.01)
Surgical Admission	0.63 (0.35–1.15, < 0.01)	0.66 (0.43–1.01, 0.05)	0.54 (0.41–0.71, < 0.01)	0.60 (0.49–0.72, < 0.01)	0.60 (0.51–0.68, < 0.01)
Moderate anemia	1.12 (0.60–2.11, 0.72)	0.81 (0.51–1.3, 0.39)	0.87 (0.64–1.19, 0.41)	0.86 (0.70–1.05, 0.14)	0.87 (0.75–1.01, 0.07)
Hypertension	0.76 (0.21–2.69, 0.67)	0.85 (0.42–1.72, 0.65)	0.89 (0.61–1.30, 0.57)	0.94 (0.74–1.18, 0.59)	0.89 (0.74–1.07, 0.20)
Malignancy	5.23 (1.47–18.61, 0.01)	2.55 (1.09–5.94, 0.02)	1.80 (1.10–2.96, 0.01)	1.52 (1.12–2.05, 0.00)	1.68 (1.32–2.14, < 0.01)
Chronic liver disease	0.61 (0.06–6.01, 0.67)	1.37 (0.57–3.25, 0.47)	1.49 (0.93–2.4, 0.09)	1.56 (1.17–2.08, 0.00)	1.47 (1.16–1.85, < 0.01)
Multiple comorbidities	1.27 (0.51–3.17, 0.60)	1.58 (0.87–2.88, 0.13)	1.18 (0.80–1.73, 0.38)	0.82 (0.63–1.06, 0.13)	1.02 (0.84–1.24, 0.84)
AUC (Q1–Q3)	0.895 (0.854–0.932)	0.8942 (0.868–0.920)	0.8855 (0.868–0.902)	0.853 (0.838–0.867)	0.875 (0.865–0.884)

RRT renal replacement therapy, *ICU* intensive care unit, *SD* standard deviation

Table 7 Multivariable logistic regression of risk factors for 1-year mortality by age categories (years)

Outcome	Age 16–25 OR (95% CI p value)	Age 26–35 OR (95% CI p value)	Age 36–45 OR (95% CI p value)	Age 46–55 OR (95% CI p value)	All OR (95% CI p value)
Age	1.04 (0.94–1.16, 0.47)	1.03 (0.96–1.10, 0.34)	1.04 (0.99–1.09, 0.06)	1.04 (1.01–1.07, 0.01)	1.04 (1.03–1.04, < 0.01)
AKI	2.25 (1.14–4.45, 0.02)	2.50 (1.50–4.15, < 0.01)	1.98 (1.45–2.70, < 0.01)	1.90 (1.54–2.36, < 0.01)	2.03 (1.74–2.39, < 0.01)
Race[a]	0.63 (0.23–1.73, 0.37)	0.53 (0.25–1.11, 0.09)	0.62 (0.39–0.99, 0.05)	0.745 (0.55–1.02, 0.07)	0.67 (0.53–0.84, < 0.01)
APACHE III score	1.02 (1.01–1.03, < 0.01)	1.02 (1.02–1.03, < 0.01)	1.02 (1.02–1.03, < 0.01)	1.02 (1.02–1.03, < 0.01)	2.04 (1.73 –2.39, < 0.01)
BMI	0.98 (0.94–1.01, 0.20)	1.01 (0.99–1.03, 0.56)	0.99 (0.98–1.01, 0.46)	0.99 (0.98–0.99, 0.02)	0.99 (0.99–0.99, 0.02)
Hypotensive Index	1.01 (1.00–1.02, 0.06)	1.00 (0.99–1.01, 0.44)	1.01 (1.00–1.01, < 0.01)	1.00 (1.00–1.01, 0.01)	1.00 (1.00–1.01, < 0.01)
Vasopressors	1.99 (0.94–4.20, 0.07)	2.41 (1.54 –3.81, < 0.01)	1.62 (1.20–2.18, < 0.01)	1.35 (1.11–1.64, < 0.01)	1.54 (1.33–1.80, < 0.01)
Surgical admission	0.80 (0.44–1.46, 0.47)	0.52 (0.36–0.77, < 0.01)	0.53 (0.42– 0.69, < 0.01)	0.52 (0.44–0.62, < 0.01)	0.54 (0.47–0.61, < 0.01)
Hypertension	1.17 (0.42–3.27, 0.77)	0.80 (0.42–1.52, 0.50)	0.85 (0.61–1.19, 0.35)	0.85 (0.69–1.05, 0.13)	0.82 (0.69–0.97, 0.02)
Malignancy	17.84 (4.66–68.35, < 0.01)	2.43 (1.08–5.45, 0.03)	1.08 (0.62–1.88, 0.08)	2.04 (1.48–2.80, < 0.01)	1.91 (1.49–2.46, < 0.01)
Chronic liver disease	2.65 (0.77 –8.92, 0.12)	0.90 (0.43–1.88, 0.76)	1.26 (0.83 –1.92, 0.27)	1.70 (1.30–2.20, < 0.01)	1.48 (1.21–1.82, < 0.01)
History of COPD	13.96 (0.73 – 268.49, 0.08)	1.31 (0.40–4.46, 0.66)	1.21 (0.68 –2.17, 0.52)	1.41 (1.06–1.89, 0.02)	1.30 (1.01–1.68, 0.04)
Multiple comorbidities	2.00 (0.87–4.61, 0.10)	3.22 (1.88–5.54, < 0.01)	2.07 (1.45 –2.95, < 0.01)	1.06 (0.84–1.36, 0.61)	1.53 (1.28–1.83, < 0.01)
AUC (Q1–Q3)	0.862 (0.816–0.907)	0.848 (0.818–0.878)	0.816 (0.794–0.837)	0.799 (0.783–0.814)	0.823 (0.812–0.834)

AKI acute kidney injury, *APACHE* Acute Physiology and Chronic Healthy Evaluation, *BMI* Body Mass Index, *COPD* chronic obstructive pulmonary disease

[a] Black compared to white

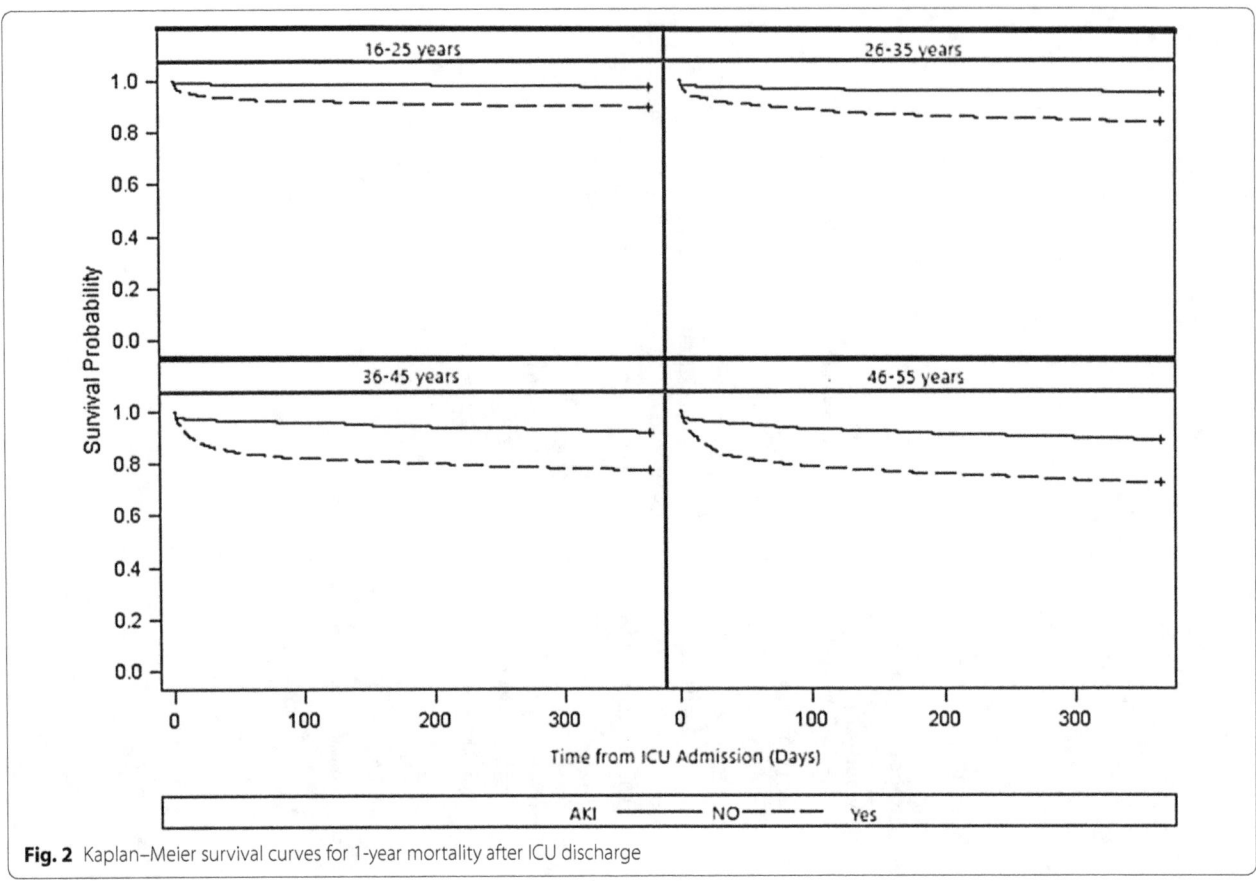

Fig. 2 Kaplan–Meier survival curves for 1-year mortality after ICU discharge

The significant association of nephrotoxic medications and AKI in the 16–25-year-old age group suggests the need for future studies exploring the effect of different drug combinations in young adults on AKI development. At the bedside, frequent evaluations for transitioning medications to less nephrotoxic alternatives along with the use of therapeutic drug monitoring when available should be initiated.

The multivariable logistic regression demonstrates a "protective effect" of NSAID use on AKI risk across all of the age groups. NSAIDs are frequently withheld from patients in the ICU due to the concern of nephrotoxicity [29]. We speculate that our study results are due to a possible healthy user bias whereby patients without CKD and/or less comorbid conditions may have been more likely to receive NSAIDs during their ICU stay than patients with an elevated creatinine values and more comorbidities. However, given that increased NSAID use was not found to be positively associated with AKI in this critically ill patient cohort, intermittent NSAID use in patients without underlying renal disease who are euvolemic should be considered for analgesia given the low risk of renal side effects, as discussed in previous investigations [30, 31]. This may be particular important given recent attention to opiate use in the critically ill.

In this study, which did not include patients over 55 years of age, we show a similar ability to predict AKI when comparing the four age strata. Also using the HiDenIC database, but including ICU patients 55 years and older, Kane-Gill et al. [20] demonstrated that the ability of similar variables used in our study to predict AKI decreases with age. Specifically, they report that for patients greater than or equal to 75 years of age an AUC for predicting AKI of 0.673 [20]. This is in contrast to the higher AUC values determined in this study for younger adults, which demonstrates the superior ability to predict and, therefore, potentially prevent AKI in patients less than 55 years of age. Notably, the risk factors between those age 16–55 in our study and those > 75 in the previously published study varied with different drugs, history of hypertension, and sepsis in the older adult group [20].

Our models for mortality were also quite robust with all AUCs of at least 0.80 and some approaching 0.90 (Tables 6, 7). While our intent was not to develop a risk prediction model for mortality with AKI, and our

Acute kidney injury epidemiology, risk factors, and outcomes in critically ill patients 16–25 years of age treated...

81

models are likely overtrained, these results are far better than most reports in the literature [32]. Use of younger patients and stratification by age group may have led to significantly better predicative value. While the AUC values appear to increase with decreasing age, the confidence intervals overlap. Future studies are needed to validate these models in independent populations.

Our study has important limitations. The identified risk factors for AKI may be surrogates of other variables. For example, the association of calcineurin inhibitor use and AKI may reflect the association of AKI with transplant status. Notably, surgical as opposed to medical admission was an increasingly powerful risk factor for AKI in younger patients, especially those 16–25 years of age. However, it could not be determined from the database if surgeries were elective versus emergent. APACHE III scores and the MDRD equation for estimating GFR have not been validated in patients less than 18 years of age. Importantly, the MDRD equation was derived from patients with CKD, and its use in patients with critical illness is unclear. All of the young adults in this study were treated in adult intensive care units at a single institution. Given the single-center nature of this study, the comorbidities of a young adult patient group treated at other institutions may be different from our cohort of patients. Therefore, the results should be validated at other centers.

Conclusions

Using the KDIGO criteria for both serum creatinine and urine output to define AKI, 39.8% of patients between the ages of 16–25 met AKI criteria during admission to an adult tertiary care center, indicating that AKI is a common event in this patient group. The diagnosis of AKI during hospital admission independently contributed toward increased hospital mortality, increased ICU mortality and increased mortality 90 days and 1 year after hospital discharge in the young adult patients. Potentially modifiable risk factors for AKI were identified, most notably nephrotoxic medication exposure. Risk factors identified in this younger population varied from published data in older adults (> 75 years old).

Abbreviations
AKI: acute kidney injury; CKD: chronic kidney disease; AWARE: Assessment of Worldwide Acute Kidney Injury, Renal Angina, and Epidemiology; ICU: intensive care unit; HiDenIC: High-Density Intensive Care; eGFR: estimated glomerular filtration rate; APACHE: Acute Physiology and Chronic Health Evaluation; NSAID: nonsteroidal anti-inflammatory drug; KDIGO: Kidney Disease Improving Global Outcomes.

Authors' contributions
DYF, JAK, and SLG contributed to study concept and design; DYF, JAK, and PP analyzed the data; DYF, JAK, SLK-G, and SLG interpreted the data; DYF and PP performed statistical analysis; JAK helped in procurement of funding. Each author contributed important intellectual content during manuscript drafting or revision and accepted accountability for the overall work by ensuring that questions pertaining to the accuracy or integrity of any portion of the work are appropriately investigated and resolved. All authors read and approved the final manuscript.

Author details
[1] Children's Hospital of Pittsburgh, 4401 Penn Avenue, Children's Hospital Drive, Faculty Pavilion Suite 2000, Pittsburgh, PA 15224, USA. [2] School of Pharmacy, University of Pittsburgh, 638 Salk Hall, 3501 Terrace Street, Pittsburgh, PA 15261, USA. [3] Center for Acute Care Nephrology, Cincinnati Children's Hospital Medical Center, 3333 Burnet Avenue, Cincinnati, OH 45229, USA. [4] The Center for Critical Care Nephrology, 3347 Forbes Avenue, Ste 220, Pittsburgh, PA 15213, USA.

Acknowledgements
None.

Competing interests
The authors declare that they have no competing interests.

Funding
This work was funded by the University of Pittsburgh Medical Center and the University of Pittsburgh; and additional support was provided by R01DK083961 from the National Institute of Diabetes, and Digestive, and Kidney Diseases (NIDDK) to JAK. The content of this paper is solely the responsibility of the authors and does not necessarily represent the official views of the NIDDK or National Institutes of Health.

References
1. Uchino S, Kellum JA, Bellomo R, et al. Acute renal failure in critically ill patients: a multinational, multicenter study. JAMA. 2005;294(7):813–8.
2. Liano F, Pascual J. Epidemiology of acute renal failure: a prospective, multicenter, community-based study. Madrid Acute Renal Failure Study Group. Kidney Int. 1996;50(3):811–8.
3. Ali T, Khan I, Simpson W, et al. Incidence and outcomes in acute kidney injury: a comprehensive population-based study. J Am Soc Nephrol. 2007;18(4):1292–8.
4. Kidney Disease: Improving Global Outcomes (KDIGO) Work Group. KDIGO clinical practice guildeline for acute kidney injury. Kidney Int Suppl. 2012;2:1–138.
5. Kaddourah A, Basu RK, Bagshaw SM, Goldstein SL, Investigators A. Epidemiology of acute kidney injury in critically ill children and young adults. N Engl J Med. 2017;376(1):11–20.
6. Sutherland SM, Byrnes JJ, Kothari M, et al. AKI in hospitalized children: comparing the pRIFLE, AKIN, and KDIGO definitions. Clin J Am Soc Nephrol. 2015;10(4):554–61.
7. Bailey D, Phan V, Litalien C, et al. Risk factors of acute renal failure in critically ill children: a prospective descriptive epidemiological study. Pediatr Crit Care Med. 2007;8(1):29–35.
8. Schneider J, Khemani R, Grushkin C, Bart R. Serum creatinine as stratified in the RIFLE score for acute kidney injury is associated with mortality and length of stay for children in the pediatric intensive care unit. Crit Care Med. 2010;38(3):933–9.
9. Zappitelli M, Parikh CR, Akcan-Arikan A, Washburn KK, Moffett BS, Goldstein SL. Ascertainment and epidemiology of acute kidney injury varies with definition interpretation. Clin J Am Soc Nephrol. 2008;3(4):948–54.
10. Akcan-Arikan A, Zappitelli M, Loftis LL, Washburn KK, Jefferson LS, Goldstein SL. Modified RIFLE criteria in critically ill children with acute kidney injury. Kidney Int. 2007;71(10):1028–35.
11. Basu RK, Zappitelli M, Brunner L, et al. Derivation and validation of the renal angina index to improve the prediction of acute kidney injury in critically ill children. Kidney Int. 2014;85(3):659–67.

12. Groeneveld AB, Tran DD, van der Meulen J, Nauta JJ, Thijs LG. Acute renal failure in the medical intensive care unit: predisposing, complicating factors and outcome. Nephron. 1991;59(4):602–10.

13. de Mendonca A, Vincent JL, Suter PM, et al. Acute renal failure in the ICU: risk factors and outcome evaluated by the SOFA score. Intensive Care Med. 2000;26(7):915–21.

14. Brivet FG, Kleinknecht DJ, Loirat P, Landais PJ. Acute renal failure in intensive care units–causes, outcome, and prognostic factors of hospital mortality; a prospective, multicenter study. French Study Group on Acute Renal Failure. Crit Care Med. 1996;24(2):192–8.

15. Wilkins RG, Faragher EB. Acute renal failure in an intensive care unit: incidence, prediction and outcome. Anaesthesia. 1983;38(7):628–34.

16. Edwards JD, Houtrow AJ, Vasilevskis EE, Dudley RA, Okumura MJ. Multi-institutional profile of adults admitted to pediatric intensive care units. JAMA Pediatr. 2013;167(5):436–43.

17. Janse AJ, Uiterwaal CS, Gemke RJ, Kimpen JL, Sinnema G. A difference in perception of quality of life in chronically ill children was found between parents and pediatricians. J Clin Epidemiol. 2005;58(5):495–502.

18. Hui-Stickle S, Brewer ED, Goldstein SL. Pediatric ARF epidemiology at a tertiary care center from 1999 to 2001. Am J Kidney Dis. 2005;45(1):96–101.

19. Cartin-Ceba R, Kashiouris M, Plataki M, Kor DJ, Gajic O, Casey ET. Risk factors for development of acute kidney injury in critically ill patients: a systematic review and meta-analysis of observational studies. Crit Care Res Pract. 2012;2012:691013.

20. Kane-Gill SL, Sileanu FE, Murugan R, Trietley GS, Handler SM, Kellum JA. Risk factors for acute kidney injury in older adults with critical illness: a retrospective cohort study. Am J Kidney Dis. 2015;65(6):860–9.

21. Levey AS, Stevens LA, Schmid CH, et al. A new equation to estimate glomerular filtration rate. Ann Intern Med. 2009;150(9):604–12.

22. WHO. World Health Organization: Haemoglobin concentrations for the diagnosis of anaemia and assessment of severity. http://www.who.int/vmnis/indicators/haemoglobin.pdf (2011). Accessed 5 April 2016.

23. Sutherland SM, Zappitelli M, Alexander SR, et al. Fluid overload and mortality in children receiving continuous renal replacement therapy: the prospective pediatric continuous renal replacement therapy registry. Am J Kidney Dis. 2010;55(2):316–25.

24. Knaus WA, Wagner DP, Draper EA, et al. The APACHE III prognostic system. Risk prediction of hospital mortality for critically ill hospitalized adults. Chest. 1991;100(6):1619–36.

25. Hoste EA, Clermont G, Kersten A, et al. RIFLE criteria for acute kidney injury are associated with hospital mortality in critically ill patients: a cohort analysis. Crit Care. 2006;10(3):R73.

26. Zavada J, Hoste E, Cartin-Ceba R, et al. A comparison of three methods to estimate baseline creatinine for RIFLE classification. Nephrol Dial Transpl. 2010;25(12):3911–8.

27. DaL Hosmer S. Applied logistic regression. 2nd ed. New York: Wiley; 2000.

28. Hoste EA, Bagshaw SM, Bellomo R, et al. Epidemiology of acute kidney injury in critically ill patients: the multinational AKI-EPI study. Intensive Care Med. 2015;41(8):1411–23.

29. Whelton A. Nephrotoxicity of nonsteroidal anti-inflammatory drugs: physiologic foundations and clinical implications. Am J Med. 1999;106(5B):13S–24S.

30. Mann JF, Goerig M, Brune K, Luft FC. Ibuprofen as an over-the-counter drug: is there a risk for renal injury? Clin Nephrol. 1993;39(1):1–6.

31. Musu M, Finco G, Antonucci R, et al. Acute nephrotoxicity of NSAID from the foetus to the adult. Eur Rev Med Pharmacol Sci. 2011;15(12):1461–72.

32. Uchino S, Bellomo R, Morimatsu H, et al. External validation of severity scoring systems for acute renal failure using a multinational database. Crit Care Med. 2005;33(9):1961–7.

9

The safety and efficacy of nicotine replacement therapy in the intensive care unit

Ben de Jong[1]*●, Anne Sophie Schuppers[2], Arriette Kruisdijk-Gerritsen[2], Maurits Erwin Leo Arbouw[3], Hubertus Laurentius Antonius van den Oever[2] and Arthur R. H. van Zanten[1]

Abstract

Background: Studies evaluating nicotine replacement therapy (NRT) to prevent nicotine withdrawal symptoms in ICU patients have yielded conflicting results. We performed a randomised controlled double-blind pilot study to assess the safety and efficacy of NRT in critically ill patients. Mechanically ventilated patients admitted to two medical–surgical intensive care units and smoking more than 10 cigarettes per day before ICU admission were enrolled in this study. Participants were randomised to transdermal NRT (14 or 21 mg per day) or placebo until ICU discharge or day 30. Smoking status was confirmed by the biomarkers serum cotinine and urinary NNAL. The primary endpoint was 30-day mortality. Among secondary endpoints and post hoc endpoints, 90-day mortality, safety, time spent without delirium, sedation and coma, and patient destination at day 30 were addressed.

Results: We enrolled 47 patients. No differences were found between NRT and control group patients concerning 30-day mortality (9.5 vs. 7.7%, $p = 0.84$) and 90-day mortality (14.3 vs. 19.2%, $p = 0.67$). The number of serious adverse events was comparable between groups (NRT: 4, control: 11, $p = 0.13$). At day 20, average time alive without delirium, sedation and coma was 16.6 days among NRT patients versus 12.6 days among control patients ($p = 0.03$). At day 30, more NRT group patients were discharged from the ICU or hospital compared with controls ($p = 0.03$).

Conclusions: NRT did not affect mortality or the number of (serious) adverse events compared with placebo. Time alive without delirium, sedation and coma at day 20 in NRT patients was longer than in control patients. An adequately powered randomised controlled trial to further study safety and efficacy of NRT in ICU patients seems feasible and is warranted.

Keywords: Smoking, NNAL, Cotinine, Delirium, Agitation, Withdrawal

Background

Tobacco use is the leading cause of preventable deaths worldwide, killing 6 million people annually and reducing life expectancy by an average of 10 years [1, 2]. In 2015, 19% of the Dutch and 11% of the US population were daily smokers [3, 4]. For patients admitted to the intensive care unit (ICU), this is even higher and 25–47% are active smokers [5–7].

Active smokers admitted to an ICU, present more agitation, self-removal of devices, need for physical restraint and receive higher doses of sedatives, neuroleptics and analgesics [5]. Agitated behaviour might be a consequence of nicotine withdrawal, but may also be due to delirium or abstinence of concomitant alcohol and/or drug use. Until now it is unclear whether tobacco use confers higher risk of delirium during ICU stay [8].

Neuroadaptation leads to withdrawal symptoms in the abstinence of nicotine. Furthermore, smoking itself may

*Correspondence: benjongde@gmail.com
[1] Department of Intensive Care Medicine, Gelderse Vallei Hospital, Willy Brandtlaan 10, 6716 RP Ede, The Netherlands
Full list of author information is available at the end of the article

also lead to a variety of pathological changes in organ systems (e.g. cardiovascular diseases) and affect multiple biological pathways, potentially increasing the risk for agitated behaviour [9, 10].

Nicotine replacement therapy (NRT) has been shown to reduce withdrawal symptoms in nicotine-dependent subjects who quit smoking [11, 12]. Research addressing the efficacy of NRT during critical illness shows conflicting results [13–22]. However, irrespective of its potential side effects and in the presence of inconsistent data on safety and efficacy, NRT is prescribed to prevent withdrawal symptoms or to treat agitated behaviour in smoking patients admitted to the ICU [23].

We designed a randomised controlled double-blind pilot study to assess the safety and efficacy of NRT in mechanically ventilated and actively smoking ICU patients.

Methods

Trial design

We performed a randomised, controlled, double-blind, pilot study between July 2012 and June 2016 that was approved by the Medical Research Ethics Committee (MREC) of the University Medical Centre of Utrecht and registered at ClinicalTrials.gov, number NCT01362959.

Participants

Mechanically ventilated and actively smoking patients admitted to the medical–surgical ICU of two University-affiliated teaching hospitals, Gelderse Vallei Hospital (17 beds, GVH) and Deventer Hospital (12 beds, DH) were eligible for inclusion.

Exclusion criteria were: age < 18 years, last smoking > 72 h before inclusion, smoking ≤ 10 cigarettes/ day, > 48 h after hospital admission admitted to the ICU, expected duration of mechanical ventilation ≤ 48 h, pregnant or breastfeeding, history of dementia or psychosis, neurologic disease on admission such as traumatic brain injury, intracranial haemorrhage, seizures, meningitis, encephalitis, intracranial tumour, cerebrovascular accident, NRT < 2 weeks before ICU admission, acute myocardial infarction, severe cardiac arrhythmia, unstable angina pectoris, generalised skin diseases, severe hearing deficiency, hypersensibility to nicotine or patches, insufficient Dutch language skills, imminent death or participation in another intervention study. Apart from regular exclusion criteria, we excluded factors interfering with the trial assessments and/or outcome or being a contraindication as mentioned in the Summary of Product Characteristics of the nicotine patches.

Written informed consent was obtained from all patients or their legal representatives. Retrospective written informed consent was obtained from the patient once mental capacity had regained.

Procedures and interventions

After inclusion and before the start of study drugs, blood and urine samples were taken to determine serum cotinine levels (Immulite 2000 nicotine metabolite assay, Siemens Healthcare Diagnostics Limited) and urine 4-(methylnitrosamino)-1-(3-pyridyl)-1-butanol (NNAL) concentrations (analysis according to Xia et al. [24]) to confirm inclusion of actively smoking patients [25, 26]. For women of fertile age, a pregnancy test was performed. Patient characteristics were recorded including age, sex, weight, length, medical history including medication and allergies, Charlson Comorbidity Index (CCI), patient type (surgical/medical), Sequential Organ Failure Assessment (SOFA) score, Acute Physiology and Chronic Health Evaluation (APACHE) II and IV scores.

Treatment allocation was performed using restricted randomisation with blocks of four, with a 1:1 ratio to NRT or placebo. Patients were stratified to patient type (medical or surgical), nicotine exposure (< 21 cigarettes or ≥ 21 cigarettes/day) and study site (GVH or DH). After enrolment, healthcare workers not involved in ICU patient care performed randomisation. Randomisation codes were unknown to the investigators, ICU staff, patients and relatives.

Patients were treated with nicotine patches (Nicotinell® TTS 20 and 30, Novartis Consumer Health) or similar size and shape, placebo patches (DuoDerm® Extra Thin, ConvaTec), both subsequently covered by an opaque plaster (Fixomull® stretch, BSN medical). Patches and covers were applied and replaced every 24 h until ICU discharge or day 30 by nurses not involved in ICU patient care, while ICU staff was not present. Patients smoking < 21 cigarettes/day received patches delivering 14 mg nicotine/24 h those smoking ≥ 21 cigarettes/day received patches delivering 21 mg nicotine/24 h.

Both hospitals involved in this study used sedation and agitation management protocols.

Trial assessments

After inclusion, patients or legal representatives completed the Alcohol Use Disorders Identification Test (AUDIT) and the Fagerström Test of Nicotine Dependence (FTND) to assess alcohol consumption and nicotine dependency.

Part of routine ICU care was the daily assessment of the Richmond Agitation and Sedation Scale (RASS) score, Confusion Assessment Method for the ICU (CAM-ICU) score, Delirium Observation Scale (DOS) score, Behaviour Pain Scale (BPS) and the Numeric Rating Scale (NRS) at 08:00, 14:00 and 21:00. During the intervention period (day 1 until discharge from the ICU or day 30), hours of physical restraint was recorded as well as self-removal of catheters, self-extubations, nosocomial infections according to CDC-criteria [27], medication prescribed and hours of mechanical ventilation.

At day 30 and day 90, patient destination and survival status was confirmed by reviewing the electronic medical record (EMR) or by telephone interviews with the patient or their representatives.

Serious adverse events (SAEs) were reported by attending physicians to the principal investigator (PI). Potential relationships to the treatment were determined according to the definitions from the Guideline for Good Clinical Practice (version November 2016). All EMRs were screened for adverse events by the investigators.

Outcomes

The primary endpoint was 30-day mortality. Secondary endpoints were 90-day mortality, ICU and in-hospital mortality, ICU and hospital length of stay (LOS), patient destination at day 30 and 90 (home, ICU, general hospital ward, nursing home, rehabilitation centre, deceased), hours with delirium assessed by the CAM-ICU or DOS-score, number of nosocomial infections, number of (serious) adverse events, number of self-removed catheters (i.e. arterial lines, peripheral and central venous catheters, nasogastric tubes, drains, urinary catheters), number of self-extubations, hours of physical restraint, hours without mechanical ventilation at day 30 (defined as persistent (non)invasive ventilation disconnection for at least 48 h), total dose of antipsychotics (i.e. haloperidol, olanzapine, quetiapine), RASS score and hours with RASS score outside the optimal range (score less than -3 and greater than $+1$).

A composite post hoc endpoint, reflecting return of normal brain function, was defined and assessed before unblinding the results comprising the number of hours alive without delirium, and without sedation (RASS ≥ 3) or coma. This endpoint was modified from a study addressing ICU sedation [28]. At day 10, 20 and 30, the average time spent with normal brain function between groups was compared.

Statistical analysis

In order to evaluate the feasibility of an adequately powered trial to study the safety and efficacy of NRT among mechanically ventilated patients and actively smoking before ICU admission, a pilot study was conducted, assessing time investment, safety and effect size on a smaller scale. The initial sample size was set at 70, accepting lack of statistical power for the primary outcome parameter. No interim analyses were planned.

Results and baseline characteristics were described as medians with interquartile ranges (IQR), means with standard deviations (SD) or as numbers and percentages (%) when appropriate. Continuous variables were analysed using Student's t test or the Mann–Whitney U test for normally distributed and non-normally distributed data, respectively. To analyse categorical variables Fisher's exact or Chi-Square tests were used.

Kaplan–Meier survival plots were generated for the 30-day and 90-day mortality, and the survival curves were compared with log-rank tests.

The primary outcome parameter was subjected to logistic multivariate analysis, in which the stratification variables (patient type, nicotine dosage and study site) were included.

A p value < 0.05 was considered statistically significant.

Data were collected in a database using Microsoft Office Access 2007 and were analysed using IBM SPSS Statistics 22 on an intention-to-treat basis.

Results

Between July 2012 and June 2016, eligibility was determined for 2715 admitted and mechanically ventilated ICU patients of whom 48 patients were enrolled: 27 patients at GVH and 21 at DH. As many patients met exclusion criteria, the inclusion rate was low. Therefore, after 4 years the study was stopped. The main reason for recruitment failure was elevated cardiac enzymes, often interpreted as a sign of instable angina pectoris or acute myocardial infarction, defined as exclusion criteria.

As one patient was excluded due to withdrawal of informed consent, 21 patients received NRT (of whom 62% a dose of 21 mg/day) and 26 patients received placebo. Baseline characteristics and serum cotinine and urinary NNAL concentrations were similar between groups and are shown in Table 1.

Primary endpoint

The 30-day mortality rates for patients in the NRT and control groups were 9.5 and 7.7%, respectively ($p = 0.84$, Fig. 1). Multiple logistic regression analysis using the 3 predefined stratification groups as independent variables showed no effect of NRT on 30-day mortality [OR 0.96 (0.11–8.23)].

Secondary clinical endpoints

The 90-day mortality rates for patients in the NRT and control groups were 14.3 and 19.2%, respectively ($p = 0.67$, Fig. 1). In the NRT group, fewer patients were still in the ICU or hospital at day 30 compared with the control group (1 vs. 11, $p = 0.03$), but not at day 90 (Fig. 2).

Table 1 Baseline characteristics of the patients

Characteristic	Nicotine replacement therapy (N = 21)	Control group (N = 26)
Age, years, mean (SD)	60.1 (10.55)	65. 2 (9.13)
Male sex, n (%)	12 (57)	16 (62)
BMI (m²/kg), mean (SD)	26.4 (6.75)	27.8 (5.95)
Charlson Comorbidity Index, median (IQR)	1 (0–1)	1 (0–2.25)
APACHE-II score, mean (SD)	19.0 (5.03)	21.1 (8.60)
APACHE-IV score, mean (SD)	69.7 (19.01)	75.9 (34.20)
Admission SOFA score, mean (SD)	6.5 (2.94)	6.9 (2.94)
Patient type (medical), n (%)	16 (76)	15 (58)
Smoking (cigarettes/day), median (IQR)	20 (12.5–27.5)	15 (14.5–25.0)
Alcohol (units/day), median (IQR)	2 (0–4)	2 (0–4)
FTND score, median (IQR)	5.5 (4–7.75)	5.0 (4–7)
AUDIT score, median (IQR)	5.5 (0.75–12)	5.0 (1–10.75)
Receiving nicotine 21 mg/day, n (%)	13 (62)	NA
Serum cotinine (ng/ml), median (IQR)	70.6 (25.8–110)	80.7 (37.5–126)
Urine NNAL (pg/ml), median (IQR)	117.6 (62.5–156.4)	177.9 (116.9–325.4)
Inclusion GVH, n (%)	12 (57)	14 (54)

BMI body mass index, *APACHE* Acute Physiology and Chronic Health Evaluation, *SOFA* Sequential Organ Failure Assessment Score, *FTND* Fagerström Test of Nicotine Dependence [0–4 (very) low, 5 medium, 6–7 high and 8–10 very high dependence], *AUDIT* Alcohol Use Disorders Identification Test (score ≥ 8 hazardous and harmful alcohol use), *NA* not applicable, *NNAL* 4-(methylnitrosamino)-1-(3-pyridyl)-1-butanol, *GVH* Gelderse Vallei Hospital

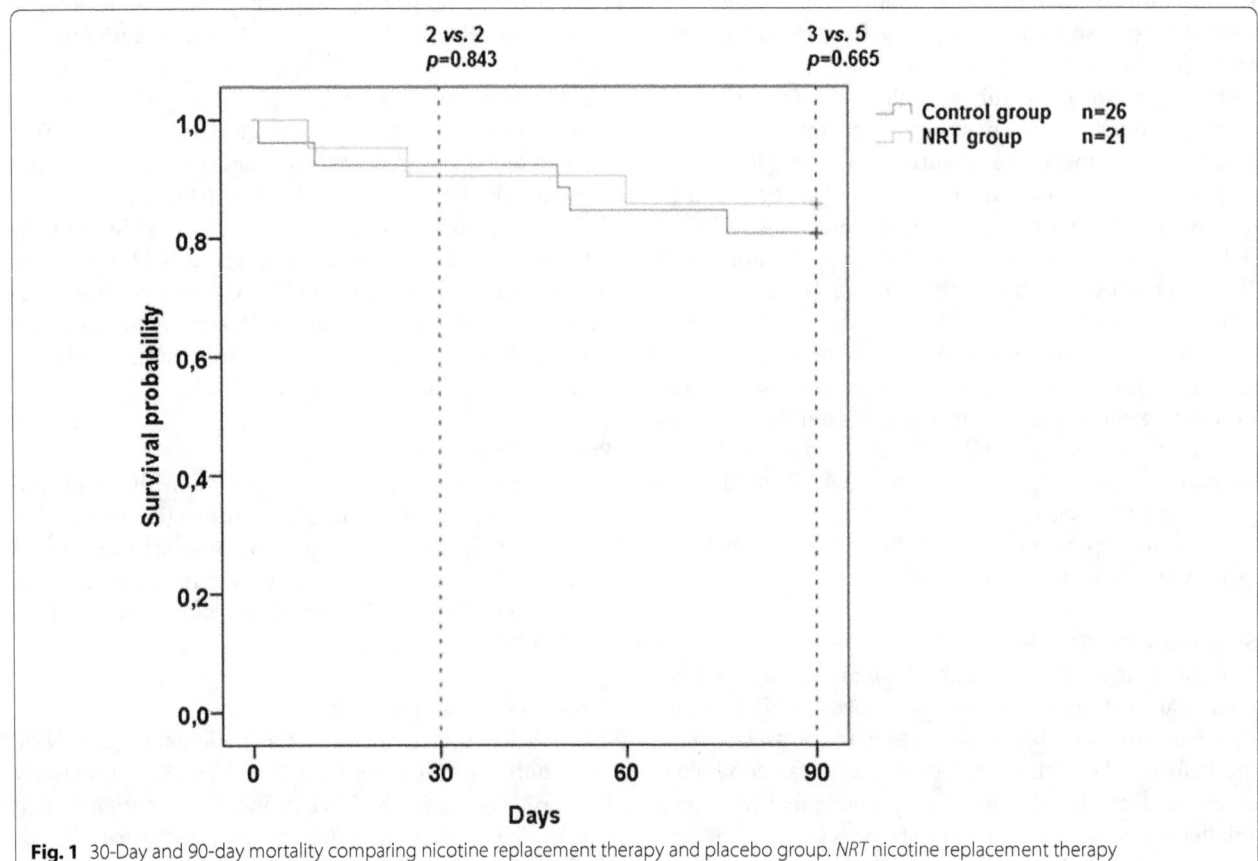

Fig. 1 30-Day and 90-day mortality comparing nicotine replacement therapy and placebo group. *NRT* nicotine replacement therapy

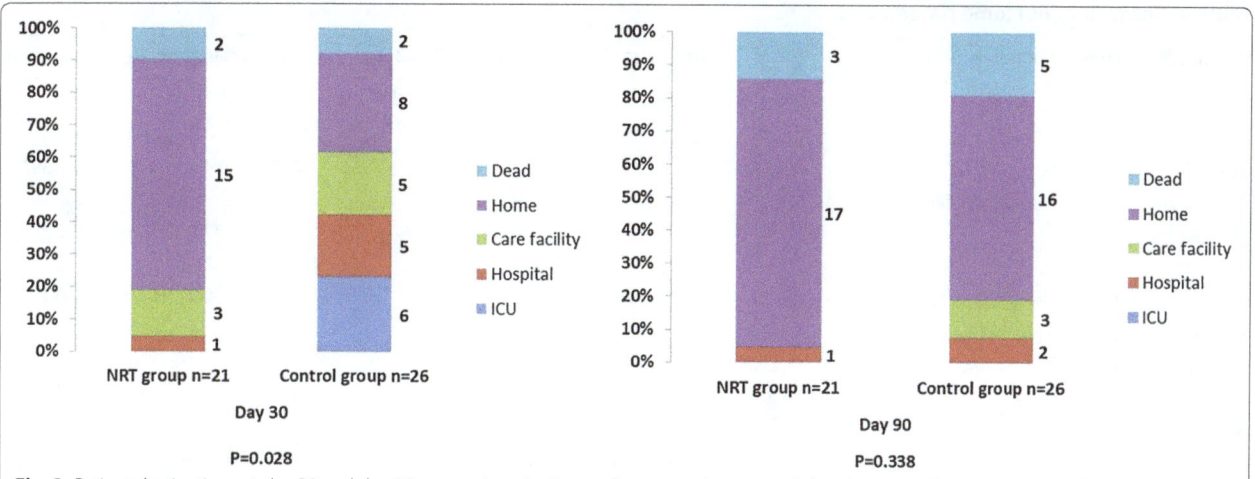

Fig. 2 Patient destinations at day 30 and day 90 comparing nicotine replacement therapy and placebo group. Data are presented as numbers. *ICU* intensive care unit, *NRT* nicotine replacement therapy

No differences were observed between NRT and control patients concerning in ICU and hospital LOS, hours without mechanical ventilation at day 30, total number of nosocomial infections, hours with delirium, time outside optimal sedation range, hours with physical restraint, number of self-removed devices and total dose of antipsychotics (Table 2).

Composite endpoint of normal brain function

During the first 10 days, patients receiving NRT on average were alive without delirium and without sedation or coma for 160 h, versus 88 h in the placebo group. The difference in time with normal brain function was 72 h, which was statistically significant ($p = 0.04$). At day 20, this difference had increased to 104 h (i.e. >4 days; $p = 0.03$). After 30 days, the difference was still 86 h, which was at that moment no longer significant (Fig. 3).

Adverse events

In total, 15 SAEs were reported during the study period: 4 in the NRT group and 11 in the control group. In the NRT group, two patients died due to respiratory failure after extubation, but with do-not-reintubate orders. The other SAEs were reintubation due to respiratory insufficiency after extubation and a spontaneous haemothorax in a patient admitted with a pneumonia and congestive heart failure. No SAEs were thought to be related to NRT.

The number of adverse events in the NRT group compared with the control group was similar (102 vs. 177, $p = 0.10$, Table 2) as well as the number of cardiovascular adverse events (16 vs. 43).

Discussion

This pilot randomised controlled trial provides data on the efficacy and safety of nicotine replacement therapy from mechanically ventilated patients, who were actively smoking before admission. Using biomarkers to distinguish active from passive smokers (serum cotinine ≥ 3.1 ng/ml or urinary NNAL ≥ 47.3 pg/ml), all patients were classified as actively smoking [25, 26].

We could not demonstrate differences between NRT and placebo groups with respect to mortality and (serious) adverse events. However, NRT was associated with more patients being discharged from the ICU or hospital at day 30. Moreover, patients receiving NRT spent more time alive without delirium and without sedation or coma during the first 20 days. This beneficial effect lost significance at day 30.

Available cohort and case–control studies assessing the role of NRT in supposed actively smoking ICU patients have shown conflicting results. Some studies suggested that NRT was associated with clinical benefits such as less agitation or decreased mortality, while others linked NRT to adverse effects such as increased ICU and hospital LOS, more delirium and need for physical restraining, increased duration of mechanical ventilation and more use of antipsychotics and even increased hospital mortality [13–19, 21]. Due to the retrospective design of all studies except one, selection bias and confounders may have influenced the reported results. In addition, varying inclusion and exclusion criteria were used, relevant differences in baseline characteristics were observed within some studies and heterogeneous populations were studied. Furthermore, smoking history obtained from patients or their legal representatives in general underestimates tobacco use in critically ill patients and there are

Table 2 Secondary outcome parameters

Secondary outcome parameters	Nicotine replacement therapy ($N=21$)	Control group ($N=26$)	p value
ICU length of stay (h), median (IQR)			
Day 30	186 (127 to 278)	246 (88 to 694)	0.41
Day 90	186 (127 to 278)	246 (88 to 694)	0.392
Hospital length of stay (h), median (IQR)			
Day 30	313 (226 to 528)	408 (220 to 720)	0.356
Day 90	313 (226 to 528)	408 (220 to 885)	0.369
Mechanical ventilation-free hours at day 30, median (IQR)	559 (494 to 605)	515 (135 to 606)	0.152
Mechanical ventilation >48 h, n (%)	17 (81)	20 (77)	–
Only non-invasive ventilation, n (%)	2 (10)	1 (4)	–
Nosocomial infections, n (%)	7 (24)	22 (76)	0.285
Hours with delirium, median (IQR)	8 (0 to 44)	16 (0 to 86)	0.152
RASS score, median (IQR)	−1.0 (−2.1 to −0.2)	−1.3 (−2.3 to −0.7)	0.266
Highest score	1 (0 to 1)	1 (0 to 1)	0.615
Lowest score	−4 (−5 to −2.5)	−5 (−5 to −4)	0.132
Outside optimal range (h)	40 (0 to 64)	48 (14 to 122)	0.202
Physical restraint (h), median (IQR)	12.0 (0 to 85.5)	44.5 (0 to 123)	0.417
Self-removed devices, n (%)			
Self-extubations	1 (20)	4 (80)	0.245
Catheters	24 (40)	36 (60)	0.886
Total dose of haloperidol (mg), median (IQR)	9 (0 to 24.5)	19.5 (3.25 to 31)	0.185
Serious adverse events, n	4	11	0.129
Adverse events, n			
Electrolyte disturbances	36	49	
Gastrointestinal	27	40	
Cardiovascular	16	43	
Arrhythmia	5	19	
Hypo-/hypertension	10	18	
Cardiac ischaemia	1	5	
Elevated cardiac enzymes	0	1	
Pulmonary	5	8	
Renal	1	6	
Others[a]	17	31	
Total adverse events, n (%)	102 (37)	177 (63)	0.096

NRT nicotine replacement therapy, *RASS* Richmond Agitation Sedation Scale, *mg* milligram, *h* hours, catheters are urinary and vascular catheters and nasogastric tubes

[a] Others: fever, fungal infection, sinusitis, allergic reaction, skin lesion, subcutaneous emphysema, thrombocytopenia, anaemia, pancytopenia, bleeding, hypo-/hyperthermia, hypothyroidism, ICU-acquired weakness, hypoventilation (hypercapnia), hemiplegia, anxiety

no validated tools or questionnaires available to detect active smoking in ICU patients [25]. None of these studies used biomarkers such as cotinine or NNAL to confirm active smoking. Moreover, in case delirium was an outcome parameter, most studies did not use validated delirium instruments [13, 14, 19–21].

The only prospective pilot study that has addressed the effect of NRT in ICU patients ($n=40$) demonstrated no effect of NRT on the use of sedatives and analgesics or ventilator free days compared with placebo [22]. However, there was a trend towards shorter ICU stay in the NRT group compared with the control group [4.5 (±3.8) vs 7.0 (±5.8) days, $p=0.08$]. This study and our study suggested that NRT may lead to a shorter ICU and hospital LOS.

At study entry, brain dysfunction could be demonstrated in around 80% of patients in both groups. However, between admission and day 20, significantly more patients in the NRT group had regained normal brain function compared with the control group. This positive effect of NRT on brain function is in accordance with the time course of nicotine withdrawal symptoms, which peaks in the first week after abstinence and lasts for 2–4 weeks [29].

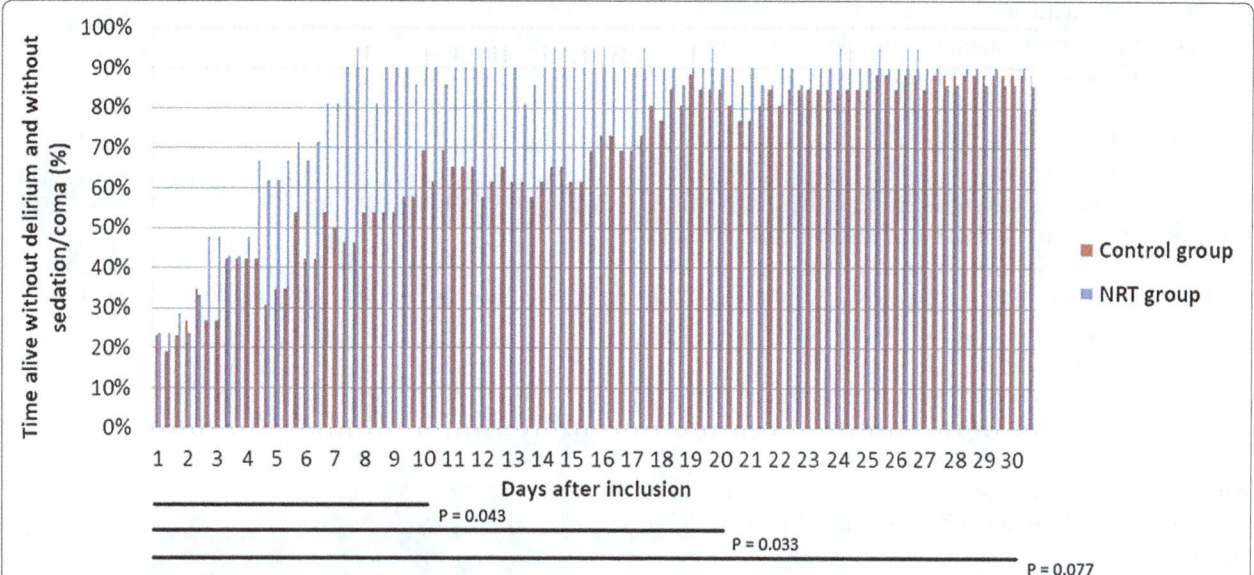

Fig. 3 Patients alive without delirium and without sedation or coma comparing nicotine replacement therapy and placebo group. Data presented as the percentage of time patients were alive without delirium and without sedation or coma (RASS ≥ − 3). *NRT* nicotine replacement therapy

Our observation that the difference between groups disappeared after 3 weeks suggests that nicotine withdrawal symptoms may have vanished during the study period, and no beneficial effect of NRT on the withdrawal syndrome may be expected any longer after 3 weeks.

Strengths and limitations

Proper patient selection is essential to evaluate the safety and efficacy of NRT in critically ill patients. In our study, the smoking status had to be confirmed by a questionnaire and had to be at a minimum of 10 cigarettes per day. The FTND classified patients as smokers with medium nicotine dependency. Serum cotinine or urinary NNAL confirmed that all patients were active smokers. Thorough patient selection with subsequent biomarker confirmation assured the inclusion of actively smoking patients and increased the validity of our study.

The main limitation of the study is the sample size with increased likelihood of type-1 or type-II errors. The small number of patients in the treatment arm ($n = 21$) precludes strong conclusions on safety and efficacy of NRT.

Recommendations for further research on NRT in critically ill patients

When a similar design to our study would be used, a RCT with mortality as the primary endpoint would need a sample size of at least 6000 participants to detect a 20% difference between NRT and placebo (alpha 0.05, power 80%). With respect to feasibility, we suggest to use a composite endpoint of time alive without delirium, sedation or coma as the primary endpoint in future trials.

This would necessitate inclusion of around 200 patients to detect a 48-h difference (alpha 0.05, power 80%). We suggest an intervention period as long as the withdrawal syndrome lasts (3–4 weeks).

An important reason for recruitment failure was the clinical indistinctness between myocardial infarction or ischaemia and increased cardiac enzymes for other reasons. When in doubt, attending physicians chose to exclude these patients. For future research, we advise clear definitions of cardiovascular events and no exclusion in the absence of a clear diagnosis by using 12-lead ECGs, repeated measurements of troponins, echocardiography to identify regional wall movement abnormalities and eventually angiography [30].

Although in our study clear effects of the present NRT could be demonstrated, in general the dosages of NRT to be used in future research and the route of administration are still unclear. In non-ICU patients, NRT is used to maintain some of the nicotine effects, but also to reduce the addiction potential by reducing the dosage and speed of delivery. Higher doses of NRT seem to be more effective in achieving smoking abstinence compared with lower doses [31]. However, during critical illness the main reason for prescribing NRT is to prevent or treat agitated behaviour. As ICU patients might have subcutaneous oedema or are treated with vasopressors, absorption of transdermal NRT may be compromised. Thus, nicotine inhalation or an oral or nasal spray and administration at a higher dose may better mimic smoking behaviour and potentially be more effective and could be considered in future studies [9, 11]. At present, there are no scientific data on the use of non-nicotine products to treat or prevent presumed nicotine withdrawal in critically ill patients (Additional file 1).

Conclusions

Among patients, actively smoking before ICU admission and mechanically ventilated after ICU admission, transdermal nicotine replacement therapy had no effect on mortality compared with placebo, although our pilot study was underpowered to detect such difference. The numbers of (serious) adverse events between groups were comparable.

Patients in the nicotine replacement therapy group spent more time with normal brain function during the first 20 days after ICU admission compared with control patients. Moreover, at day 30, more patients in this group were discharged from the ICU or hospital compared with controls.

An adequately powered RCT to study safety and efficacy of NRT in ICU patients seems feasible and is warranted.

Abbreviations
APACHE: Acute Physiology and Chronic Health Evaluation; AUDIT: Alcohol Use Disorders Identification Test; BPS: Behaviour Pain Scale; CAM-ICU: Confusion Assessment Method for the ICU; CCI: Charlson Comorbidity Index; DH: Deventer Hospital; DOS: Delirium Observation Scale; EMR: electronic medical record; FTND: Fagerström Test of Nicotine Dependence; GVH: Gelderse Vallei Hospital; ICU: intensive care unit; IQR: interquartile ranges; LOS: length of stay; MREC: Medical Research Ethics Committee; NNAL: 4-(methylnitrosamino)-1-(3-pyridyl)-1-butanol; NRS: Numeric Rating Scale; NRT: nicotine replacement therapy; PI: principal investigator; RASS: Richmond Agitation and Sedation Scale; RCT: randomised controlled trial; SAEs: serious adverse events; SD: standard deviations; SOFA: Sequential Organ Failure Assessment.

Authors' contributions
BJ and AZ were involved in conception and design of the study. BJ, AS, HO, AK-G contributed to data collection. BJ, AS, HO, MA, AZ collected data analysis and interpretation. BJ, AS, HO, MA, AZ were involved in drafting the article. All authors were involved in critical revision of the article. All authors were involved in final approval of the version for publication. All authors agree to be accountable for all aspects of the study and manuscript. All authors read and approved the final manuscript.

Author details
[1] Department of Intensive Care Medicine, Gelderse Vallei Hospital, Willy Brandtlaan 10, 6716 RP Ede, The Netherlands. [2] Department of Intensive Care Medicine, Deventer Hospital, Nico Bolkesteinlaan 75, 7416 SE Deventer, The Netherlands. [3] Department of Clinical Pharmacy, Deventer Hospital, Nico Bolkesteinlaan 75, 7416 SE Deventer, The Netherlands.

Competing interests
All authors declare that they have no competing interests.

Funding
Not applicable.

References
1. World Health Organization. WHO report on the global tobacco epidemic, 2011: warning about the dangers of tobacco. Geneva: World Health Organization; 2011. p. 8.
2. Jha P, Ramasundarahettige C, Landsman V, et al. 21st-Century hazards of smoking and benefits of cessation in the united states. N Engl J Med. 2013;368:341–50.
3. Trend in roken volwassenen, 1990–2015. https://www.volksgezondheid enzorg.info/onderwerp/roken/cijfers-context/trends#definities. Accessed 11 Jan 2018.
4. Burden of tobacco use in de U.S.: current cigarette smoking among U.S. adults aged 18 years and older. https://www.cdc.gov/tobacco/campaign/tips/resources/data/cigarette-smoking-in-united-states.html. Accessed 11 Jan 2018.
5. Lucidarme O, Seguin A, Daubin C, et al. Nicotine withdrawal and agitation in ventilated critically ill patients. Crit Care. 2010;14(2):R58.
6. Van Rompaey B, Elseviers MM, Schuurmans MJ, et al. Risk factors for delirium in intensive care patients: a prospective cohort study. Crit Care. 2009;13(3):R77.
7. Moller AM, Pedersen T, Villebro N, et al. A study of the impact of long-term tobacco smoking on postoperative intensive care admission. Anaesthesia. 2003;58(1):55–9.
8. Zaal IJ, Devlin JW, Peelen LM, et al. A systematic review of risk factors for delirium in the ICU. Crit Care Med. 2015;43(1):40–7.
9. Benowitz NL. Nicotine addiction. N Engl J Med. 2010;362(24):2295–303.
10. National Center for Chronic Disease Prevention and Health Promotion (US) office on smoking and health. The health consequences of smoking—50 years of progress: a report of the surgeon general. Atlanta (GA): Centers for Disease Control and Prevention (US); 2014. Chapter 5 (Nicotine) and Chapter 8 (Cardiovascular Diseases).
11. Hatsukami DK, Stead LF, Gupta PC. Tobacco addiction. Lancet. 2008;371(9629):2027–38.
12. Fagerström KO, Schneider NG, Lunell E. Effectiveness of nicotine patch and nicotine gum as individual versus combined treatment for tobacco withdrawal symptoms. Psychopharmacology. 1993;111(3):271–7.
13. Mayer SA, Chong JY, Ridgway E, et al. Delirium from nicotine withdrawal in neuro-ICU patients. Neurology. 2001;57(3):551–3.
14. Honisett TD. Nicotine replacement therapy for smokers admitted to intensive care. Intensive Crit Care Nurs. 2001;17(6):18–21.
15. Lee AH, Afessa B. The association of nicotine replacement therapy with mortality in a medical intensive care unit. Crit Care Med. 2007;35(6):1517–21.
16. Paciulio CA, Short MR, Steinke DT, et al. Impact of nicotine replacement therapy on postoperative mortality following coronary artery bypass graft surgery. Ann Pharmacother. 2009;43(7):1197–202.
17. Panos NG, Tesoro EP, Kim KS, et al. Outcomes associated with transdermal nicotine replacement therapy in a neurosurgery intensive care unit. Am J Health Syst Pharm. 2010;67(16):13571361.
18. Cartin-Ceba R, Warner DO, Hays JT, et al. Nicotine replacement therapy in critically ill patients: a prospective observational cohort study. Crit Care Med. 2011;39(7):1635–40.
19. Seder DB, Schmidt JM, Badjatia N, et al. Transdermal nicotine replacement therapy in cigarette smokers with acute subarachnoid hemorrhage. Neurocrit Care. 2011;14(1):77–83.
20. Gillies MA, McKenzie CA, Whiteley C, et al. Safety of nicotine replacement therapy in critically ill smokers: a retrospective cohort study. Intensive Care Med. 2012;38(10):1683–8.
21. Kerr A, McVey JT, Wood AM, et al. Safety of nicotine replacement therapy in critically ill smokers: a retrospective cohort study. Anaesth Intensive Care. 2016;44(6):758–61.
22. Pathak V, Rendon ISH, Lupu R, et al. Outcome of nicotine replacement therapy in patients admitted to ICU: a randomized controlled double-blind prospective pilot study. Respir Care. 2013;58(10):1625–9.
23. Kowalski M, Udy AA, McRobbie HJ, et al. Nicotine replacement therapy for agitation and delirium management in the intensive care unit: a systematic review of the literature. J Intensive Care. 2016;15(4):69.
24. Xia Y, McGuffey JE, Bhattacharyya S, et al. Analysis of the tobacco-specific nitrosamine 4-(methylnitrosamino)-1-(3-pyridyl)-1-butanol in urine by extraction on a molecularly imprinted polymer column and liquid chromatography/atmospheric pressure ionization tandem mass spectrometry. Anal Chem. 2005;77(23):7639–45.

25. Hsieh SJ, Ware LB, Eisner MD, et al. Biomarkers increase detection of active smoking and secondhand smoke exposure in critically ill patients. Crit Care Med. 2011;39(1):40–5.
26. Goniewicz ML, Eisner MD, Lazcano-Ponce E, et al. Comparison of urine cotinine and the tobacco-specific nitrosamine metabolite 4-(methylnitrosamino)-1-(3-pyridyl)-1-butanol (NNAL) and their ratio to discriminate active from passive smoking. Nicotine Tob Res. 2011;13(3):202–8.
27. Horan TC, Andrus M, Duceck MA. CDC/NHSN surveillance definition of health care-associated infection and criteria for specific types of infections in the acute care setting. Am J Infect Control. 2008;36(5):309–32.
28. Pandharipande PP, Pun BT, Herr DL, et al. Effect of sedation with dexmedetomidine vs lorazepam on acute brain dysfunction in mechanically ventilated patients: the MENDS randomized controlled trial. JAMA. 2007;298(22):2644–53.
29. Hughes JR. Effects of abstinence from tobacco: valid symptoms and time course. Nicotine Tob Res. 2007;9(3):315–27.
30. Carroll I, Mount T, Atkinson D. Myocardial infarction in intensive care units: a systematic review of diagnosis and treatment. J Intensive Care Soc. 2016;17(4):314–25.
31. Stead LF, Perera R, Bullen C, et al. Nicotine replacement therapy for smoking cessation. Cochrane Database Syst Rev. 2012. https://doi.org/10.1002/14651858.cd000146.pub4.

10

Pharmacogenomic biomarkers do not predict response to drotrecogin alfa in patients with severe sepsis

Djillali Annane[1], Jean-Paul Mira[2], Lorraine B. Ware[3], Anthony C. Gordon[4], Charles J. Hinds[5], David C. Christiani[6], Jonathan Sevransky[7], Kathleen Barnes[8], Timothy G. Buchman[7], Patrick J. Heagerty[9], Robert Balshaw[10], Nadia Lesnikova[10], Karen de Nobrega[10], Hugh F. Wellman[11], Mauricio Neira[11], Alexandra D. J. Mancini[11], Keith R. Walley[12] and James A. Russell[12]*

Abstract

Purpose: To explore potential design for pharmacogenomics trials in sepsis, we investigate the interaction between pharmacogenomic biomarkers and response to drotrecogin alfa (activated) (DrotAA). This trial was designed to validate whether previously identified improved response polymorphisms (IRPs A and B) were associated with an improved response to DrotAA in severe sepsis.

Methods: Patients with severe sepsis at high risk of death, who received DrotAA or not, with DNA available were included and matched to controls adjusting for age, APACHE II or SAPS II, organ dysfunction, ventilation, medical/surgical status, infection site, and propensity score (probability that a patient would have received DrotAA given their baseline characteristics). Independent genotyping and two-phase data transfer mitigated bias. The primary analysis compared the effect of DrotAA in IRP+ and IRP− groups on in-hospital 28-day mortality. Secondary endpoints included time to death in hospital; intensive care unit (ICU)-, hospital-, and ventilator-free days; and overall DrotAA treatment effect on mortality.

Results: Six hundred and ninety-two patients treated with DrotAA were successfully matched to 1935 patients not treated with DrotAA. Genotyping was successful for 639 (DrotAA) and 1684 (nonDrotAA) matched patients. The primary hypothesis of a genotype-by-treatment interaction (assessed by conditional logistic regression analysis) was not significant (P = 0.30 IRP A; P = 0.78 IRP B), and there was no significant genotype by treatment interaction for any secondary endpoint.

Conclusions: Neither IRP A nor IRP B predicted differential response to DrotAA on in-hospital 28-day mortality.

ClinicalTrials.gov registration NCT01486524

Keywords: Drotrecogin alfa (activated), Activated protein C, Pharmacogenomics biomarker, Propensity score, Severe sepsis

Background

Pharmacogenomic biomarkers identify patients who have altered drug response according to their genotype. For example, use of pharmacogenomics of warfarin decreases risk of adverse events (severe hemorrhage) and increases efficacy [1–3]. Similarly, pharmacogenomics could be used to predict how patients with sepsis may respond to adjunctive therapies.

Treatment with DrotAA led to variable clinical responses in patients with sepsis. Then, one trial conducted in both severe sepsis and septic shock found a significant absolute

*Correspondence: jrussell@mrl.ubc.ca
[12] Critical Care Research Laboratories, Centre for Heart Lung Innovation, St. Paul's Hospital, University of British Columbia, Burrard Building, Rm 166 - 1081 Burrard St, Vancouver, BC V6Z 1Y6, Canada
Full list of author information is available at the end of the article

risk reduction (ARR) of 6.1% in the 28-day mortality rate [4]. Other trials including only severe sepsis [5] or only septic shock [6, 7] failed to find survival benefit. One reason for the highly variable responses to DrotAA treatment observed in clinical trial may be related to genetic predisposition. In previous analyses, a combination of single nucleotide polymorphisms (SNPs) that defined two improve response polymorphisms (IRPs) was associated with a significant genotype-by-treatment interaction for effect of DrotAA on mortality.

Though DrotAA was withdrawn from the market by Ely Lilly, our overarching goal was to elaborate a pharmacogenomic approach using DrotAA as a practical example. Accordingly, the primary hypothesis was that IRP A and/ or IRP B predict a differential DrotAA treatment effect in patients with severe sepsis and high risk of death.

Methods

This is an abbreviated presentation of the methods of the current study because the details were published prior to undertaking analyses [8].

Prior studies—background on selection of pharmacogenomic biomarkers for current study

To screen for genomic biomarkers, a Genome Wide Association Study (GWAS) of the PROWESS study [4] was performed (unpublished data) using DNA from 1446 patients to genotype approximately 1.2 million SNPs (Illumina® Human1 M-Duo BeadChip). These results were taken forward to an independent cohort of patients who had septic shock, some of whom were treated with DrotAA and some of whom were not. This small replication cohort was drawn from St. Paul's Hospital (SPH) and the Vasopressin and Septic Shock Trial (VASST) [9].

The replication cohort was used to confirm two IRPs. Two-SNP composite improved response polymorphisms (IRPs), A and B, were constructed. Patients were classified as IRP A+ or − and IRP B+ or − if they had one of both of the responsive genotype. For each IRP, individual patients were considered biomarker positive if they had the responsive genotype for either of the SNPs or for both of the SNPs in the IRP. The individual SNPs in each IRP were associated with a differential DrotAA treatment effect in PROWESS (derivation cohort) and replicated in the replication cohort (unpublished).

The two SNPs comprising IRP A were chosen based first on the alignment of direction and strength of their signals by analyzing the interaction of SNP and treatment effect on mortality in both the PROWESS study and the replication cohort. Secondly, these two SNPs were chosen based on biological plausibility linking the proteins coded by these genes to pathways of sepsis or pathways regarding mechanisms of action of DrotAA. The two SNPs of IRP A

are RYR2 (ryanodine receptor 2 gene) rs684923 on chromosome 1 and ACIN1 (apoptotic chromatin condensation inducer 1 gene) rs3751501 on chromosome 14. The SNP of RYR2 could act to enhance efficacy of activated protein C on protection of endothelial permeability via its effects on endothelial protein C receptor and sphingosine-1-phosphate receptor 1 (S1P). When activated protein C (APC) binds to PAR1, this triggers more conversion of sphingosine to S1P, and this could decrease the amount of sphingosine and thus disinhibit the ryanodine receptor. We also suggest that this disinhibition of the ryanodine receptor by the actions of APC varies according to the genotype of the ryanodine receptor.

Phosphorylation of a residue (S422) inACIN1 (Acinus-S variant) by AKT (prosurvival kinase) completely inhibits cleavage of Acinus-S by caspase-3, abrogating the formation of fragment p17 which is essential for chromatin condensation during apoptosis. Apoptosis is increased in some tissues and cells (lymphocytes, dendritic cells, pulmonary and gut epithelial cells) and is decreased in other tissues and cells (neutrophils) in sepsis. This gene modulates apoptosis and activated protein C has anti-apoptotic actions apoptosis so we suggest that there could be an interaction between polymorphisms of ACIN1 and response to DrotAA. More specifically, the genetic variants rs3751501 (AA|AG), associated with increased ARR (absolute risk reduction) and coding for amino acid 478 F in ACIN1, would render ACIN1 constitutively nonphosphorylated at residue 478 F and hence constitutively nonphosphorylated at S422, leading to AKT-independent regulation of chromatin condensation by Acinus-S during apoptosis, because nonphosphorylated acinus-S would be constitutively cleavable by caspase-3.

The two SNPs comprising IRP B were chosen based solely on the strength of their signals in the PROWESS and replication cohorts. These two SNPs are SPATA7 (spermatogenesis associated 7 gene) rs3179969 on chromosome 14 and FLI1 (Friend leukemia virus integration 1 gene) rs640098 on chromosome 11.

For the replication cohort, the ARR was 19.7% for IRP A+ patients (95% confidence interval (CI) 2.2–37.1%), whereas for the IRP A − patients the ARR was −8.9% (95% CI −22.6–4.9%)($p = 0.018$ unadjusted). The ARR was 21.2% for IRP B+ patients (95% CI 3.2–39.2%), whereas for the IRP B − patients the ARR was −5% (95% CI −18.2–8.2%)($p = 0.04$ unadjusted).

The current study—overall design

This was an international, multicenter, retrospective, controlled, outcome-blinded, genotype-blinded, and matched-patients study [8]. Retrospectively accessed DNA and clinical data were analyzed to validate the prespecified IRPs. Prospective aspects of this study were the genotyping of patients with regard to the IRPs and the statistical testing of the prespecified genotype hypothesis. Eight academic centers contributed the data and DNA from 10 cohorts (5 EU, 4 US, 1 Canada).

Study population and treatment groups

Patients included in the current study (the INDICATED population) met prespecified eligibility criteria [8] and DrotAA-treated patients were matched to DrotAA-free patients. Eligibility criteria (aligned with the approved use of DrotAA in the USA and EU) were used to select the primary study population (INDICATED). Such patients with high risk of death represented common practice for use of DrotAA [10–14]. No patient in this study was part of a prospective randomized trial of DrotAA. Patients were treated according to standard care at their sites, and data and DNA samples collected at that time were retrospectively accessed for this study. All patients were enrolled after the Food and Drug Administration (FDA) or European Medicines Agency (EMA) approval of DrotAA.

Matching DrotAA-treated to control patients

The current study incorporated a robust, well-accepted matching strategy. A propensity score of the estimated probability that a patient would have received DrotAA given their key baseline characteristics was calculated, and patients were selected as matches had to be within a prespecified tolerance on this score. Combining the use of propensity scores with covariate matching is superior to the use of either strategy alone [15]. The intended clinical variables for the calculation of the Mahalanobis distance and the reasons why these variables were chosen were described previously [8].

Syreon Corporation (a clinical research organization) conducted the study. A two-phase transfer of data from each center was performed to ensure that the selection of matched control patients was blinded and unbiased. Data transfer 1 included variables to confirm eligibility and to conduct the matching. Once the matching was achieved, the matched sets of treated and control patients were "locked" together. Then data transfer 2 (outcomes and genotypic data) was sent to Syreon.

Genotyping

Genotyping for the IRP SNPs was done using a validated Taqman®-based analytical method and the laboratory was blinded to treatment and outcome. A 91-SNP ancestry informative marker (AIM) panel was genotyped by the GoldenGate® analytical method.

Statistical analysis

As previously noted [8], this study had 90% power to detect a treatment-by-IRP interaction assuming an absolute mortality reduction of 15% in the DrotAA-treated group compared to control in IRP + patients and with 1–2% difference in mortality between the treated and control groups in IRP- patients.

The primary analysis was done on the Matched-INDICATED population (comparing the effect of treatment in the IRP + and IRP- groups) by testing for the effect of the interaction between IRP and DrotAA treatment on the primary endpoint in a conditional logistic regression model, conditioning on the matching while incorporating the principal component scores from the 91-SNP AIM panel data (as covariates to control for potential population stratification). The primary endpoint was in-hospital mortality through Day 28 (i.e., patients were followed until hospital discharge or Day 28, whichever came first). Each of the primary analyses, one for IRP A and one for IRP B, was done as a two-sided test with $\alpha = 2.5\%$ for an overall, Bonferroni-corrected, type I error rate of 5%.

Results

Prior to matching patients treated with DrotAA differed significantly from nonDrotAA patients in many important baseline clinical respects (Additional file 1: Supplement Tables 1–6). After applying the eligibility criteria for the INDICATED population, there were 11,018 patients not treated with DrotAA from whom to choose matched controls for the 738 DrotAA-treated patients (ratio 15:1) (Fig. 1). Suitable matches were not available for 46 (6.2%) of the 738 INDICATED DrotAA-treated patients. Thus, after matching, the number of matched-INDICATED DrotAA-treated patients was 692. Overall the matched ratio was 2.8 control patients for every DrotAA-treated patient. Baseline clinical characteristics of the matched 692 DrotAA patients were similar to the 1,935 matched control patients (Table 1). The DrotAA group had higher proportion of coagulation dysfunction and a higher use of vasopressors (Table 1). Matching was done before genotype was known so it is relevant to observe that within the IRP A + and IRP A- and the IRP B+ and IRP B− genotype subgroups, DrotAA-treated patients were similar to matched control patients (Additional file 1: Supplement Tables 8–19). The Primary Analysis Population (PAP) included 639 DrotAA-treated patients and 1684 matched controls. The primary reasons why patients could not be included in the PAP were insufficient quantity of DNA or unsuccessful genotyping (Fig. 1, Additional file 1: Supplement Table 7).

Effect of DrotAA on mortality

Irrespective of genotype, the ARR was in favor of DrotAA (estimated weighted mortality: DrotAA 25.1%, nonDrotAA 30.5%) ($P = 0.006$, Additional file 1: Supplement Table 21).

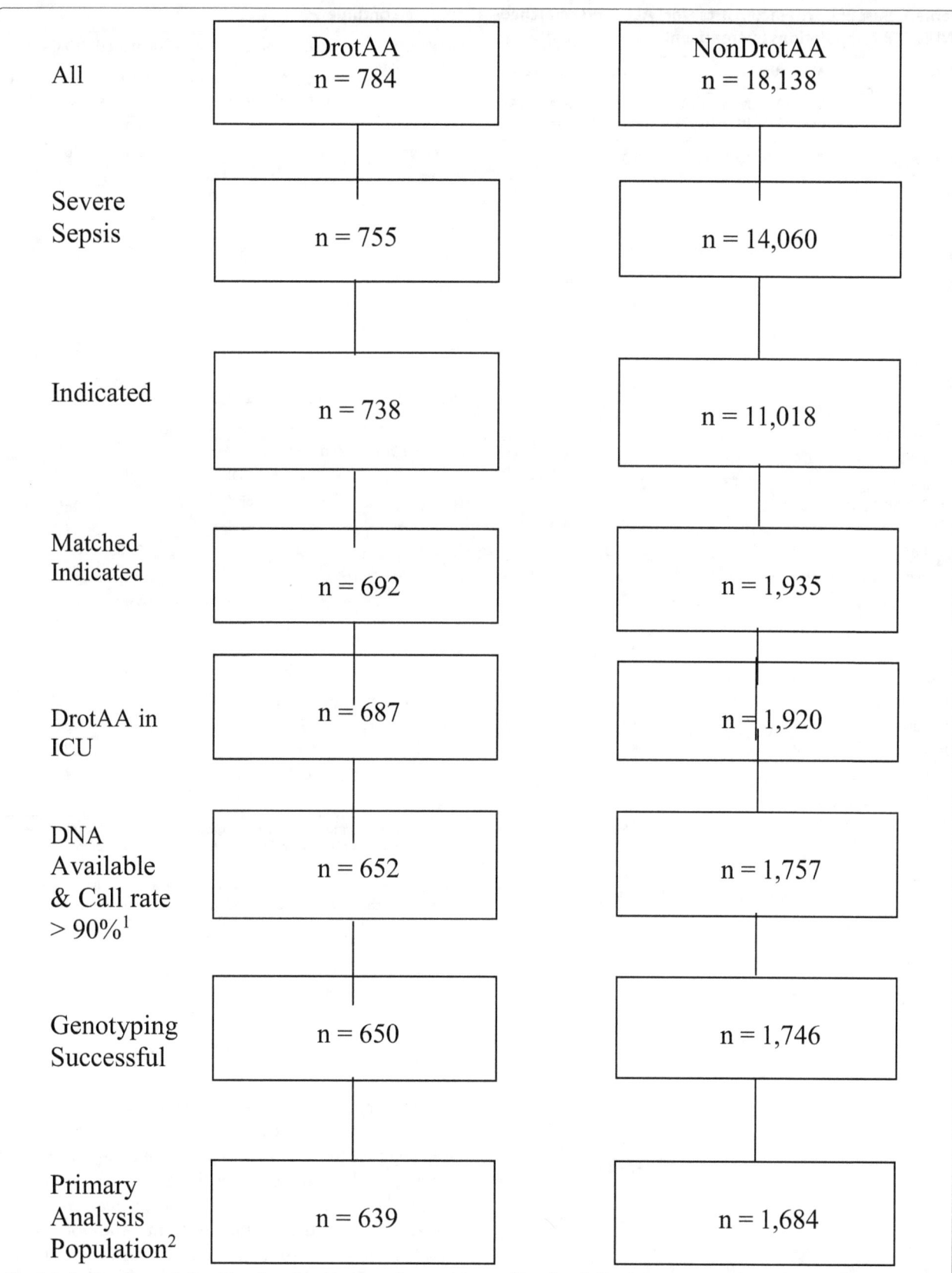

Fig. 1 Patient enrollment in DrotAA and nonDrotAA groups. Superscript notes: [1]Based on GoldenGate genotyping for AIM panel SNPs and research SNPs. [2]Each matched set required 1 DrotAA-treated patient and 1–3 nonDrotAA-treated patients

Table 1 Baseline characteristics for ALL and matched-INDICATED populations by treatment

Table 1 continued

Baseline characteristics[a]	ALL patients		Matched-INDICATED	
	DrotAA (n = 784)	NonDrotAA (n = 18,138)	DrotAA (n = 692)	NonDrotAA (n = 1935)
Age (Mean)	58.4	60.4	59.0	59.1
SD	16.1	16.9	15.4	9.2
P value[b]	0.001		0.69	
Male (%)	59.7	59.9	60.1	61.2
P value	0.93		0.65	
APACHE II (mean)	26.1	21.1	25.8	25.5
SD	8.2	7.7	7.9	4.7
P value	< 0.0001		0.02	
SAPS II (mean)	58.1	47.8	59.1	58.5
SD	19.2	19.1	18.8	10.9
P value	< 0.0001		0.77	
Origin of sepsis (%)				
Nosocomial	8.4	4.7	7.2	12.3
Community acquired	38.6	14.3	39.7	34.7
Unknown	52.9	81.0	53.0	53.0
P value	0.003		< 0.0001	
Anatomic site of primary infection (%)				
Lung	51.5	23.4	52.9	46.8
Abdomen	12.2	6.9	13.2	12.7
CNS	1.3	0.6	0.9	0.7
Blood	3.4	2.0	3.0	3.5
Urinary tract	4.1	2.7	3.8	3.3
Unknown	22.1	60.2	21.1	29.0
Other	5.4	4.2	5.2	4.1
P value	0.0004		0.55	
Use of vasopressors (%)				
Yes	91.2	54.7	91.8	81.2
No	8.3	39.2	7.8	17.8
Unknown	0.5	6.1	0.4	1.0
P value	< 0.0001		< 0.0001	
Mechanical ventilation (%)				
Yes	76.3	72.3	75.7	76.4
No	6.4	19.5	6.2	5.2
Unknown	17.3	8.2	18.1	18.4
P value	< 0.0001		0.08	
Number of organ systems with dysfunction (%)				
0	1.4	9.9	0.0	0.0
1	2.2	23.8	0.1	0.8
2	20.7	30.8	21.0	22.0
3	33.0	19.4	35.1	34.0
4	24.9	11.3	26.3	29.4
5	13.6	4.1	13.9	11.7
6	4.2	0.7	3.6	2.2
P value	< 0.0001		0.82	
Cardiovascular dysfunction (%)				
Yes	96.0	66.9	98.7	98.3
No	2.4	30.2	1.0	1.0
Unknown	1.5	2.9	0.3	0.7
P value	< 0.0001		0.36	
Pulmonary dysfunction (%)				
Yes	92.6	69.5	95.4	95.3
No	5.1	18.8	3.9	3.4
Unknown	2.3	11.7	0.7	1.3
P value	< 0.0001		0.34	
CNS dysfunction (%)				
Yes	28.4	21.0	27.7	31.4
No	33.2	34.5	33.8	30.9
Unknown	38.4	44.5	38.4	37.7
P value	0.0003		0.01	
Coagulation dysfunction (%)				
Yes	31.4	14.0	31.8	25.0
No	65.4	68.7	66.3	72.6
Unknown	3.2	17.3	1.9	2.4
P value	< 0.0001		< 0.0001	
Renal dysfunction (%)				
Yes	63.3	29.4	65.6	61.7
No	33.9	54.1	32.4	36.6
Unknown	2.8	16.6	2.0	1.7
P value	< 0.0001		< 0.01	
Hepatic dysfunction (%)				
Yes	23.9	13.0	24.4	23.8
No	66.8	66.7	67.6	68.5
Unknown	9.3	20.3	7.9	7.7
P value	< 0.0001		0.71	

[a] Summary statistics for the NonDrotAA group were weighted to reflect the unequal numbers of DrotAA and NonDrotAA patients in each of the matched sets

[b] Descriptive P values are from clustered regression analysis using linear regression (numeric variables) or binary logistic regression (categorical variables) comparing the proportion of patients in the most frequent category between DrotAA vs NonDrotAA, clustering on the matched sets and with weights based on the number of patients in DrotAA and NonDrotAA matched sets. Patients in the unknown categories were excluded from the tests. No adjustments were made to account for multiple inference

Primary endpoint: genotype-by-DrotAA treatment interaction

The primary hypothesis of a genotype by DrotAA treatment interaction assessed by conditional logistic regression analysis for IRP A was not significant ($P = 0.30$, Table 2), and the direction of the effect was opposite to what had been expected as shown by the negative parameter estimate for the interaction term (Additional file 1: Supplement Tables 20–21). The IRP B result was also not significant ($P = 0.78$, Table 2), and the direction of effect was opposite to what had been expected. There was a

Table 2 Primary efficacy analysis—conditional logistic regression model including AIM Panel PCs

Factor/effect	Estimate	SE	Odds ratio (OR) estimate	OR 95% CI		P value[c]
				Lower	Upper	
Primary efficacy analysis for IRP A						
IRP A*Treatment Interaction[a]	− 0.31	0.303	0.731	0.403	1.324	0.30
IRP A+: DrotAA versus NonDrotAA	0.11	0.245	1.112	0.688	1.799	0.66
IRP A−: DrotAA versus NonDrotAA	0.42	0.145	1.522	1.145	2.024	< 0.01
DrotAA: IRP A+ versus IRP A−	− 0.30	0.258	0.740	0.446	1.228	0.24
NonDrotAA: IRP A+ versus IRP A−	0.01	0.150	1.013	0.755	1.359	0.93
AIM Panel PCs[b]						0.14
Primary efficacy Analysis for IRP B						
IRP B*Treatment Interaction[a]	− 0.09	0.325	0.912	0.482	1.722	0.78
IRP B+: DrotAA versus NonDrotAA	0.23	0.277	1.257	0.730	2.162	0.41
IRP B−: DrotAA versus NonDrotAA	0.32	0.138	1.379	1.052	1.807	0.02
DrotAA: IRP B+ versus IRP B−	− 0.19	0.285	0.829	0.475	1.449	0.51
NonDrotAA: IRP B+ versus IRP B−	− 0.09	0.156	0.910	0.670	1.236	0.55
AIM Panel PCs[b]						0.14

Analysis for IRP A involved 376 discordant matched sets from a total of 637 matched sets

Analysis for IRP B involved 372 discordant matched sets from a total of 634 matched sets

[a] The interaction odds ratio is a ratio of odds ratios

[b] A total of 10 AIM Panel PCs were included which accounted for 33.9% of the variance in the AIM Panel data for the Matched-INDICATED Primary Analysis Population based on all cohorts

[c] P values from conditional logistic regression partial likelihood ratio tests for the IRP*Treatment Interaction and the combined AIM Panel PCs; all other P values are from Wald Chi-square tests

therapeutic benefit of DrotAA treatment in IRP A- negative and IRP B- negative patients.

Neither IRP A nor IRP B predicted ICU and hospital survival rates or the destination at hospital discharge. At hospital discharge, the mortality rates were 32.2 and 36.2% for DrotAA group and nonDrotAA groups, respectively. Approximately 19% of patients were discharged home, 13% went to long-term care facilities, 9% went to another acute care hospital, and discharge location was unknown for the remainder (24–27%).

Sensitivity analyses with common matching variables included as covariates

The inclusion of the common matching variables as covariates in the conditional logistic regression model did not change any of the conclusions regarding IRP A, IRP B, or the overall DrotAA effect (Table 3). We used conditional logistic regression and included common matching variables (age, APACHE II score or SAPS II score, and respiratory dysfunction (yes/no)) as covariates to correct for residual imbalances across IRP genotype subgroups. Neither self-reported race nor genetically determined continent of origin impacted the overall DrotAA treatment effect or the IRP*Treatment interactions in conditional logistic regression models.

Sensitivity analyses according to high APACHE II/SAPS II scores

As in PROWESS [4] the overall effect of DrotAA differed according to severity of illness (Table 4). Greater severity of illness was defined by APACHE II ≥25 and by SAPS II ≥54. ARR based on crude mortality rates was 10.3% in the high severity of illness and—1.8% in the low severity of illness subgroups.

Sensitivity analyses of individual IRP A and IRP B SNPs

None of the IRP A nor IRP B SNPs was significantly associated with treatment effect when analyzed individually.

Secondary endpoints

Time to death in hospital analyses showed a beneficial DrotAA treatment effect but no additional benefit to knowing IRP A or IRP B genotype (Fig. 2). None of the secondary efficacy endpoints analyses (time to death in hospital, ICU-free days, hospital-free days, and mechanical-ventilator-free days) showed a significant genotype-by-treatment interaction (Additional file 1: Supplement Tables 22–26).

Discussion

This international, multicenter, retrospective, non-randomized, controlled, outcome-blinded, genotype-blinded, and matched-patients study found that neither

Table 3 Secondary analysis with common matching variables included as covariates—conditional logistic regression for differential treatment effects of IRP A and IRP B on mortality

Factor/effect	Estimate	SE	Odds Ratio (OR) estimate	OR 95% CI		P value[c]
				Lower	Upper	
Analysis for IRP A						
IRP A*Treatment Interaction[a]	−0.34	0.304	0.710	0.391	1.289	0.26
IRP A+ : DrotAA versus NonDrotAA	0.08	0.246	1.087	0.671	1.761	0.74
IRP A−: DrotAA versus NonDrotAA	0.43	0.146	1.532	1.151	2.039	< 0.01
DrotAA: IRP A+ versus IRP A−	−0.32	0.259	0.725	0.436	1.205	0.22
NonDrotAA: IRP A+ versus IRP A−	0.02	0.150	1.022	0.761	1.372	0.89
AIM Panel PCs[b]						0.13
Common covariates used in matching						0.74
Age (per year)	−0.02	0.024	0.976	0.930	1.023	0.30
APACHE II (per point)[d]	0.05	0.080	1.054	0.901	1.233	0.51
SAPS II (per point)[d]	0.01	0.041	1.006	0.929	1.091	0.88
Respiratory dysfunction (Yes vs. No)	0.86	0.778	2.371	0.515	10.90	0.27
Analysis for IRP B						
IRP B*Treatment Interaction[a]	−0.10	0.325	0.908	0.480	1.719	0.77
IRP B+: DrotAA versus NonDrotAA	0.22	0.278	1.251	0.726	2.155	0.42
IRP B−: DrotAA versus NonDrotAA	0.32	0.138	1.377	1.050	1.806	0.02
DrotAA: IRP B+ vs IRP B−	−0.19	0.285	0.826	0.472	1.443	0.50
NonDrotAA: IRP B+ vs IRP B−	−0.10	0.157	0.909	0.668	1.236	0.54
AIM panel PCs[b]						0.15
Common covariates used in matching						0.75
Age (per year)	−0.02	0.024	0.976	0.931	1.024	0.32
APACHE II (per point)[d]	0.04	0.080	1.045	0.894	1.223	0.58
SAPS II (per point)[d]	−0.00	0.041	0.997	0.919	1.081	0.94
Respiratory dysfunction (Yes vs. No)	0.12	0.935	1.127	0.180	7.050	0.90

Analysis for IRP A involved 376 discordant matched sets from a total of 637 matched sets

Analysis for IRP B involved 372 discordant matched sets from a total of 634 matched sets

[a] The interaction odds ratio is a ratio of odds ratios

[b] A total of 10 AIM Panel PCs were included which account for 33.9% of the variance in the AIM Panel data for the Matched-INDICATED Primary Analysis Population based on all cohorts

[c] P values from conditional logistic regression partial likelihood ratio tests for the IRP*Treatment Interaction and the combined AIM Panel PCs; all other P values are from Wald Chi-square tests

[d] Sites with APACHE II scores were analyzed with 0's for SAPS II scores, and vice versa

IRP A nor IRP B predicted differential DrotAA treatment effects on in-hospital mortality through Day 28 in patients with severe sepsis. Furthermore, there was no significant genotype by treatment interaction for any of the secondary endpoints. Nonetheless, as yet undiscovered, other genotypes might accurately predict response to DrotAA.

Despite the negative results of the genotype by DrotAA treatment interaction, we suggest that this study provided a potential design for future evaluations of pharmacogenomic biomarkers of drugs and devices for use in sepsis. Most recent and ongoing sepsis trials include DNA biobanking. We propose that these trials systematically explore potential experimental treatment interaction with genomic biomarkers. If any positive interaction,

a confirmatory RCT with biomarker-based stratification of randomization would then be conducted.

The possible explanations for the negative findings are that the prior discovery studies were false positive results that did not validate because the biology assumptions were incorrect for the biology SNPs and that the statistics were misleading for the statistically chosen SNPs. The lessons to be learned for future biomarker trials include need for greater validation in prior studies before the pivotal trials are done, perhaps focus only on statistically chosen SNPs, and access to prior trials in which SNPs were assessed (such as PROWESS in the current example).

We believe that this is the largest study of predictive genomic biomarkers for any drug used in sepsis. DrotAA

Table 4 Secondary analyses for effects of high APACHE II/SAPS II scores on differential treatment effects of IRP A and IRP B on mortality—conditional logistic regression models including AIM panel PCs

Factor/effect	Estimate	SE	Odds Ratio (OR) estimate	OR 95% CI		P value[c]
				Lower	Upper	
Analysis for IRP A						
Treatment	−0.15	0.258	0.861	0.519	1.427	0.56
IRP A	−0.08	0.278	0.926	0.537	1.597	0.78
IRP A by treatment interaction[a]	−0.01	0.535	0.989	0.347	2.819	0.98
High APACHE II/SAPS II Scores	−0.06	0.352	0.940	0.472	1.872	0.86
High APACHE II/SAPS II scores by treatment interaction[a]	0.82	0.315	2.273	1.226	4.215	< 0.01
High APACHE II/SAPS II scores by IRP A Interaction[a]	0.15	0.329	1.164	0.611	2.218	0.65
IRP A by treatment by high APACHE II/SAPS II Scores	−0.42	0.651	0.659	0.184	2.360	0.52
AIM Panel PCs[b]						< 0.01
Analysis for IRP B						
Treatment	−0.13	0.251	0.880	0.538	1.438	0.61
IRP B	0.14	0.280	1.153	0.666	1.999	0.61
IRP B by treatment interaction[a]	−0.09	0.541	0.912	0.316	2.635	0.87
High APACHE II/SAPS II Scores	0.10	0.344	1.100	0.561	2.157	0.78
High APACHE II/SAPS II Scores by Treatment[a]	0.63	0.302	1.869	1.033	3.379	0.04
High APACHE II/SAPS II Scores by IRP B Interaction[a]	−0.35	0.338	0.704	0.363	1.366	0.30
IRP B by treatment by high APACHE II/SAPS II Scores	0.09	0.677	1.092	0.290	4.118	0.90
AIM Panel PCs[b]						< 0.01

Analysis for IRP A involves 376 discordant matched sets from a total of 637 matched sets. Analysis for IRP B involves 372 discordant matched sets from a total of 634 matched sets

[a] The interaction odds ratio is a ratio of odds ratios

[b] A total of 10 AIM Panel PCs have been included which account for 33.9% of the variance in the AIM Panel data for the Matched-INDICATED Primary Analysis Population based on all cohorts

[c] P values are from Wald Chi-square tests; the test of the combined AIM Panel PCs is the sum of the individual Wald Chi-square tests

treatment was associated with similar survival benefit in the IRP + and IRP- genotype subgroups. Self-reported ethnicity, genetically assigned continent of origin, and high APACHE II/SAPS II analyses did not show predictive genetic IRP effects in any subgroup. Exploratory analyses of the four individual IRP SNPs also did not show any predictive biomarker effects. Similarly, neither IRP A nor IRP B was predictive of differential DrotAA treatment effects on secondary efficacy endpoints. Only the IRP B + genotype was associated with significantly longer duration in hospital in DrotAA-treated patients compared with the IRP B- genotype.

Strengths of this study were first, identification of a well-defined and clinically appropriate patient population (on-label as defined by the approved indications for DrotAA in both the EU and the USA). Secondly, we minimized patient selection bias by using matching to select appropriate patients for the control group to overcome the lack of randomization to DrotAA treatment. DrotAA was typically given to younger patients with greater severity of disease in clinical practice. Therefore, simply comparing the mortality rates in all DrotAA-treated patients to all nonDrotAA-treated patients in the 10

cohorts would have been invalid. The considerations in designing this study were to use either design-based or analysis-based methods to control for characteristics that differed at baseline between treatment groups. We chose to use a design-based approach of matching to tightly control for key measures, so that the control group was comparable to the treated group. This also permitted efficient use of resources since only a subsample of all possible controls would be needed for detailed genotypic evaluation. The low use of DrotAA in clinical practice for patients with severe sepsis in the included cohorts permitted this matched-patients study to be conducted. If the drug had been used most of the time in the eligible patients, then it would have been very difficult to match appropriate nonDrotAA-treated patients as matched controls. The matching process was successful in achieving well-balanced study groups, and balance between the two study groups was achieved across IRP genotype subgroups (IRP+, IRP−), thus minimizing confounding of any biomarker effects (IRP*treatment interaction) by baseline differences.

The third strength of the study was quality of data, genotyping, and ancestry-control. Extensively reviewed

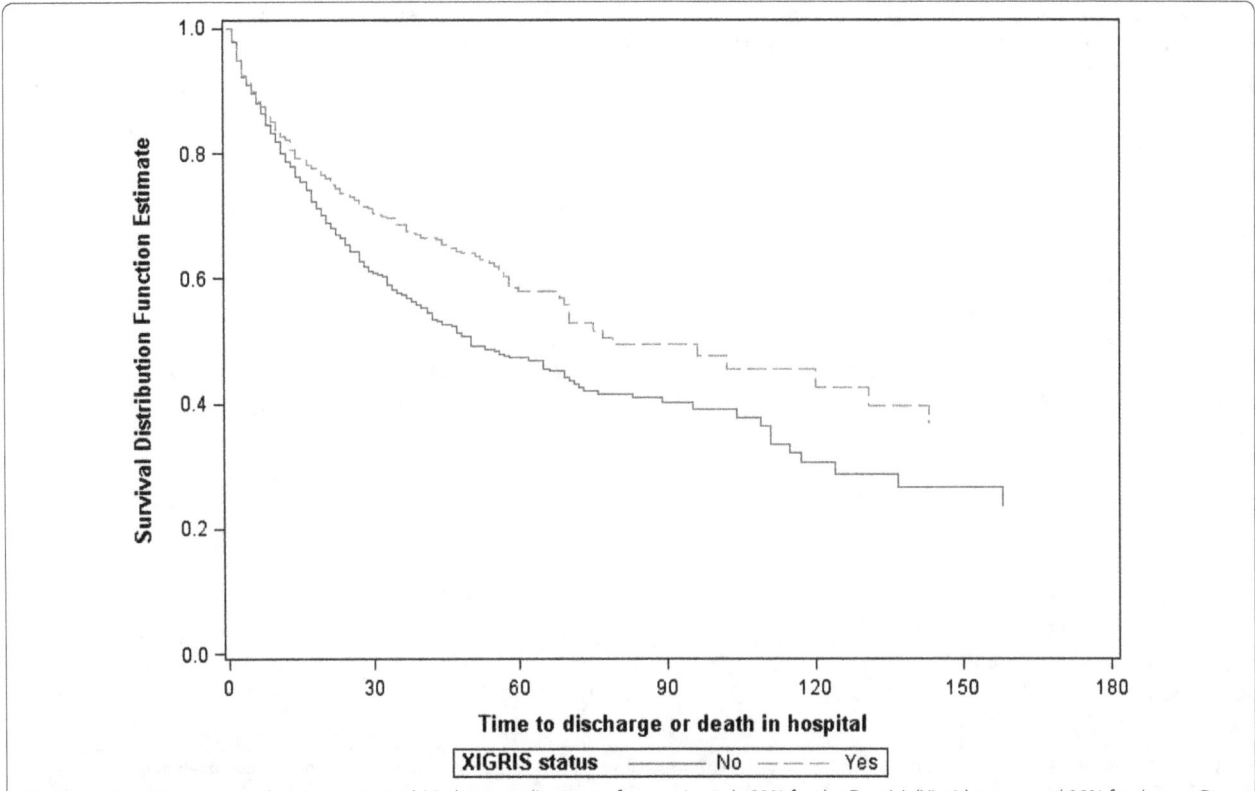

Fig. 2 Kaplan–Meier curves showing estimated 28-day mortality rates of approximately 28% for the DrotAA (Xigris) group and 38% for the nonDrotAA group

phenotypic data from all 10 cohorts were combined in a common database. Genotyping of the IRP SNPs was conducted using a validated Taqman-based method. A panel of ancestry informative markers (AIM panel with 91 SNPs) was genotyped using a qualified GoldenGate genotyping method. Quality criteria were applied to the genomic data based on per-sample and per-SNP call rates and Hardy–Weinberg equilibrium testing. These strengths are confirmed by finding similar results to PROWESS in that we were successful in overcoming the patient selection bias that can occur in a retrospective, nonrandomized study.

DrotAA has been suggested to be beneficial in the most severe patients, and especially in those with advanced coagulopathy. Coagulation dysfunction was diagnosed in only 31.8% of the treated patients, which might partly explain the negative results. However, we clarify that we chose our inclusion criteria to align with the drug label and indicated use of DrotAA. Our overall hypothesis was that a genomic marker(s) would identify responders to DrotAA and that a diagnostic kit could then be developed to help clinicians decide whom to treat with DrotAA.

The SNP selection and interaction test results of the prior studies could have been influenced by the so-called winner's curse. If adequate methods had been taken to deal with the winner's curse, then the sample size requirement for adequate power may have increased because we would not have over-estimated the assumed effect size of the IRP.

Although the present results are negative, it is useful to discuss the feasibility of IRP detection (including time and cost) and treatment allocation based on the presence of such IRPs. The genotype can be measured now in 40–60 min (Cepheid for example), even in the Emergency or ICU setting, and location(s) a time frame reasonable for IRP detection in sepsis and septic shock. The cost would depend upon the technology platform cost, the reagent costs, and the clinical value of the test results based on studies of cost–benefit of the test versus not having the test.

Limitations of our study were that the treatment assignment of DrotAA was not blinded nor randomized, outcomes were obtained retrospectively from databases, and we could not assess safety due to lack of adequate data. Examples of some confounders that we could not control for are physician and judgement regarding patient prognosis and eligibility for treatment with Dro-tAA, individual ICU or hospital policies regarding use of DrotAA, and other underlying disease that we did not capture. We did not specifically select patients that were randomized in DrotAA trials because we did not have access to the trials of DrotAA that collected DNA such as PROWESS [4, 16]. Sepsis is a complex trait, so it is likely that future research regarding better patient selection for treatment will consider several phenotypic biomarkers (not just focusing on genetic diversity) with or without genotype assessments.

Why were our IRP A and IRP B genotypes not predictive? It is possible that our method of selection of SNPs for IRP A and IRP B was inadequate. We used an under-powered replication cohort to refine SNPs of interest from the PROWESS study and we incorporated both SNPs based on pure statistical signal in the replication cohort as well as SNPs that were chosen based on both strength of signal in the replication cohort as well as bio-logical plausibility. Our study highlights the importance and difficulty of validation of predictive genotype-base biomarkers in severe sepsis.

Our finding of a beneficial treatment effect of DrotAA in the current study differs from PROWESS SHOCK [6] and from the APROCCHS trial [7] (in which there was no treatment effect) and may reflect selection bias. Additionally, our study was not randomized, included an earlier era of patients, and we found higher mortality rates than in PROWESS SHOCK.

Conclusions

Neither IRP A nor IRP B predicted a differential DrotAA treatment effect in patients with severe sepsis and high risk of death.

Abbreviations

PROWESS: prospective recombinant human activated protein C worldwide evaluation in severe sepsis; IRP: improved response polymorphism; DROTAA: drotrecogin alfa (activated); APACHE II: acute physiology and chronic health evaluation; SAPS: simplified acute physiology score; SNP: single nucleotide polymorphism; ICU: intensive care unit; ARR: absolute risk reduction; GWAS: Genome Wide Association Study; SPH: St. Paul's Hospital; VASST: vasopressin and septic shock trial; RYR2: ryanodine receptor 2 gene; ACIN1: apoptotic chromatin condensation inducer 1 gene; S1P: sphingosine-1-phosphate receptor 1; APC: activated protein C; PAR1: protease-activated receptor 1; AKT: prosurvival kinase; SPATA7: spermatogenesis associated 7 gene; FLI1: friend leukemia virus integration 1 gene; FDA: food and drug administration; EMA: European medicines agency; AIM: ancestry informative marker; PAP: primary analysis population; APROCCHS: activated protein C and corticosteroids for human septic shock.

Authors' contributions

DA, PJH, RB, NL, HFW, MN, ADJM, and JAR contributed to conception and design. DA, JP M, LBW, ACG, CJH, DCC, JS, KB, TGB, PJH, RB, NL, KN, HFW, MN,

ADJM, KRW, and JAR contributed to analysis and interpretation, and drafted the manuscript for important intellectual content. All authors read and approved the final manuscript.

Authors' information
Not applicable.

Author details
[1] Service de Reanimation Medicale, Hopital R. Poincare, 104 Bd Raymond Poincare, 92380 Garches, France. [2] Sorbonne Paris Cité, Cochin Hotel-Dieu University Hospital Medical Intensive Care Unit, AP-HP, Université Paris Descartes, 75014 Paris, France. [3] Departments of Medicine and Pathology, Microbiology and Immunology, Vanderbilt University School of Medicine, 1161 21st Avenue South T1218 MCN, Nashville, TN 37232-2650, USA. [4] Section of Anaesthetics, Pain Medicine, and Intensive Care, Charing Cross Hospital, Imperial College London, Fulham Palace Road, London W6 8RF, UK. [5] Barts and The London School of Medicine, Queen Mary University of London, London, UK. [6] Harvard Medical School and School of Public Health, 665 Huntington Avenue, Building I Room 1401, Boston, MA 02115, USA. [7] Emory Center for Critical Care, Woodruff Health Sciences Center, Emory University, Atlanta, GA, USA. [8] Division of Allergy and Clinical Immunology, Department of Medicine, Johns Hopkins University, Baltimore, MD, USA. [9] Department of Biostatistics, University of Washington, F-600, Health Sciences Building, Office: H-665D HSB, Box 357232, Seattle, WA 98195-7232, USA. [10] Syreon Corporation, Vancouver, BC, Canada. [11] Formerly with Sirius Genomics Inc, Vancouver, BC, Canada. [12] Critical Care Research Laboratories, Centre for Heart Lung Innovation, St. Paul's Hospital, University of British Columbia, Burrard Building, Rm 166 - 1081 Burrard St, Vancouver, BC V6Z 1Y6, Canada.

Acknowledgements
We thank all the patients who are part of this study and their families. We also thank the caregivers of the patients in these centers. Dr Gordon is a UK National Institute for Health Research (NIHR) Clinician Scientist award holder and is grateful for funding from the NIHR comprehensive Biomedical Research Centre funding stream. Dr. Ware is funded by an American Heart Association Established Investigator Award.

Competing interests
Dr. Russell was a consultant, founder, and shareholder of Sirius Genomics at the time of this study. Dr. Russell reports patents owned by the University of British Columbia (UBC) that are related to PCSK9 inhibitor (s) and sepsis and related to the use of vasopressin in septic shock. Dr. Russell is an inventor on these patents. Dr. Russell is a founder, Director, and shareholder in Cyon Therapeutics Inc. (developing a sepsis therapy). Dr. Russell has share options in Leading Biosciences Inc. Dr. Russell is a shareholder in Molecular You Corp. Dr. Russell reports receiving consulting fees from: (1) Cubist Pharmaceuticals (now owned by Merck; formerly was Trius Pharmaceuticals; developing antibiot-ics), (2) Leading Biosciences (developing a sepsis therapeutic), (3) Ferring Pharmaceuticals (manufactures vasopressin and is developing selepressin), (4) Grifols (sells albumin), (5) La Jolla Pharmaceuticals (developing angioten-sin II; Dr. Russell chairs the DSMB of a trial of angiotensin II), (6) CytoVale Inc. (developing a sepsis diagnostic), (7) Asahi Kesai Pharmaceuticals of America (AKPA)(developing recombinant thrombomodulin). Dr. Russell reports having received an investigator-initiated grant from Grifols that is provided to and administered by UBC. Ms. Mancini and Mr. Wellman were employees and shareholders of Sirius Genomics at the time of the study. Anthony C. Gordon and Patrick J. Heagerty were consultants to Sirius Genomics at the time of this study. Dr. Walley was a founder and shareholder of Sirius Genomics at the time of this study. Robert Balshaw, Nadia Lesnikova, and Karen de Nobrega were employees of Syreon Corp. at the time of this study.

Funding
This study was funded by Sirius Genomics Inc.

References

1. Wang L, McLeod HL, Weinshilboum RM. Genomics and drug response. N Engl J Med. 2011;364(12):1144–53.
2. Schwarz UI, Ritchie MD, Bradford Y, et al. Genetic determinants of response to warfarin during initial anticoagulation. N Engl J Med. 2008;358(10):999–1008.
3. Rieder MJ, Reiner AP, Gage BF, et al. Effect of VKORC1 haplotypes on transcriptional regulation and warfarin dose. N Engl J Med. 2005;352(22):2285–93.
4. Bernard GR, Vincent JL, Laterre PF, et al. Efficacy and safety of recombinant human activated protein C for severe sepsis. N Engl J Med. 2001;344(10):699–709.
5. Abraham E, Laterre PF, Garg R, et al. Drotrecogin alfa (activated) for adults with severe sepsis and a low risk of death. N Engl J Med. 2005;353(13):1332–41.
6. Ranieri VM, Thompson BT, Barie PS, et al. Drotrecogin alfa (activated) in adults with septic shock. N Engl J Med. 2012;366(22):2055–64.
7. Annane D, Timsit JF, Megarbane B, et al. Recombinant human activated protein C for adults with septic shock: a randomized controlled trial. Am J Respir Crit Care Med. 2013;187(10):1091–7.
8. Annane D, Mira JP, Ware LB, et al. Design, conduct, and analysis of a multicenter, pharmacogenomic, biomarker study in matched patients with severe sepsis treated with or without drotrecogin Alfa (activated). Ann Intensive Care. 2012;2(1):15.
9. Russell JA, Walley KR, Singer J, et al. Vasopressin versus norepinephrine infusion in patients with septic shock. N Engl J Med. 2008;358(9):877–87.
10. Rowan KM, Welch CA, North E, Harrison DA. Drotrecogin alfa (activated): real-life use and outcomes for the UK. Crit Care. 2008;12(2):R58.
11. Bertolini G, Rossi C, Anghileri A, Livigni S, Addis A, Poole D. Use of Drotrecogin alfa (activated) in Italian intensive care units: the results of a nationwide survey. Intensive Care Med. 2007;33(3):426–34.
12. Wheeler A, Steingrub J, Schmidt GA, et al. A retrospective observational study of drotrecogin alfa (activated) in adults with severe sepsis: comparison with a controlled clinical trial. Crit Care Med. 2008;36(1):14–23.
13. Kanji S, Perreault MM, Chant C, Williamson D, Burry L. Evaluating the use of Drotrecogin alfa (activated) in adult severe sepsis: a Canadian multicenter observational study. Intensive Care Med. 2007;33(3):517–23.
14. Vincent JL, Laterre PF, Decruyenaere J, et al. A registry of patients treated with drotrecogin alfa (activated) in Belgian intensive care units: an observational study. Acta Clin Belg. 2008;63(1):25–30.
15. Rosenbaum PR, Rubin DB. The bias due to incomplete matching. Biometrics. 1985;41(1):103–16.
16. Man M, Close SL, Shaw AD, et al. Beyond single-marker analyses: mining whole genome scans for insights into treatment responses in severe sepsis. Pharmacogenomics J. 2013;13(3):218–26.

11

Venovenous extracorporeal membrane oxygenation devices-related colonisations and infections

Guillemette Thomas[1], Sami Hraiech[1,2], Nadim Cassir[2], Samuel Lehingue[1,2], Romain Rambaud[1,2], Sandrine Wiramus[3], Christophe Guervilly[1], Fanny Klasen[1,2], Mélanie Adda[1], Stéphanie Dizier[1], Antoine Roch[2,4], Laurent Papazian[1,2] and Jean-Marie Forel[1,2]* ⓘ

Abstract

Background: Nosocomial infections occurring during extracorporeal membrane oxygenation (ECMO) support have already been reported, but few studied infections directly related to ECMO devices. This study aims to evaluate the rate of both colonisations and infections related to ECMO devices at the time of ECMO removal.

Results: We included all consecutive adult patients treated with venovenous ECMO (VV-ECMO) for at least 48 h during a 34-month study. At the time of ECMO removal, blood cultures, swab cultures on insertion cannula site and intravascular cannula extremity cultures were systematically performed. Each ECMO device was classified according to the infectious status into three groups: (1) uninfected/uncolonised ECMO device, (2) ECMO device colonisation and (3) ECMO device infection. Ninety-nine patients underwent 103 VV-ECMO, representing 1472 ECMO days. The ECMO device infection rate was 9.7% (10 events), including 7 ECMO device-related bloodstream infections (6.8%). The ECMO device colonisation rate was 32% (33 events). No difference was observed between the three groups, regarding days of mechanical ventilation, ICU length of stay, ICU mortality and in-hospital mortality. We observed a longer ECMO duration in the ECMO device colonisation group as compared to the uninfected/uncolonised ECMO device group [12 (9–20 days) vs. 5 days (5–16 days), respectively, $p < 0.05$].

Conclusions: At the time of ECMO removal, systematic blood culture and intravascular extremity cannula culture may help to diagnose ECMO device-related infection. We reported a quite low infection rate related to ECMO device. Further studies are needed to evaluate the benefits of systematic strategies of cannula culture at the time of ECMO removal.

Keywords: Venovenous extracorporeal membrane oxygenation, Device-related infections, Device-related colonisation, Infection rate, Colonisation rate

Background

Venovenous extracorporeal membrane oxygenation (VV-ECMO) has become a widely accepted treatment option for life-threatening acute respiratory failure when mechanical ventilation (MV) and adjunctive measures fail to provide adequate gas exchange or when lung rest cannot be achieved due to high ventilator requirements [1, 2]. Over the last two decades, the technique has improved significantly, and several studies have reported encouraging survival rates using VV-ECMO in adults with acute respiratory distress syndrome (ARDS) [3–6]. However, major adverse events have been described, among which infections seem to be the most frequent [1, 6]. In 2011, the Extracorporeal Life Support Organization (ELSO) reported an incidence of 11.7% proven infections in 20,741 ECMO cases for a rate of 15.4 per 1000 ECMO

*Correspondence: jean-marie.forel@ap-hm.fr
[1] Hôpital Nord, Réanimation des Détresses Respiratoires et des Infections Sévères, Assistance Publique–Hôpitaux de Marseille, 13015 Marseille, France
Full list of author information is available at the end of the article

days [7]. To date, most of the studies described nosocomial infections or bloodstream infections (BSI) occurring during ECMO support, but very few studied infections directly related to ECMO devices. Moreover, these studies often mixed venovenous and venoarterial ECMO support, which are very different devices regarding the type of patients, the duration of ECMO and the cannulation procedure [8, 9].

The main objective of this study was to evaluate the rates of both infections and colonisations related to ECMO devices in VV-ECMO adult patients at the time of ECMO removal.

Methods

Study design

An epidemiologic, prospective, observational study was conducted in the 14-bed medical intensive care unit (ICU) of a teaching hospital (Hôpital Nord, Marseille, France), a regional referral centre for the treatment of acute severe respiratory failure. The study was approved by the ethical committee of the «Société de Réanimation de Langue Française». According to French law, no consent for the study was required because it did not modify existing diagnostic or therapeutic strategies.

Patients and ECMO indications

We prospectively included all consecutive adult patients treated with VV-ECMO for at least 48 h during a 34-month study. The ECMO-based programme includes a mobile unit that is able to initiate ECMO in referring hospitals of our region (Provence-Alpes-Côte d'Azur) before transfer to our ECMO referral centre [5].

The decision to initiate ECMO is based on the following: persistent hypoxaemia, defined as $PaO_2/FiO_2 \leq 70$ mmHg for at least 6 h under FiO2 at 1 despite optimisation of mechanical ventilation or $PaO_2/FiO_2 < 100$ mmHg with a Pplat value greater than 35 cmH_2O or respiratory acidosis with pH ≤ 7.15 despite a respiratory rate greater than 35/min. Exclusion criteria for ECMO included the following: any contraindications to heparin treatment, Sequential Organ Failure Assessment (SOFA) score > 16 [10], moribund patients or those with decisions to limit therapeutic interventions.

ECMO protocol

Venovenous ECMO was instituted using percutaneous cannulation by cardiac surgeons, typically in a femoral–jugular configuration but also in femoral–femoral configuration, especially when ECMO was used as a bridge to lung transplantation. We used centrifugal pumps (Bioconsole 560; Medtronic Perfusion Systems, Minneapolis, MN, USA) with a flow of 3–5 L/min in all patients. Circuits were heparin-coated and composed of Quadrox D with Bioline Coating oxygenators (Maquet, Hirrlingen, Germany), 17–25-Fr cannulae (Edwards Lifesciences, Irvine, CA, USA) and intersept polyvinyl chloride (PVC) class VI tubing (Medtronic, Watford, Hertfordshire, UK).

All cannulas were inserted using strict sterile precautions consistent with Healthcare Infection Control Practices Advisory Committee guidelines (HICPAC guidelines) [11]. For each patient, the cannula insertion site was cleansed with 96% ethanol solution containing 5% povidone-iodine. Sterile drapes were placed over the insertion site. No specific antibioprophylaxis was used at the time of cannulation. Occlusive dressings were used.

A highly trained ICU nursing staff achieved standardised cannula care every 72 h or earlier if clinically indicated (dirty or bloody dressing). If necessary (haemolysis, fibrinolysis), the ECMO circuit was changed using strict sterile precautions as detailed above.

When the ECMO was removed, specimens were systematically collected as follows: (a) blood cultures were sampled from the central venous catheter (CVC), arterial catheter and post-membrane oxygenator. The blood culture vials used for aerobic and anaerobic cultures (Bactec; Becton–Dickinson, Sparks, MD, USA) were incubated for 5 days. After the incubation period and automatic culture detection (Bactec 9240; Becton–Dickinson, Sparks, MD, USA), Gram staining was performed, and the samples were cultured on 5% sheep blood and chocolate agar plates at 37 °C under aerobic and anaerobic atmospheric conditions for all positive blood cultures. (b) Swabs were sampled on the drainage and return cannula site skin just before cleaning with 5% povidone-iodine antiseptic. The culture technique is described as follows. (c) The intravascular extremity of the drainage and return cannula were cut in a sterile manner and analysed by a culture technique described as follows. The extremities of the cannulas, the central venous and the arterial catheter tips when removed, were mixed with tryptic soy broth; 10 μL of each mixture was then cultured on chocolate agar plates at 37 °C under aerobic atmospheric conditions. Swab samples were semi-quantitatively processed immediately by streaking the entire surface of the plates. Identification was performed when a culture yielded at least 10^3 colony-forming units (CFU)/mL. Matrix-assisted laser desorption/ionisation time-of-flight mass spectrometry (MALDI-TOF MS) was used for the bacterial identification as previously described [12].

Definition of ECMO device colonisation and infection

The definitions of ECMO device colonisation or infection were adapted from French and American central line-associated bloodstream infection guidelines [13, 14]. These definitions concern the central line defined as an intravascular catheter that terminates at or close to the heart or in one of the great vessels excluding ECMO devices. Thus, the following definitions were used: (a) cannula colonisation (CC) was defined as a positive quantitative intravascular extremity culture ($\geq 10^3$ CFU). (b) Skin colonisation (SC) was a positive quantitative swab culture ($\geq 10^3$ CFU). (c) Not related ECMO device bacteraemia was defined as one or more positive blood cultures with negative cannula colonisation and another infectious site responsible for bacteraemia. (d) Contamination was defined as one positive blood culture for common skin contaminants [14, 15]. (e) ECMO device infection (ED-I) corresponded to: (e.1) ECMO device-related blood stream infection (EDR-BSI), which was a combination of one or more positive blood cultures (from the CVC, arterial catheter or post-membrane oxygenator) sampled immediately before or within 48 h after ECMO removal, a quantitative intravascular cannula extremity positive culture for the same micro-organism(s) and no other infection explaining the positive blood culture; (e.2) cannula infection (CI), which was considered in cases of a positive quantitative intravascular cannula extremity culture, negative blood culture and systemic infectious signs in the absence of any other infection. CI was also considered in case of a positive quantitative intravascular cannula extremity culture and local infection signs (local purulence or infection signs at insertion site); (e.3) in patients with blood culture and/or quantitative intravascular cannula portion culture positive for coagulase-negative staphylococci, EDR-BSI and CI were considered depending on clinical features (fever, sepsis, septic shock) within 48 h after ECMO removal and on clinical evolution under specific treatment if introduced by the clinician.

An adjudication committee, including one infectious disease specialist and three intensivists, retrospectively classified each case into three categories: (1) uninfected/uncolonised ECMO device (U-I/C ED), including sterile samples, skin colonisation, blood culture contamination and not related ECMO device bacteraemia; (2) ECMO device colonisation (ED-C), including cannula colonisation associated or not with skin colonisation; (3) ECMO device infection (ED-I), including EDR-BSI and CI as previously defined.

Collected data
Prospectively collected data included demographic data; body mass index (BMI); severity of illness as assessed by the Simplified Acute Physiology Score (SAPS) II [16] and SOFA score at ICU admission [10]; major comorbidities; indication for ECMO; site of cannulation; site of ECMO implantation; ECMO system exchange; ECMO transfusion (blood, platelets and plasma), pre- and per-ECMO steroid use; pre- and per-ECMO antibiotics use; duration

of both ECMO and mechanical ventilation; outcome (ICU and hospital mortalities, ventilator and ECMO-free days at both day 28 and day 90, ICU length of stay); and nosocomial infections, primary bloodstream infections or fungaemia during ECMO support. Nosocomial infection definitions agreed with those of the Centers for Disease Control and Prevention National Nosocomial Infections Surveillance System [17]. Ventilator-associated pneumonia (VAP) was diagnosed according to previously published criteria [18].

End points
The primary end points were the rates of ECMO device infection or colonisation at the time of ECMO removal. Secondary end points were the rate of skin colonisation and outcomes, such as ICU length of stay, ICU mortality, in-hospital mortality and day-90 mortality, day-28 and day-90 ventilator and ECMO-free days.

Statistical analysis
Descriptive statistics included percentages for categorical variables and medians and interquartile ranges for continuous variables. Comparisons between the three categories (U-I/C ED, ED-C and ED-I) for continuous variables were made using the Kruskal–Wallis test with a post hoc method for multiple comparisons (step-up Simes method to calculate adjusted p value). Comparisons between the three categories (U-I/C ED, ED-C and ED-I) for categorical variables were made using the Pearson Chi-square test for trend. A multinomial logistic regression procedure was performed to identify factors associated with ED-I or ED-C. The U-I/C ED group was used as the reference group. All of the variables with p value < 0.20 (gender, body mass index, statin therapy, per-ECMO plasma transfusion, reason for ECMO, location of ECMO cannulation, type of cannulation, pre-ECMO antibiotic and ECMO duration) were included in the model. The Fleiss' kappa was calculated to evaluate the reliability agreement between the 4 experts regarding the classification of each ECMO case. A p value < 0.05 was considered significant. The statistical analysis was conducted using SPSS, version 20.0 (NY, USA).

Results
Patients
During the study period, 105 patients underwent 109 VV-ECMO (Fig. 1). Four patients underwent 2 VV-ECMO during the same ICU stay with an interval of at least 2 days between each ECMO implantation. Finally, 103 VV-ECMO were analysed (representing 1472 ECMO days). The median age was 49 years (38–62), and the most frequent reason for ECMO was ARDS (77.6%). Fifty-three patients were referred to our ECMO centre

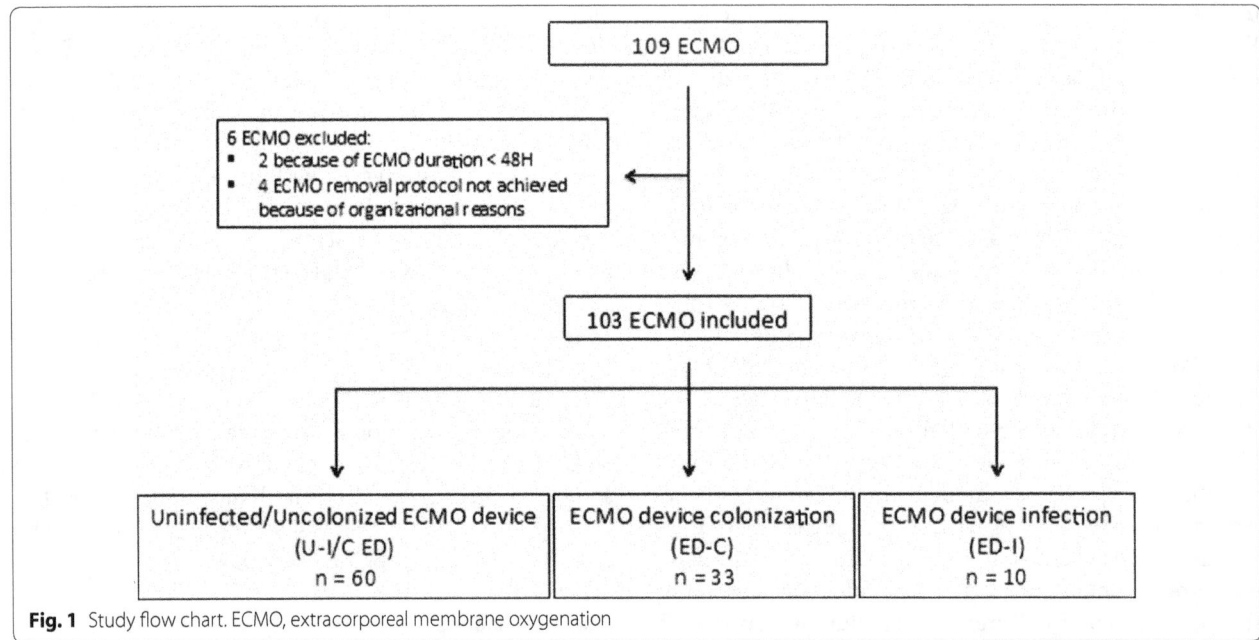

Fig. 1 Study flow chart. ECMO, extracorporeal membrane oxygenation

and transported by our mobile team. The median ECMO duration was 11 days (6–18 days). A total of 63 circuit changes were done in 38 VV-ECMO. General characteristics of each group are provided in Table 1.

ECMO device colonisation and infection (Fig. 2)

At the time of ECMO removal, the rate of ECMO device colonisation (ED-C) was 32% (33 events). The rate of ECMO device infection (ED-I) was 9.7% (10 events), including 7 ECMO device-related bloodstream infections (6.8%). No patient presented with insertion site infectious signs at any moment during ECMO support or within the 48-h period following ECMO removal. The uninfected/uncolonised ECMO device (U-I/C ED) rate was 58.3% (60 of 103). Fleiss' kappa coefficient was 0.94 (standard error, 0.04), corresponding to strong agreement between the experts regarding the classification.

A total of 127 femoral cannulas were inserted. In all, 22% (28 of 127) of the cultures were positive for at least one micro-organism compared with 35.4% of the cultures (28 of 79) regarding the jugular site ($p = 0.052$). Micro-organisms responsible for ED-C and ED-I are detailed in Fig. 3 and Additional file 1: Table S1. Coagulase-negative staphylococcus was the most frequent organism responsible for ED-I (8/10, 80%) and ED-C (20/33, 60.6%). The details of blood culture results are summarised in Additional file 2: Table S2.

We observed a longer ECMO duration in the ED-C group compared with the U-I/C ED group [12 days

(9–20 days) versus 5 days (5–16 days), respectively, $p < 0.05$]. Using multivariate analysis, we did not identify any factor associated with ED-C or ED-I (Additional file 3: Table S3).

Skin colonisation

The skin colonisation rate was 23.3% (24 events). When cannula colonisation was observed, concomitant skin colonisation was present in 42.4% of cases (14 of 33), with the same micro-organism in 71.4% of cases (10 of 14). Considering ED-I, no concomitant skin colonisation was observed. No differences were noted regarding skin colonisation between femoral and jugular sites (22/127, 17.3%; 14/79, 17.7%, respectively, $p = 0.91$).

Outcome

Fifty-two patients died in the ICU (50.5%) and 58 during hospitalisation (56.3%). No difference was observed among the three categories (U-I/C ED, ED-C and ED-I) regarding ICU length of stay, ICU mortality, in-hospital mortality and day-90 mortality (Table 2).

A total of 27 patients underwent at least one nosocomial infection other than ED-I, without differences among the three groups ($p = 0.30$). Forty-four nosocomial infections, excluding ED-I, occurred during the 103 VV-ECMO supports, corresponding to 29.9 infectious episodes per 1000 ECMO days. Ventilator-associated pneumonia (VAP) was the most frequent nosocomial infection (45.5%), followed by primary bloodstream infection (36.4%) (Additional file 4: Table S4).

Table 1 General characteristics of ECMO in patients without infected/colonised ECMO device, with ECMO device colonisation and ECMO device infection (at the time of ECMO removal)

Number of ECMO[a]	U-I/C ED 60	ED-C 33	ED-I 10	P value[b]
Age (years)	48 (37–61)	57 (47–63)	43 (41–63)	0.278
Male (n, %)	35 (58.3)	23 (69.7)	8 (80)	0.122
BMI (kg/m^2)	24 (22–29)	27 (24–31)	26 (24–27)	0.183
SOFA score[c]	10 (7–12)	9 (7–14)	9 (7–10)	0.607
SAPS II[c]	44 (39–56)	47 (38–57)	46 (36–53)	0.833
Underlying condition				
Diabetes mellitus	9 (15)	4 (12.1)	0	0.233
Renal insufficiency	0	2 (6.1)	0	0.300
Immunocompromised[d]	5 (8.3)	6 (18.2)	1 (10)	0.402
COPD	5 (8.3)	2 (6.1)	0	0.349
Solid tumour	9 (15)	4 (12.1)	2 (20)	0.906
Cirrhosis	2 (3.3)	0	0	0.272
Statin therapy	8 (13.3)	2 (6.1)	0	0.118
ICU stay before ECMO centre admission	2 (0–8)	5 (1–10)	3 (0–4)	0.237
Reason for ECMO[e]				
ARDS	42 (70)	28 (84.8)	10 (100)	0.011*
CAP	18	13	5 (50)	
NP	20	13	4 (40)	
Extrapulmonary	4	2	1 (10)	
Bridge to lung transplantation	2 (6.7)	2 (6.1)	0	0.965
Primary graft dysfunction	14 (23.3)	3 (9.1)	0	0.023*
ECMO characteristics				
Mobile ECMO team	27 (45)	21 (63.6)	5 (50)	0.272
Location of ECMO cannulation				
ICU	44 (73.3)	31 (93.9)	10 (100)	0.005#*
Operating room	16 (26.7)	2 (6.1)	0	
Per-ECMO blood transfusion	9 (4–21)	8 (5–17)	9 (6–16)	0.934
Per-ECMO platelet transfusion	1 (0–4)	1 (0–4)	1 (0–1)	0.651
Per-ECMO plasma transfusion	2 (0–10)	0 (0–4)	0 (0–4)	0.197
Pre-ECMO steroids	14 (23.3)	8 (24.2)	2 (20)	0.903
Per-ECMO steroids	31 (51.7)	15 (45.5)	3 (30)	0.214
Pre-ECMO antibiotics[f]	48 (80)	29 (87.9)	10 (100)	0.085
Per-ECMO antibiotics[g]	58 (96.7)	33 (100)	10 (100)	0.272
Antibiotics at the time of ECMO removal	48 (80)	30 (90.9)	5 (50)	0.314
BSI during ECMO[h]	10 (16.7)	8 (24.2)	2 (20)	0.525
Cannulation				
Femoro–femoral	19 (31.7)	5 (15.2)	0	0.011*
Femoro-jugular	41 (68.3)	28 (84.8)	10 (100)	

Table 1 continued

Number of ECMO[a]	U-I/C ED 60	ED-C 33	ED-I 10	P value[b]
ECMO circuit change (≥ 1)	24 (40)	12 (36.4)	2 (20)	0.278
ECMO duration (days)	7.5 (5–16)	12 (9–20)	13 (11–17)	0.021#

Data are provided as no. (%) of ECMO or median value (interquartile range)

ARDS acute respiratory distress syndrome, *BMI* body mass index, *CAP* community-acquired pneumonia, *COPD* chronic obstructive pulmonary disease, *ECMO* extracorporeal membrane oxygenation, *ICU* intensive care unit, *NP* nosocomial pneumonia, *SAPS II* Simplified Acute Physiology Score, *SOFA* sepsis-related organ failure assessment, *U-I/C ED* uninfected/uncolonised ECMO device, *ED-C* ECMO device colonisation, *ED-I* ECMO device infection

* $p < 0.05$, comparison between U-I/C ED and ED-I

# $p < 0.05$, comparison between U-I/C ED and ED-C

[a] Among the 99 patients, 4 underwent 2 ECMO during their ICU stay corresponding to 103 VV-ECMO

[b] p value corresponds to the comparison between the three categories (U-I/C ED, ED-C, ED-I)

[c] Calculated at ICU admission

[d] Includes patients with human immunodeficiency virus, solid organ transplantation or haematological malignancy and those receiving chemotherapy, immunosuppressive agents or long-term corticosteroid therapy

[e] For 2 patients, ECMO reason was thoracic surgery

[f] Pre-ECMO antibiotics correspond to antibiotics received for at least 24 h before ECMO implantation

[g] Per-ECMO antibiotics correspond to antibiotics received immediately after ECMO implantation

[h] Bloodstream infection (BSI) under ECMO includes primary and secondary bloodstream infections

Discussion

To our knowledge, this is the first study that systematically analysed ECMO devices at the time of ECMO removal, providing the rate of ECMO device-related infection and colonisation in an adult cohort of venovenous ECMO supports. Our results indicate that the ECMO device infection rate (cannula infections or ECMO device-related bloodstream infections) was 9.7%, and the ECMO device colonisation rate was 32%. Indeed, most of the studies related the incidence of nosocomial infections and bloodstream infections while on venoarterial or venovenous ECMO support, and these studies often used paediatric cohorts [7–9, 19, 20]. The originality of our work was to assess the infection and colonisation rates directly associated with the ECMO device. Schmidt et al. [9] reported a large series of 220 venoarterial ECMO support cases in adult cardiogenic shock and described 21 (9.5%) cannula infections, defined as the association of local signs of infection at the access site with a positive culture of subcutaneous needle aspirate from the cannula site. One major difference with this study is that VA-ECMO cannulation was performed

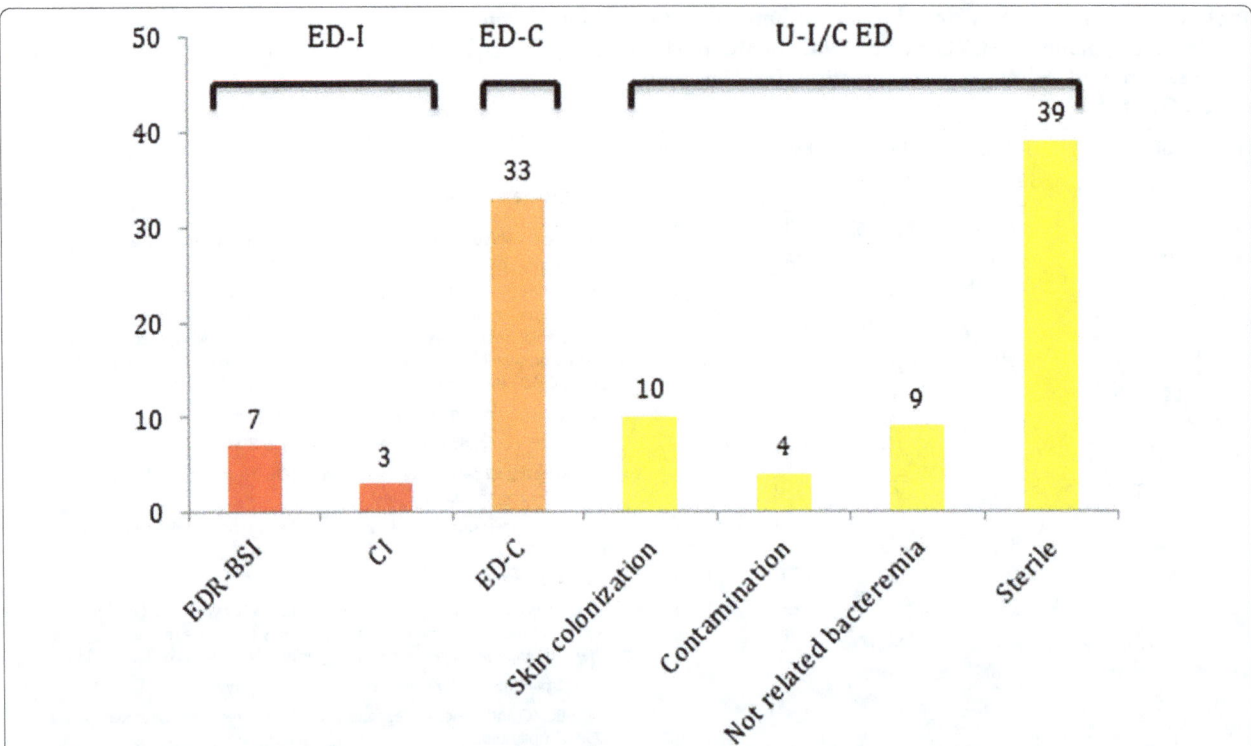

Fig. 2 Details of each ECMO samples leading to different categories: ECMO device infection (ED-I) including ECMO device-related bloodstream infections (EDR-BSI) and cannula infections (CI); ECMO device colonisation (ED-C); uninfected/uncolonised ECMO device (U-I/C ED) including skin colonisation, contamination, not related bacteremia and sterile samples

with an invasive surgical procedure, especially in the case of central VA-ECMO, whereas VV-ECMO cannulation only requires a percutaneous procedure (which was the case for all of our patients). Furthermore, the definition of cannula infection was different and could reflect surgical site infection rather than cannula infection in this study. Of note, none of our patients presented with cannula local infectious signs at any moment during ECMO support and even during the 48 following hours. Lubnow et al. described technical complications leading to system exchange in 265 adult patients treated with VV-ECMO support for acute respiratory failure. Eighty-three patients underwent at least one system change, and 4 of these cases (5%) were due to suspected infection [21]. More recently, Hahne et al. evaluated the culture results of 186 cannulae removed from 94 patients who benefited from extracorporeal circulation for lung or cardiac assistance. Fifteen patients (16%) presented cannula-related infection [22].

ECMO device-related infections may involve the drainage cannula, the return cannula or the membrane oxygenator (MO). Thus, Kuehn et al. [23] hypothesised that the artificial surfaces of the ECMO circuit, particularly the MO, could be the target of microbial adhesion and colonisation, favouring the development

of ECMO-related bloodstream infection. The overall patient-based positivity by PCR was 45%. In the present study, membrane oxygenator infection was difficult to assess. We performed post-membranous blood culture on the day of removal (Additional file 4: Table S4), which was positive in 15 cases and allowed the diagnosis of ECMO device-related bloodstream infection (EDR-BSI) in only one case.

Our results revealed a longer ECMO duration in the ED-C group compared with the U-I/C ED group. Catheter duration is a well-known risk factor for catheter colonisation or catheter-related bloodstream infection [24]. Moreover, the prevalence of nosocomial infection increases with ECMO duration [7, 9]. No difference was observed between the U-I/C ED group and ED-I, which is probably due to the small number of patients in this group. At least, skin colonisation was not observed in the 10 ED-I, suggesting that ECMO device-related infections could originate from haematogenous contamination or circuit changes although our data cannot confirm this hypothesis (Table 1).

We reported a higher proportion of primary graft dysfunction, femoro–femoral cannulation and cannulation in the operating room in the U-I/C ED group compared with the ED-C group and/or the ED-I group. This finding

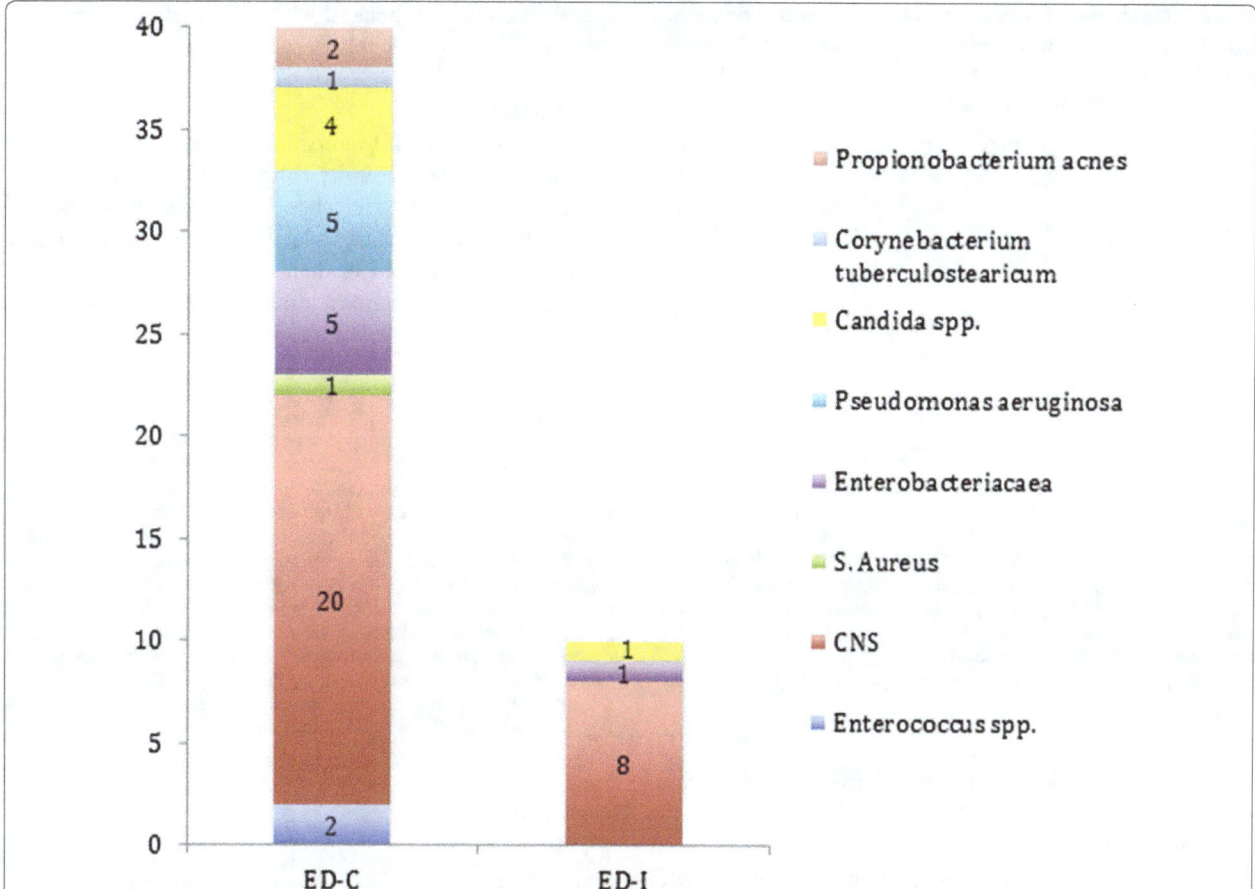

Fig. 3 Micro-organisms associated with ECMO device colonisations and infections. *CNS* Coagulase-negative staphylococci. Seven cannulas were colonised with two different micro-organisms corresponding to 33 cannula colonisations and a total number of 40 micro-organisms

can be easily explained by the fact that all patients with primary graft dysfunction benefited from ECMO cannulation at the end of the lung transplant, in the operating room, and with femoro–femoral cannulation due to surgical technical reasons. Moreover, the duration of ECMO was reduced for primary graft dysfunction indication compared with ARDS indication [5 (4–6) vs. 12 days (7–18), $p < 0.001$ data not shown]. Thus, the differences observed between the different groups are probably the result of significant differences of ECMO duration.

Our study described a very much higher rate of infection with ECMO device than with central venous catheter. During the study period, central venous catheter-related infection rate was 1.2 per 1000 catheter days. ECMO cannula size is bigger (17–25 Fr) and duration of ECMO longer than central venous catheter. Moreover, cannula change is highly problematic because of the few vascular accesses and due to patient's vital dependence on ECMO support.

Antibiotic prophylaxis to prevent nosocomial infections in ECMO patients remains highly controversial due to the emergence of resistance to antibiotics and *Clostridium difficile*-associated colitis [25]. Daily surveillance blood cultures have been proposed as an alternative to antibiotic prophylaxis and remain a routine practice in many ECMO centres, but this strategy is costly and resource consuming [9, 19, 26]. Wide variability in practice is also noted regarding the prevention of nosocomial and bloodstream infections for patients requiring ECMO. In a recent survey of the ELSO members interested in nosocomial bloodstream infection prevention practice, only one-quarter of respondents reported the use of a bundle or checklist during ECMO cannula insertion and less than half utilise a bundle or checklist for cannula maintenance [27]. In our opinion, if daily surveillance blood culture in patients with ECMO support should not be recommended, the systematic culture of vascular cannula portions associated with blood culture performed at the time of removal may help the clinician to make the diagnosis of ECMO device-related infection and guide the antibiotics prescription. Finally, we did not use chlorhexidine antiseptic protocol at the time of

Table 2 Outcome of extracorporeal membrane oxygenation in patients without infected/colonised ECMO device, with ECMO device colonisation and ECMO device infection (at the time of ECMO removal)

Number of ECMO[a]	U-I/C ED 60	ED-C 33	ED-I 10	p value
ICU LOS	25 (14–39)	24 (20–33)	30 (23–37)	0.614
ICU mortality	27 (45)	21 (63.6)	4 (40)	0.559
Day-90 mortality	28 (46.7)	22 (66.7)	4 (40)	0.622
In-hospital mortality	32 (53.3)	22 (66.7)	6 (60)	0.896
Days of MV	23 (12–37)	24 (18–32)	28 (23–30)	0.671
VFD day 28	0 (0–1)	0 (0–0)	0 (0–0)	0.385
VFD day 90	1 (0–60)	0 (0–35)	9 (0–52)	0.506
ECMOFD day 28	13 (0–21)	3 (0–18)	7 (0–14)	0.169
ECMOFD day 90	63 (0–83)	9 (0–78)	62 (0–76)	0.156
ECMO weaning	43 (71.7)	17 (51.5)	7 (70)	0.283

Data are provided as no. (%) of ECMO or median value (interquartile range)

ECMO extracorporeal membrane oxygenation, *ECMOFD* ECMO-free day, *ICU* intensive care unit, *LOS* length of stay, *MV* mechanical ventilation, *VFD* ventilator-free day, *U-I/C ED* uninfected/uncolonised ECMO device, *ED-C* ECMO device colonisation, *ED-I* ECMO device infection

[a] Among the 99 patients, 4 underwent 2 ECMO during their ICU stay corresponding to 103 VV-ECMO

cannula insertion and for the standardised cannula care. Chlorhexidine-impregnated dressing for cannula dressing was not used in our study which could be evaluated in the future to evaluate the impact on the rate of ECMO device colonisation and infection.

Our study presents several limitations. There is currently no consensus on the definition of ECMO device-related infection. Indeed, the Centers for Disease Control and Prevention (CDC) guidelines have established a clear definition of central line-related infection or blood stream infections that precisely exclude ECMO devices [14]. Moreover, the definitions that include differential time to blood culture positivity appear to be inappropriate given the impossibility and danger of performing blood culture in ECMO cannulae [13, 28]. We have decided to use the threshold of 10^3 colony-forming unit for the positivity of the device culture, which is derived from catheter infection literature but not validated for the ECMO device so far. At least, our study focused on ECMO device infection and colonisation at the time of removal and not during the ECMO support period. Moreover, the huge majority of our patients were receiving antibiotics at the time of ECMO insertion and during the ECMO run. These two last elements could have led to possible underestimation of the number of infections and colonisations. We did not collected data regarding dressing disruption or changes that might help to explain the differences between the rate of colonisation and the rate of infection. Using a multinomial logistic regression procedure, we failed to

establish factors associated with ECMO device colonisation or infection, probably because of the cohort size.

Conclusions

At the time of ECMO removal, systematic blood culture and intravascular extremity cannula culture may help to diagnose ECMO device-related infection. We reported a quite low infection rate related to the devices. Further studies are needed to evaluate the benefits of systematic strategies of cannula culture at the time of ECMO removal.

Abbreviations
ARDS: acute respiratory distress syndrome; BC: blood culture; BMI: body mass index; BSI: bloodstream infections; CC: cannula colonisation; CI: cannula infection; CFU: colony-forming units; CVC: central venous catheter; ELSO: Extracorporeal Life Support Organization; ECMO: extracorporeal membrane oxygenation; ED-C: ECMO device colonisation; ED-I: ECMO device infection; EDR-BSI: ECMO device-related blood stream infection; HICPAC Guidelines: Healthcare Infection Control Practices Advisory Committee Guidelines; ICU: intensive care unit; MALDI-TOF MS: matrix-assisted laser desorption/ionisation time-of-flight mass spectrometry; MV: mechanical ventilation; PEEP: positive end-expiratory pressure; Pplat: plateau pressure; SAPS: Simplified Acute Physiology Score; SK: akin colonisation; SOFA: Sequential Organ Failure Assessment; U-I/C ED: uninfected/uncolonised ECMO device; VAP: ventilator-associated pneumonia; VT: tidal volume; VV-ECMO: venovenous extracorporeal membrane oxygenation.

Authors' contributions
JMF and GT designed the work. SL, RR, SW, FK and SD collected the data. GT, JMF, LP analysed, interpreted the patient data and wrote the manuscript. SH, NC, MA and CG examined the data to class the type of infection. AR revised the manuscript. All authors read and approved the final manuscript.

Author details
[1] Hôpital Nord, Réanimation des Détresses Respiratoires et des Infections Sévères, Assistance Publique–Hôpitaux de Marseille, 13015 Marseille, France. [2] URMITE, UMR CNRS 7278, Faculté de Médecine, Aix-Marseille Université, 13005 Marseille, France. [3] Hôpital de la Conception, Réanimation des brulés Assistance Publique–Hôpitaux de Marseille, 13005 Marseille, France. [4] Hôpital Nord, Service des Urgences, Assistance Publique–Hôpitaux de Marseille, 13015 Marseille, France.

Acknowledgements
This manuscript was edited for proper English language, grammar, punctuation, spelling and overall style by one or more of the highly qualified native English-speaking editors at American Journal Experts.

Competing interests
The authors declare that they have no competing interests.

Funding
Not applicable.

References
1. Brodie D, Bacchetta M. Extracorporeal membrane oxygenation for ARDS in adults. N Engl J Med. 2011;365:1905–14. https://doi.org/10.1056/NEJMct1103720.

2. Rehder KJ, Turner DA, Cheifetz IM. Extracorporeal membrane oxygenation for neonatal and pediatric respiratory failure: an evidence-based review of the past decade (2002–2012). Pediatr Crit Care Med J Soc Crit Care Med World Fed Pediatr Intensive Crit Care Soc. 2013;14:851–61. https://doi.org/10.1097/PCC.0b013e3182a5540d.

3. Australia and New Zealand Extracorporeal Membrane Oxygenation (ANZ ECMO) Influenza Investigators. Extracorporeal Membrane Oxygenation for 2009 Influenza A(H1N1) Acute Respiratory Distress Syndrome. JAMA. 2009; 302:1888–1895; https://doi.org/10.1001/jama.2009.1535.

4. Camboni D, Philipp A, Lubnow M, Bein T, Haneya A, Diez C, Schmid C, Müller T. Support time-dependent outcome analysis for veno-venous extracorporeal membrane oxygenation. Eur J Cardio Thorac Surg Off J Eur Assoc Cardio Thorac Surg. 2011;40:1341-1346-1347. https://doi.org/10.1016/j.ejcts.2011.03.062.

5. Roch A, Hraiech S, Masson E, Grisoli D, Forel J-M, Boucekine M, Morera P, Guervilly C, Adda M, Dizier S, Toesca R, Collart F, Papazian L. Outcome of acute respiratory distress syndrome patients treated with extracorporeal membrane oxygenation and brought to a referral center. Intensive Care Med. 2014;40:74–83. https://doi.org/10.1007/s00134-013-3135-1.

6. Fan E, Gattinoni L, Combes A, Schmidt M, Peek G, Brodie D, Muller T, Morelli A, Ranieri VM, Pesanti A, Brochard L, Hodgson C, Van Kiersbilck C, Roch A, Quintel M, Papazian L. Venovenous extracorporeal membrane oxygenation for acute respiratory failure: a clinical review from an international group of experts. Intensive Care Med. 2016;42:712–24. https://doi.org/10.1007/s00134-016-4314-7.

7. Bizzarro MJ, Conrad SA, Kaufman DA, Rycus P. Infections acquired during extracorporeal membrane oxygenation in neonates, children, and adults. Pediatr Crit Care Med J Soc Crit Care Med World Fed Pediatr Intensive Crit Care Soc. 2011;12:277–81. https://doi.org/10.1097/PCC.0b013e3181e28894.

8. Sun H-Y, Ko W-J, Tsai P-R, Sun C-C, Chang Y-Y, Lee C-W, Chen Y-C. Infections occurring during extracorporeal membrane oxygenation use in adult patients. J Thorac Cardiovasc Surg. 2010;140(1125–1132):e2. https://doi.org/10.1016/j.jtcvs.2010.07.017.

9. Schmidt M, Bréchot N, Hariri S, Guiguet M, Luyt C-E, Makri R, Leprince P, Trouillet J-L, Pavie A, Chastre J, Combes A. Nosocomial infections in adult cardiogenic shock patients supported by venoarterial extracorporeal membrane oxygenation. Clin Infect Dis Off Publ Infect Dis Soc Am. 2012;55:1633–41. https://doi.org/10.1093/cid/cis783.

10. Vincent JL, Moreno R, Takala J, Willatts S, De Mendoça A, Bruining H, Reinhart CK, Suter PM, Thijs LG. The SOFA (Sepsis-related Organ Failure Assessment) score to describe organ dysfunction/failure. On behalf of the Working Group on Sepsis-Related Problems of the European Society of Intensive Care Medicine. Intensive Care Med. 1996;22:707–10.

11. O'Grady NP, Alexander M, Burns LA, Dellinger EP, Garland J, Heard SO, Lipsett PA, Masur H, Mermel LA, Pearson ML, Raad II, Randolph AG, Rupp ME, Saint S. Summary of recommendations: guidelines for the prevention of intravascular catheter-related infections. Clin Infect Dis Off Publ Infect Dis Soc Am. 2011;52:1087–99. https://doi.org/10.1093/cid/cir138.

12. Seng P, Drancourt M, Gouriet F, La Scola B, Fournier PE, Rolain JM, Raoult D. Ongoing revolution in bacteriology: routine identification of bacteria by matrix-assisted laser desorption ionization time-of-flight mass spectrometry. Clin Infect Dis Off Publ Infect Dis Soc Am. 2009;49:543–51. https://doi.org/10.1086/600885.

13. Comité technique des infections nosocomiales et des infections liées aux soins, Ministère de la santé, de la jeunesse et des sports DGS/DHOS. http://socialsante.gouv.fr/IMG/pdf/rapport_complet.pdf. Accessed 15 June 2015

14. Centers of Disease Control and Prevention, Healthcare Infection Control Practices Advisory Committee (CDC/HIPAC). http://www.cdc.gov/hicpac/pubs.html. Accessed 15 June 2015.

15. Hall KK, Lyman JA. Updated review of blood culture contamination. Clin Microbiol Rev. 2006;19:788–802. https://doi.org/10.1128/CMR.00062-05.

16. Le Gall JR, Lemeshow S, Saulnier F. A new Simplified Acute Physiology Score (SAPS II) based on a European/North American multicenter study. JAMA. 1993;270:2957–63.

17. Garner JS, Jarvis WR, Emori TG, Horan TC, Hughes JM. CDC definitions for nosocomial infections, 1988. Am J Infect Control. 1988;16:128–40.

18. Papazian L, Roch A, Charles PE, Penot-Ragon C, Perrin G, Roulier P, Goutorbe P, Lefrant JY, Wiramus S, Jung B, Perbet S, Hernu R, Nau A, Baldesi O, Allardet-Servent J, Baumstarck K, Jouve E, Moussa M, Hraiech S, Guervilly C, Forel JM, STATIN-VAP Study Group. Effect of statin therapy on mortality in patients with ventilator-associated pneumonia: a randomized clinical trial. JAMA. 2013;310:1692–700. https://doi.org/10.1001/jama.2013.280031.

19. Kaczala GW, Paulus SC, Al-Dajani N, Jang W, Blondel-Hill E, Dobson S, Cogswell A, Singh AJ. Bloodstream infections in pediatric ECLS: usefulness of daily blood culture monitoring and predictive value of biological markers. The British Columbia experience. Pediatr Surg Int. 2009;25:169–73. https://doi.org/10.1007/s00383-008-2299-1.

20. Burket JS, Bartlett RH, Vander Hyde K, Chenoweth CE. Nosocomial infections in adult patients undergoing extracorporeal membrane oxygenation. Clin Infect Dis Off Publ Infect Dis Soc Am. 1999;28:828–33. https://doi.org/10.1086/515200.

21. Lubnow M, Philipp A, Foltan M, Enger TB, Lunz D, Bein T, Haneya A, Schmid C, Riegger G, Müller T, Lehle K. Technical complications during veno-venous extracorporeal membrane oxygenation and their relevance predicting a system-exchange–retrospective analysis of 265 cases. PLoS ONE. 2014;9:e112316. https://doi.org/10.1371/journal.pone.0112316.

22. Hahne K, Horstmann C, Fischer D, Kock R, Peters G, Lebiedz P. Cannula-related infection in adult medical intensive care unit patients undergoing extracorporeal life support and extracorporeal membrane oxygenation. J Hosp Infect. 2015;91:372–4. https://doi.org/10.1016/j.jhin.2015.08.022.

23. Kuehn C, Orszag P, Burgwitz K, Marsch G, Stumpp N, Stiesch M, Haverich A. Microbial adhesion on membrane oxygenators in patients requiring extracorporeal life support detected by a universal rDNA PCR test. ASAIO J Am Soc Artif Intern Organs. 2013;59:368–73. https://doi.org/10.1097/MAT.0b013e318299fd07.

24. Polderman KH, Girbes ARJ. Central venous catheter use. Part 2: infectious complications. Intensive Care Med. 2002;28:18–28. https://doi.org/10.1007/s00134-001-1156-7.

25. Paterson DL. "Collateral damage" from cephalosporin or quinolone antibiotic therapy. Clin Infect Dis Off Publ Infect Dis Soc Am. 2004;38(Suppl 4):S341–5. https://doi.org/10.1086/382690.

26. Kao LS, Fleming GM, Escamilla RJ, Lew DF, Lally KP. Antimicrobial prophylaxis and infection surveillance in extracorporeal membrane oxygenation patients: a multi-institutional survey of practice patterns. ASAIO J Am Soc Artif Intern Organs. 2011;57:231–8. https://doi.org/10.1097/MAT.0b013e31820d19ab.

27. Glater-Welt LB, Schneider JB, Zinger MM, Rosen L, Sweberg TM. Nosocomial bloodstream infections in patients receiving extracorporeal life support: variability in prevention practices: a survey of the Extracorporeal Life Support Organization members. J Intensive Care Med. 2015;. https://doi.org/10.1177/0885066615571540.

28. Mermel LA, Allon M, Bouza E, Craven DE, Flynn P, O'Grady NP, Raad II, Rinjders BJA, Sherertz RJ, Warren DK. Clinical practice guidelines for the diagnosis and management of intravascular catheter-related infection: 2009 Update by the Infectious Diseases Society of America. Clin Infect Dis Off Publ Infect Dis Soc Am. 2009;49:1–45. https://doi.org/10.1086/599376.

12

My patient has received fluid: How to assess its efficacy and side effects?

Xavier Monnet[1,2]* and Jean-Louis Teboul[1,2]

Abstract

Many efforts have been made to predict, before giving fluid, whether it will increase cardiac output. Nevertheless, after fluid administration, it is also essential to assess the therapeutic efficacy and to look for possible adverse effects. Like for any drug, this step should not be missed. Basically, volume expansion is aimed at improving tissue oxygenation and organ function. To assess this final result, clinical signs are often unhelpful. The increase in urine output in case of acute kidney injury is a poor marker of the kidney perfusion improvement. Even if oxygen delivery has increased with fluid, the increase in oxygen consumption is not constant. Assessing this response needs to measure markers such as lactate, central/mixed venous oxygen saturation, or carbon dioxide-derived indices. If tissue oxygenation did not improve, one should check that cardiac output has actually increased with fluid administration. To assess this response, changes in arterial pressure are not reliable enough, and direct measurements of cardiac output are required. In cases where cardiac output did not increase with fluid, one should check that it was not due to an insufficient volume of fluid administered. For this purpose, volume markers of cardiac preload sometimes lack precision. The central venous pressure, in theory at least, should not augment to a large extent in fluid responders. The worst adverse effect of fluids is the increase in the cumulative fluid balance. In patients with acute respiratory distress syndrome (ARDS), the risk of aggravating pulmonary oedema should be systematically assessed by looking for increases in extravascular lung water, or, more indirectly, increases in central venous or pulmonary artery occlusion pressure. In ARDS patients receiving fluid, one should always keep in mind the risk of inducing/aggravating right ventricular dilation, which should be confirmed through echocardiography. The risk of increasing the intra-abdominal pressure should be carefully sought in patients at risk. Finally, fluid-induced haemodilution should not be neglected. Like for any drug which has inconsistent effectiveness and may exert significant harm, the correct fluid management should include a cautious and comprehensive assessment of fluid-induced benefits and side effects.

Keywords: Fluid responsiveness, Pulse pressure variation, Passive leg raising, Fluid challenge, Cardiac output, Extravascular lung water

Introduction

Despite its trivial aspect, administration of fluid in critically ill patients poses several complex problems. Many efforts have been made to determine, before giving fluid, whether it will increase cardiac output. Nevertheless, after fluid administration, like for any treatment which has inconsistent effectiveness and which might induce significant side effects, it is essential to ask: was volume expansion effective? Was it harmful? Fluids are drugs. Assessing their efficiency and their adverse side effects should be part of good clinical practice. It seems to us that this step is often missed. In this review, based on the published data, we will attempt to show how essential it is to carefully evaluate the positive and negative effects of volume expansion once it has been administered and which evaluation criteria might be useful for this purpose.

Was volume expansion efficient?
What is fluid efficiency?

When fluid is administered in case of acute circulatory failure, it is with the final goal of increasing tissue

*Correspondence: xavier.monnet@aphp.fr
[1] Hôpital de Bicêtre, Service de Réanimation Médicale, Hôpitaux Universitaires Paris-Sud, 78, rue du Général Leclerc, 94270 Le Kremlin-Bicêtre, France
Full list of author information is available at the end of the article

oxygenation and, if it was previously impaired, of improving organ function. Nevertheless, between volume expansion and the resolution of organ failure, multiple steps are to be crossed (Fig. 1). At each one, issues might explain why fluid administration is eventually not effective.

Basically, fluid is administered in order to increase the mean systemic pressure, which is the forward pressure of venous return. Nevertheless, capillary leak or vasodilation may impede that fluid actually increases the stressed blood volume [1]. If it occurs, the raise in mean systemic filling pressure leads to an increase in cardiac output if both ventricles are preload dependent. In such a case, the right atrial pressure does not change or increases to a lesser extent than the mean systemic filling pressure, so that the pressure gradient of venous return increases [2]. If it happens, the increase in cardiac output leads to the increase in the oxygen delivery, i.e. the flow of oxygen that is sent towards the tissues, though the fluid-induced haemodilution tends to smoothen this effect [3]. The increase in cardiac output might increase the mean arterial pressure (Fig. 1). Nevertheless, this is not constant, since the sympathetic system physiologically tends to maintain the mean arterial pressure constant when cardiac output varies [4].

The increase in arterial flow and/or pressure increases the blood flow through the microcirculation and, sometimes, this is accompanied by a significant increase in the proportion of perfused vessels [5]. This step might be impeded by microvascular failure, especially in case of sepsis [5]. Provided that microcirculation is intact, the increase in microcirculatory flow leads to an increased oxygen availability for the tissues, which might be attenuated by tissue oedema. The aerobic metabolism increases in response. Nevertheless, mitochondrial dysfunction, as it may occur during sepsis, might explain why tissue hypoxia persists in spite of increased oxygen availability [6] (Fig. 1).

Finally, the reduction in tissue hypoxia should improve organ function. Nevertheless, this becomes impossible if organ function has been structurally injured by prolonged hypoperfusion. For instance, tubular necrosis explains that acute kidney injury persists in spite of resolution of the acute phase of shock (Fig. 1).

Did tissue oxygenation improve?

Basically, the decision to infuse fluids should be triggered by obvious signs of tissue hypoperfusion. In particular, it should never be taken only for increasing cardiac output, for instance, on the basis of positive tests of fluid responsiveness. The harmful effects of fluid infusion are today clearly demonstrated, and strategies aiming at systematically maximising oxygen delivery and cardiac output have been shown to be useless or even deleterious [7].

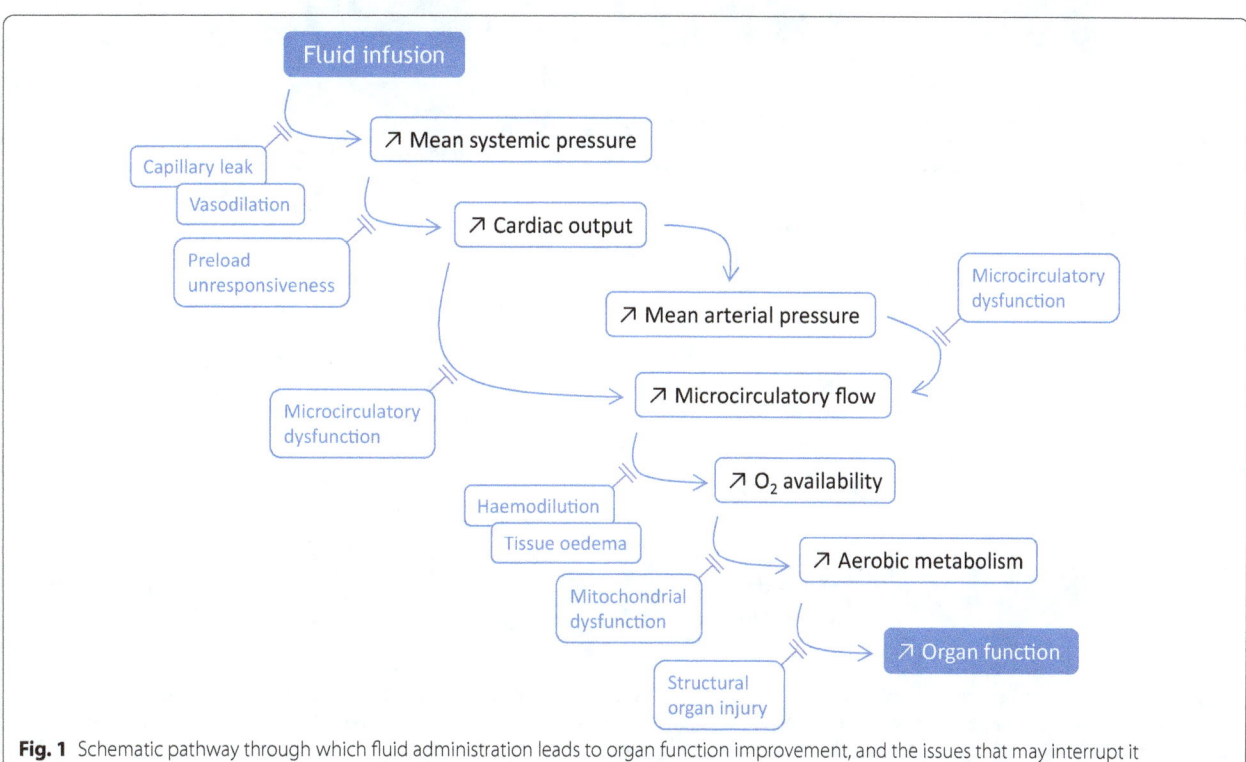

Fig. 1 Schematic pathway through which fluid administration leads to organ function improvement, and the issues that may interrupt it

The resolution of organ dysfunction that has been induced by shock, like acute kidney injury, obviously indicates that tissue perfusion occurred. Nevertheless, as stated above, the increase in urine output is unhelpful in the numerous cases in which tubular necrosis has already occurred. Even if this is not the case, the increase in diuresis is very poorly correlated with the simultaneous changes in cardiac output [8]. Moreover, when it occurs, the increase in urine output is delayed compared to the improvement in renal perfusion [9].

In general, looking for the improvement in tissue oxygenation likely requires more sophisticated indices (Fig. 1). In a study performed in critically ill patients, in the subgroup in which cardiac output increased, oxygen consumption improved significantly (by more than 15%) in only 56% of patients [3]. In the other ones, the increase in cardiac output was not accompanied by any beneficial effect on oxygen consumption. In fact, these results are in agreement with the physiology of the relationship between oxygen delivery and consumption. In patients in whom increased cardiac output was accompanied by an increase in oxygen consumption, oxygen consumption and delivery were likely working on the dependent part of their relationship.

These results do not mean that volume expansion was unnecessary in cases where oxygen consumption did not increase. The increase in oxygen delivery profitably moves the patient away from the dangerous zone where oxygen consumption becomes dependent on delivery. Nevertheless, it must be kept in mind that aiming at achieving supranormal values for cardiac output or normal values for mixed venous oxygen saturation does not reduce morbidity or mortality among critically ill patients [7].

What these results suggest is that the effects of fluid administration on tissue oxygenation should be monitored. To do this, several indices might be considered. Mixed or central venous saturation of oxygen (SvO_2 and $ScvO_2$, respectively) might be useful. When it is low and when it increases with volume expansion, it means that tissue oxygenation improved [10, 11] (Fig. 2). Nevertheless, if the oxygen delivery/consumption relationship is in its dependent zone, an increase in oxygen delivery does not induce a substantial increase in $SvO_2/ScvO_2$ because oxygen extraction is maximal until oxygen delivery increases above its critical value. Another limitation in $SvO_2/ScvO_2$ might appear in patients with septic shock with tissue oxygen extraction impairment, since the

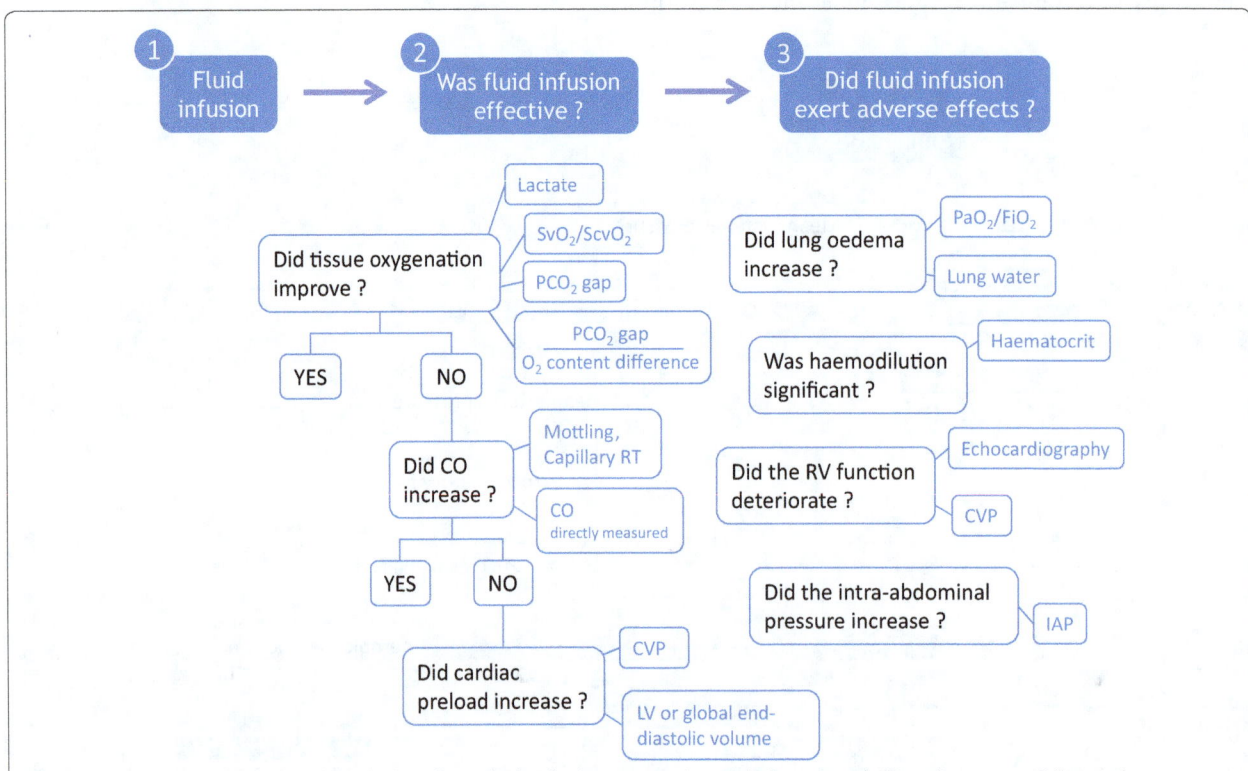

Fig. 2 Summary of the criteria on which the benefits and risks of volume expansion might be assessed. *CO* cardiac output, *CVP* central venous pressure, *FiO_2* oxygen inspired fraction, *IAP* intra-abdominal pressure, *LV* left ventricular, *PCO_2* carbon dioxide partial pressure, *PaO_2* arterial oxygen partial pressure, *RT* refill time, *SvO_2/ScvO_2* mixed/central venous oxygen saturation

$SvO_2/ScvO_2$ value remains in the normal range and constant in spite of anaerobic metabolism.

Biochemical markers of anaerobic metabolism might be useful in these cases. Lactate, the most commonly used, will decrease if oxygen delivery increases under the effect of fluid. Its main drawback is that its changes are slow. A decrease in the veno-arterial difference in carbon dioxide (CO_2) pressure (PCO_2 gap) will indicate that the cardiac output increase is enough to bring more CO_2 towards the lungs (Fig. 2). Nevertheless, it is not a marker of anaerobic metabolism. By contrast, the ratio of PCO_2 gap over the arteriovenous difference in oxygen content, an estimate of the respiratory quotient, more directly reflects anaerobic metabolism [12]. It is as reliable as lactate to indicate that tissue oxygenation increases with fluid administration, but its potential advantage is that it will decrease more rapidly [3] (Fig. 2).

Did cardiac output increase?

If fluid administration has not improved tissue oxygenation, one should check that it has actually increased cardiac output. Indeed, a significant increase in cardiac output in response to fluid administration happens inconstantly because the shape of the Frank–Starling curve, that relies stroke volume and cardiac preload, is flat [13]. This justifies predicting fluid responsiveness before performing volume expansion, but also to assess the fluid response once it has been performed.

The first way to evidence a fluid-induced increase in cardiac output might be to look for the decrease in the sympathetic reflex-induced vasoconstriction in territories which perfusion has been "sacrificed" for the benefit of more vital organs. In practice, one may look for the disappearance of skin mottling or the increase in the capillary refill time. Of course, these signs are unhelpful if they are absent at baseline. Moreover, they are hardly precisely quantified, though methods have been developed for this purpose [14].

In fact, to estimate the effects of fluid infusion on cardiac output, there is no other way than... to measure cardiac output! Unfortunately, simple changes in blood pressure cannot accurately estimate the effects of fluid loading. In a study in which 228 patients received volume expansion, changes in arterial pulse pressure, measured via a femoral catheter, were very roughly correlated with those of cardiac output [4]. The changes in arterial *pulse* pressure detected fluid responders—in terms of cardiac output—with 22% false negatives. The changes in *mean* arterial pressure were even less reliable [4]. In another study, in which arterial pressure was measured at the radial site, there was no correlation at all between changes in arterial pulse pressure and cardiac output [15]. These findings are easily explained by the basic cardiovascular physiology. Mean arterial pressure is regulated by the sympathetic system which tends to keep it constant while cardiac output varies. It is the value of arterial pressure that is the worst to reflect changes in cardiac output, and its changes during volume expansion are systematically damped compared to those of cardiac output. Arterial pulse pressure is physiologically related to stroke volume [16], but this relationship is not linear because it is influenced by the arterial compliance and the pulse wave amplification [4].

In practice, this likely means that in complex patients, in which a precise assessment of treatments effectiveness is mandatory, effects of fluid administration should be monitored by direct measurements of cardiac output. Of note, all the techniques that measure cardiac output are not equivalent for this purpose. Some techniques (pulmonary artery catheter, transpulmonary thermal or lithium dilution devices, oesophageal Doppler and echocardiography) provide a more direct estimation of cardiac output than some other ones (pulse contour analysis, bioreactance). They also differ in terms of precision. The least change in cardiac output that can be deemed as significant is, for instance, as low as 5% for pulse contour analysis, but only 15% when the pulmonary artery catheter, transpulmonary thermodilution devices or echocardiography are used [17].

If cardiac output did not increase: did cardiac preload increase?

If cardiac output did not increase with fluid infusion, two reasons might be invoked. Either cardiac preload increased but the patient was not preload responsive, or the volume of fluid administered was not enough to significantly increase cardiac preload (Fig. 1) [1]. This may occur if the dose of fluid was too small or if fluid has diluted in a large, dilated, venous compartment.

In order to rule out the latter hypothesis, one may look at the fluid-induced changes in the markers of cardiac preload. Among them, the cardiac end-diastolic volume might be estimated through echocardiography or transpulmonary thermodilution [17]. In theory, they should increase with volume expansion. Nevertheless, one must admit that these measurements are not very precise, such that small but significant increases in cardiac preload might be missed. For instance, the least significant change of transpulmonary thermodilution for measuring the global end-diastolic volume is only 12% [18].

The measurement of central venous pressure is more precise. Nevertheless, central venous pressure does not necessarily increase significantly, even in cases where volume expansion has increased cardiac preload. Indeed, in patients who respond to volume expansion by an increase in cardiac output—and thus in venous return, which equals cardiac output at steady state—the increase in venous return is provoked by an increase in its pressure gradient (mean systemic pressure—right atrial pressure). For this to happen, right atrial pressure—and thus central venous pressure—must increase to a lesser extent than the mean systemic pressure. Thus, in theory, fluid administration might be effective and cardiac output might increase although the central venous pressure did not change to a large extent. This limitation might be overcome by measuring the mean systemic pressure, but this is not possible in routine practice. Nevertheless, it remains that in fluid non-responders, central venous pressure increases as much as the mean systemic pressure. Then, in theory, if cardiac output does not increase with volume expansion, a reliable way to ascertain that this was due to fluid unresponsiveness, and not to an insufficient fluid volume, is to look for an increase in the central venous pressure. Nevertheless, increasing the central venous pressure is not per se a goal of fluid administration.

Did volume expansion induce adverse side effects?
Like any other drug, whatever its efficacy, the adverse side effects that may result from fluid administration must be carefully searched. Continuously balancing their weight against haemodynamic benefits helps decide to go on with fluid administration or to choose another therapeutic strategy.

Did lung oedema appear/worsen?
Volume expansion might increase the total cumulative fluid balance in case of renal failure. As it has been now very clearly established, the higher the cumulative fluid balance, the higher the mortality of critically ill patients, especially in case of acute respiratory distress syndrome (ARDS) [19] and/or septic shock [20]. The increase in fluid balance is due both to the facts that copious amounts of fluids are administered and that fluids in excess cannot be normally eliminated through the kidneys. This is due to a potential renal failure and to the accumulation of fluid in the interstitial compartment. This capillary leak syndrome is favoured by systemic inflammation and hypoalbuminemia.

Besides the cumulative fluid balance, more specific signs of fluid overload must be sought. An increase in the peripheral subcutaneous oedema clearly indicates that fluid has leaked out of the vessels. Obviously, the highest risk is to aggravate lung oedema. Chest X-ray is not sensitive enough since it can detect only large increases in lung oedema. High values of central venous pressure or of pulmonary artery occlusion pressure could be more specific. Nevertheless, they do not take into account a key

parameter, which is pulmonary capillary permeability. If pulmonary capillary permeability is much increased, lung oedema might have appeared even though the values of pulmonary artery occlusion pressure and central venous pressure are not much increased.

Extravascular lung water, which is the volume of fluid accumulated in the interstitium and alveoli, is a much more direct reflection of lung oedema created by fluid accumulation (Fig. 2). Then, it is likely one of the most meaningful variables of the adverse side effects of volume expansion, especially in patients with ARDS [21]. Extravascular lung water can be estimated at the bedside through transpulmonary thermodilution [22]. This is likely the most interesting aspect of that technique, and the estimation can now be considered as reliable [17, 22]. In a randomised study including critically ill patients, it has been shown that the cumulative fluid balance was better maintained if clinicians guided their fluid strategy by measuring extravascular lung water rather than the pulmonary artery occlusion pressure [23]. This was associated with a decrease in the duration of ventilation and of the stay in the intensive care unit [23].

Has the right ventricular function deteriorated?
In case of right ventricular failure, as during ARDS, a specific risk of fluid infusion is to aggravate the right ventricular dilation. The right ventricle is very sensitive to changes in its afterload, which explains the risk that it dilates in case of ARDS. In addition, in case of right ventricular preload unresponsiveness, any fluid administration might further increase the right ventricular overload, and finally the right ventricular dilation. The septal shift it induces should reduce the left ventricular filling and contribute to the decrease in cardiac output.

The right ventricular impairment should be assessed if several fluid infusions have been repeated in a few hours. There is no doubt that echocardiography is the gold standard to assess the right ventricular failure. Nevertheless, it cannot be easily repeated over the day. A faster and easier means is to look for increases in the central venous pressure [24]. This emphasises the value of central venous pressure (Fig. 2), which should not be used to decide to give fluid, since it is not a reliable marker of fluid responsiveness, but which is a reliable marker of the right heart function. An elevation in central venous pressure should prompt to confirm the right ventricular dysfunction by echocardiography (Fig. 2).

Did volume expansion increase the intra-abdominal pressure?
Worsening of prior intra-abdominal hypertension (IAH) is likely one of the adverse effects of fluid resuscitation that is often neglected in practice. One should always

keep in mind that the incidence of IAH in critically ill patients is around 20–30% on admission, while as many as 50–70% of patients (depending on the condition) may develop IAH during the first week of stay in the intensive care unit [25].

One of the most important risk factors for IAH is fluid resuscitation [26]. There is a meaningful correlation between IAH, extravascular lung water kinetics and fluid balance in critically ill patients [27]. In fact, IAH may induce organ dysfunction through two major pathways: firstly, by decreasing the perfusion pressure gradient of the intra-abdominal organs; secondly, by impairing systemic haemodynamics. Typically, organ dysfunction appears when intra-abdominal pressure is higher than 20–25 mmHg [25]. This should spur us to assess the effects of volume expansion on the intra-abdominal pressure in patients with suspected or established IAH (Fig. 2).

Did volume expansion induce haemodilution?

Administration of crystalloids or colloids unavoidably results in haemodilution, and the degree of this haemodilution is far from negligible. One must keep in mind that the normal total blood volume is 65–70 mL/kg and that it is even reduced in many conditions associated with circulatory failure. A volume expansion of even only 500 mL is significant.

In a study in which critically ill patients received a 500-mL volume expansion, our group showed that this resulted in a decrease in haemoglobin concentration by 8%. More importantly, in patients who did not respond to fluid by an increase in cardiac output (non-responders), this led to a significant decrease in oxygen delivery [3]. Clearly, these results once more emphasise how volume expansion is deleterious in fluid non-responders.

Conclusion

Fluids should be considered as a drug, which positive effects are inconstant and which carries a significant risk of adverse effects. Like for any drug, one should not miss after having administered fluids to ask two questions: has it been effective and has it been harmful? Who would administer antibiotics without assessing the body temperature or the biological markers of inflammation? Who would administer aminosides without checking the renal function? The correct fluid management should not be limited to the prediction of fluid responsiveness, but should include a cautious assessment of fluids benefits and side effects.

Abbreviations
ARDS: acute respiratory distress syndrome; IAH: intra-abdominal pressure; CO_2: carbon dioxide; PCO_2 gap: veno-arterial difference in carbon dioxide tension; SvO_2/$ScvO_2$: central/mixed venous oxygen saturation.

Authors' contributions
XM and J-LT both prepared the manuscript. Both authors read and approved the final manuscript.

Author details
[1] Hôpital de Bicêtre, Service de Réanimation Médicale, Hôpitaux Universitaires Paris-Sud, 78, rue du Général Leclerc, 94270 Le Kremlin-Bicêtre, France. [2] Université Paris-Sud, Inserm UMR S_999, 94270 Le Kremlin-Bicêtre, France.

Acknowledgements
Not applicable.

Competing interests
Xavier Monnet and Jean-Louis Teboul are members of the Medical Advisory Board of Pulsion Medical Systems.

Funding
Not applicable.

References
1. Aya HD, Rhodes A, Chis Ster I, Fletcher N, Grounds RM, Cecconi M. Hemodynamic effect of different doses of fluids for a fluid challenge: a quasi-randomized controlled study. Crit Care Med. 2017;45:e161–8.
2. Guerin L, Teboul JL, Persichini R, Dres M, Richard C, Monnet X. Effects of passive leg raising and volume expansion on mean systemic pressure and venous return in shock in humans. Crit Care. 2015;19:411.
3. Monnet X, Julien F, Ait-Hamou N, Lequoy M, Gosset C, Jozwiak M, et al. Lactate and venoarterial carbon dioxide difference/arterial-venous oxygen difference ratio, but not central venous oxygen saturation, predict increase in oxygen consumption in fluid responders. Crit Care Med. 2013;41:1412–20.
4. Monnet X, Letierce A, Hamzaoui O, Chemla D, Anguel N, Osman D, et al. Arterial pressure allows monitoring the changes in cardiac output induced by volume expansion but not by norepinephrine. Crit Care Med. 2011;39:1394–9.
5. Ospina-Tascon G, Neves AP, Occhipinti G, Donadello K, Buchele G, Simion D, et al. Effects of fluids on microvascular perfusion in patients with severe sepsis. Intensive Care Med. 2010;36:949–55.
6. Ronco JJ, Fenwick JC, Wiggs BR, Phang PT, Russell JA, Tweeddale MG. Oxygen consumption is independent of increases in oxygen delivery by dobutamine in septic patients who have normal or increased plasma lactate. Am Rev Respir Dis. 1993;147:25–31.
7. Gattinoni L, Brazzi L, Pelosi P, Latini R, Tognoni G, Pesenti A, et al. A trial of goal-oriented hemodynamic therapy in critically ill patients. SvO_2 Collaborative Group. N Engl J Med. 1995;333:1025–32.
8. Legrand M, Dupuis C, Simon C, Gayat E, Mateo J, Lukaszewicz AC, et al. Association between systemic hemodynamics and septic acute kidney injury in critically ill patients: a retrospective observational study. Crit Care. 2013;17:R278.
9. Moussa MD, Scolletta S, Fagnoul D, Pasquier P, Brasseur A, Taccone FS, et al. Effects of fluid administration on renal perfusion in critically ill patients. Crit Care. 2015;19:250.
10. Giraud R, Siegenthaler N, Gayet-Ageron A, Combescure C, Romand JA, Bendjelid K. $ScvO_2$ as a marker to define fluid responsiveness. J Trauma. 2011;70:802–7.
11. Kuiper AN, Trof RJ, Groeneveld AB. Mixed venous O_2 saturation and fluid responsiveness after cardiac or major vascular surgery. J Cardiothorac Surg. 2013;8:189.
12. Mekontso-Dessap A, Castelain V, Anguel N, Bahloul M, Schauvliege F, Richard C, et al. Combination of venoarterial PCO_2 difference with arteriovenous O_2 content difference to detect anaerobic metabolism in patients. Intensive Care Med. 2002;28:272–7.
13. Monnet X, Marik PE, Teboul JL. Prediction of fluid responsiveness: an update. Ann Intensive Care. 2016;6:111.

14. Ait-Oufella H, Bourcier S, Alves M, Galbois A, Baudel JL, Margetis D, et al. Alteration of skin perfusion in mottling area during septic shock. Ann Intensive Care. 2013;3:31.

15. Pierrakos C, Velissaris D, Scolletta S, Heenen S, De Backer D, Vincent JL. Can changes in arterial pressure be used to detect changes in cardiac index during fluid challenge in patients with septic shock? Intensive Care Med. 2012;38:422–8.

16. Chemla D, Hebert JL, Coirault C, Zamani K, Suard I, Colin P, et al. Total arterial compliance estimated by stroke volume-to-aortic pulse pressure ratio in humans. Am J Physiol. 1998;274:H500–5.

17. Monnet X, Teboul JL. Transpulmonary thermodilution: advantages and limits. Crit Care. 2017;21:147.

18. Monnet X, Persichini R, Ktari M, Jozwiak M, Richard C, Teboul JL. Precision of the transpulmonary thermodilution measurements. Crit Care. 2011;15:R204.

19. Jozwiak M, Silva S, Persichini R, Anguel N, Osman D, Richard C, et al. Extravascular lung water is an independent prognostic factor in patients with acute respiratory distress syndrome. Crit Care Med. 2013;41:472–80.

20. Vincent JL, Sakr Y, Sprung CL, Ranieri VM, Reinhart K, Gerlach H, et al. Sepsis in European intensive care units: results of the SOAP study. Crit Care Med. 2006;34:344–53.

21. Schuster DP, Stark T, Stephenson J, Royal H. Detecting lung injury in patients with pulmonary edema. Intensive Care Med. 2002;28:1246–53.

22. Jozwiak M, Teboul JL, Monnet X. Extravascular lung water in critical care: recent advances and clinical applications. Ann Intensive Care. 2015;5:38.

23. Mitchell JP, Schuller D, Calandrino FS, Schuster DP. Improved outcome based on fluid management in critically ill patients requiring pulmonary artery catheterization. Am Rev Respir Dis. 1992;145:990–8.

24. Vieillard-Baron A, Matthay M, Teboul JL, Bein T, Schultz M, Magder S, et al. Experts' opinion on management of hemodynamics in ARDS patients: focus on the effects of mechanical ventilation. Intensive Care Med. 2016;42:739–49.

25. De Waele JJ, De Laet I, Malbrain ML. Understanding abdominal compartment syndrome. Intensive Care Med. 2016;42:1068–70.

26. Holodinsky JK, Roberts DJ, Ball CG, Blaser AR, Starkopf J, Zygun DA, et al. Risk factors for intra-abdominal hypertension and abdominal compartment syndrome among adult intensive care unit patients: a systematic review and meta-analysis. Crit Care. 2013;17:R249.

27. Cordemans C, De Laet I, Van Regenmortel N, Schoonheydt K, Dits H, Huber W, et al. Fluid management in critically ill patients: the role of extravascular lung water, abdominal hypertension, capillary leak, and fluid balance. Ann Intensive Care. 2012;2:S1.

13

Transcutaneous electromyographic respiratory muscle recordings to quantify patient–ventilator interaction in mechanically ventilated children

Alette A. Koopman[1], Robert G. T. Blokpoel[1*], Leo A. van Eykern[2], Frans H. C. de Jongh[3], Johannes G. M. Burgerhof[4] and Martin C. J. Kneyber[1,5,6]

Abstract

Background: To explore the feasibility of transcutaneous electromyographic respiratory muscle recordings to automatically quantify the synchronicity of patient–ventilator interaction in the pediatric intensive care unit.

Methods: Prospective observational study in a tertiary paediatric intensive care unit in an university hospital. Spontaneous breathing mechanically ventilated children < 18 years of age were eligible for inclusion. Patients underwent a 5-min continuous recording of ventilator pressure waveforms and transcutaneous electromyographic signal of the diaphragm. To evaluate patient–ventilator interaction, the obtained neural inspiration and ventilator pressurization timings were used to calculate trigger and cycle-off errors of each breath. Calculated errors were displayed in the dEMG-phase scale.

Results: Data of 23 patients were used for analysis. Based on the dEMG-phase scale, the median rates of synchronous, dyssynchronous and asynchronous breaths as classified by the automated analysis were 12.2% (1.9–33.8), 47.5% (36.3–63.1), and 28.9% (6.6–49.0).

Conclusions: The dEMG-phase scale quantifying patient–ventilator breath synchronicity was demonstrated to be feasible and a reliable scale for mechanically ventilated children, reflected by high intra-class correlation coefficients. As this non-invasive tool is not restricted to a type of ventilator, it could easily be clinical implemented in the ventilated pediatric population. However; correlation studies between the EMG signal measured by surface EMG and esophageal catheters have to be performed.

Keywords: Child, Mechanical ventilation, Asynchrony, Electromyography, Patient–ventilator interaction, Paediatric intensive care

Background

Patient–ventilator asynchrony (PVA) in mechanically ventilated adults is associated with prolonged duration of mechanical ventilation (MV), increased use of sedatives and longer intensive care unit (ICU) and hospital stay

[1–3]. Although the occurrence of PVA in mechanically ventilated children is common as we and others have shown, the relationship between PVA and clinical outcome is unclear for this group of patients [4–6].

Previously, we have shown in a heterogeneous group of mechanically ventilated children that one out of every three breaths was out of sync when the airway pressure and flow waveforms were visually inspected [4]. However, such inspection is cumbersome and may not reflect the true prevalence of PVA as the neural breathing drive is not taken into consideration. Alternatively, electrical

*Correspondence: r.g.t.blokpoel@umcg.nl

[1] Division of Paediatric Intensive Care, Department of Paediatrics, Beatrix Children's Hospital, University Medical Center Groningen, The University of Groningen, Internal Postal Code CA 62, P.O. Box 30.001, 9700 RB Groningen, The Netherlands

Full list of author information is available at the end of the article

activity of the diaphragm measured with a specific nasogastric catheter (EAdi) or the esophageal pressure signal can be used and is in fact more accurate signals for identifying PVA [6–11].

So far, use of these methods has been restricted to research purposes mainly because of the lack of ability to provide the clinician with real-time feedback of the level of PVA. In order to truly understand the clinical relevance of PVA in mechanically ventilated children, there needs to be a system that provides such feedback on both the occurrence and type of PVA. Recent advances have been made in the development of tools to automatically identify PVA [2, 12–15]. Such real-time automatic analyses are needed for clinical trials investigating the efficacy of interventions targeted at reducing PVA and on patient outcome. Sinderby et al. [16] developed an automated, objective and standardized neural index to quantify patient–ventilator interaction (NeuroSync) based on the measurements of EAdi and ventilator pressure waveforms. Determining patient–ventilator interaction by this method had a higher inter-rater reliability and proved to be more sensitive than manual analysis.

However, this new approach is only limited to ventilators capable of measuring EAdi. Furthermore, it mandates the insertion of an esophageal catheter which may be a disadvantage especially in the pediatric context. Transcutaneous recording of the electromyographic signals of the diaphragm (dEMG) may be considered as a suitable alternative [17–19]. Although at this moment no correlation studies between dEMG and EAdi have been performed, this non-invasive, easy-to-perform technique provides reproducible electromyographic signals of the diaphragm [17]. We therefore tested the hypothesis that it would be feasible to automatically detect, quantify and display patient–ventilator interactions using a modified NeuroSync index (dEMG-phase scale) in mechanically ventilated children when analyzing dEMG together with ventilator pressure and flow versus time waveform.

Methods

Study population

This study was performed at the pediatric intensive care unit (PICU) of the Beatrix Children's Hospital, University Medical Center Groningen between February and July 2015. The Institutional Review Board approved the study. Signed informed consent was obtained from both parents or legal caretakers. Mechanically ventilated children < 18 years of age were eligible for inclusion. Patients with congenital or acquired neuromuscular disorders, premature birth with gestational age corrected for post-conceptional age < 40 weeks, severe traumatic brain injury (i.e. Glasgow Coma Scale < 8), congenital or acquired damage to the phrenic nerve, congenital or acquired paralysis of

the diaphragm, use of neuromuscular blockade, chronic lung disease (i.e. tracheostomy ventilation), severe pulmonary hypertension, contra-indication for placement of electrodes on the skin and patients unable to trigger the ventilator from any other cause were excluded.

Study procedure

During the study, all patients remained subjected to standard-of-care of the intensive care. Measurements took place within the 24 h prior to extubation. The attending physician defined the ventilator mode and settings in agreement with our local guideline. Expiratory tidal volume (V_T) was targeted at 6–8 mL/kg actual bodyweight. The flow trigger was set at 1.0 L/min. A proximal flow-sensor was used in patients < 15 kg. In cases of decreased respiratory system compliance, permissive hypercapnia was applied (pH > 7.20). The level of pressure support ventilation (PSV) was routinely set as PSV = peak inspiratory pressure (PIP) minus positive end-expiratory pressure (PEEP). Ventilator settings were fixed during the measurement unless the clinical condition of a patient required an adjustment of the setting made by the attending physician. Patients were ventilated in a time-cycled, pressure-limited synchronized mode of ventilation with PSV, pressure controlled/synchronized intermittent mandatory ventilation (PC/SIMV + PSV), pressure-limited mode with preset tidal volume (V_T), i.e. pressure regulated volume controlled with PSV (PRVC/SIMV + PSV) or pressure controlled assist control (PC/AC) using the AVEA ventilator (CareFusion, Yorba Linda, CA, USA). Continuous infusion of midazolam, oral lorazepam and morphine or fentanyl intravenously was given for analgesia–sedation. The COMFORT behavior scale was used to titrate the level of sedation [20, 21]. Ten minutes prior to the recordings, patients were suctioned and the circuit was cleared from any water. Patients were in a 30 degrees anti-Trendelenburg supine position.

Ventilator pressure waveforms and dEMG acquisition

Patients underwent a 5-min continuous recording of ventilator pressure waveforms and dEMG. Ventilator pressure tracings were acquired through the ventilator's RS232 interface (Ventilator Open XML Protocol, VOXP) at a sampling frequency of 100 Hz. The dEMG was derived from one pair of single Ag/AGCl electrodes (EasyTrode TM Pre gelled Electrodes, Multi Bio Sensors Inc, El Paso, USA) bilaterally placed at the costo-abdominal margin in the nipple line. A common electrode was placed at the sternal level [17]. The dEMG was recorded at a sampling frequency of 500 Hz using the Dipha (Inbiolab, Groningen, The Netherlands). Polybench software (Applied Biosignals GmbH, Weener, Germany) was used to record the pre-processed data from the ventilator and the EMG recording device. The ventilator pressure waveforms and electrical activity of the diaphragm were analyzed offline.

Data processing

The recorded dEMG needed to be processed for reliable assessment of the respiratory neural drive. The electrical activity of the heart and other peak artifacts were isolated from the raw dEMG data by means of an extended version of the gating technique [22]. The gates were filled with the running average of the processed dEMG signal. A 50 Hz notch filter was used to minimize electrical interference from electronic devices on the intensive care. After filtering and gating, the running root mean square (RMS) (time window $T = 0.2$ s) of the processed dEMG signal was calculated. The calculated dEMG was used for analysis.

Description of patient–ventilator interaction

To evaluate patient–ventilator interaction, the computed dEMG activity was both manually and automatically compared to the ventilator's waveforms to calculate the dEMG-phase scale (dEMG-phase scale$_{MANU}$ and dEMG-phase scale$_{AUTO}$, respectively), using the modified Neuro-Sync method previously described by Sinderby et al. [16]. Two investigators (AK and RB) manually analyzed the ventilator pressure and dEMG tracings using a graphical interface designed in Polybench (Applied Biosignals GmbH, Weener, Germany). Each investigator individually placed markers in the interface at the onset of neural inspiration (NA$_{ON}$), at 1/3 decline in the dEMG from its peak, i.e. the termination of neural inspiration (NA$_{OFF}$), at the beginning of ventilator pressurization (MV$_{ON}$) and at the end of ventilator pressurization (MV$_{OFF}$). The obtained neural inspiration and ventilator pressurization timings: NA$_{ON}$, NA$_{OFF}$, MV$_{ON}$ and MV$_{OFF}$ were used to calculate trigger and cycle-off errors of each breath. The algorithm for automated analysis was designed according to the same rules as for manual analysis. Early trigger and cycle-off errors as well as late trigger and cycle-off errors could range between 0 and 100%. Limits whether a breath is synchronous, dyssynchronous were set, accordingly to Sinderby et al. [16], at $\pm$ 33% difference between NA$_{ON}$ and MV$_{ON}$ and NA$_{OFF}$ and MV$_{OFF}$. Neural inspirations not related to ventilator pressurizations or vice versa were considered as asynchronous breaths and assigned 100%. Cases of asynchronous breaths included ventilatory pressurization without neural activity (MV without NA), neural activity without ventilatory pressurization (NA without MV), multiple ventilatory pressurizations with one neural activity (multiple MV with NA) and multiple neural activities within one ventilatory pressurization (multiple NA with MV). Obtained data are shown

in a graphical representation of the dEMG-phase scale; the intra-breath patient–ventilator interaction diagram. The dEMG-phase scale was defined as the mean absolute error of all breaths. The dEMG-phase scale$_{MANU}$, which was obtained by both experts, was compared with the dEMG-phase scale$_{AUTO}$.

Baseline characteristics

Patient baseline demographics included age, gender, weight, admission diagnosis, Pediatric Index of Mortality (PIM) II and 24-h Pediatric RISk of Mortality (PRISM) II score, time of recordings and admission diagnosis. Before initiation of the measurements, ventilator settings including mode, pressure above peep (PAP), PEEP, mean airway pressure (P_{mean}), PSV, expiratory tidal volume (V_T), frequency of set breaths, fraction of inspired oxygen (FiO$_2$) and inspiratory time were recorded. Clinical data included prior use of neuromuscular blockade, tube size, air leakage around the endotracheal tube (ETT), end tidal CO$_2$ and received amount of analgesia-sedation in the last 4 h preceding the registration. The COMFORT score was evaluated during the recording [20, 21].

Statistical analysis

The Shapiro–Wilk test was used to test data for normal distribution. Descriptive data were expressed as median [first quartile; third quartile] or percentage (%) of total. The breath-by-breath inter-rater agreement, defined as the agreement between errors obtained by the two investigators, and inter-method agreement, defined as the agreement between errors obtained by automated analysis and the average errors obtained by the two investigators, were evaluated by means of the intra-class correlation coefficient (ICC). Reliability was considered to be acceptable if the ICC was greater than 0.75 and excellent if the ICC was greater than 0.90 [23, 24]. After confirmation of a good breath-by-breath inter-rater and inter-method reproducibility, the agreement between dEMG-phase scale$_{MANU}$ and dEMG-phase scale$_{AUTO}$ was evaluated. All statistical analyses were performed using SPSS version 24 (IBM, Armonk, USA).

Results
Study population

Patient characteristics are summarized in Table 1. At the time of analysis, one patient was excluded because she developed meningitis with severe neurologic impairment on the measurement day. Thus, data of $N = 23$ (17 boys and 6 girls) patients were used for analysis. Seventeen (74%) patients were ventilated for respiratory failure of any cause; five patients (22%) were admitted after corrective cardiac surgery for congenital heart disease. One patient was ventilated for circulatory failure (4%).

Table 1 Baseline demographics, mode of ventilation and ventilator settings

Variable	
N	23
Gender (male, n)	17
Pulmonary diagnosis (n)	17
Surgical diagnosis (n)	5
PIM II	− 2.9 [− 3.3; − 2.5]
PRISM II	11.0 [9.0; 15.0]
Age (months)	3.6 [1.4; 9.8]
Duration MV (days)	4.7 [2.9; 7.0]
Cuffed ETT (n)	14
Air leakage uncuffed ETT (%)	2.0 [0.0; 8.0]
End tidal pCO_2 (kPa)	6.1 [5.7; 6.5]
COMFORT scale	14 [11; 15]
Expiratory V_T/kg (ml)	7.2 [6.1; 8.3]
Patient triggered breaths (%)	96 [61; 99]
PC/AC (N)	21
PC/SIMV + PSV (N)	2
PAP (cm H_2O)	13 [12; 14]
PEEP (cm H_2O)	6 [5; 6]
Set frequency (/min)	25 [20; 30]
FiO_2	0.35 [0.25; 0.40]
Inspiratory time (s)	0.55 [0.50; 0.65]
PSV (cm H_2O)	13 [13]

PIM II, Pediatric Index of Mortality score II; PRISM II, Pediatric Risk of Mortality score II; MV, mechanical ventilation; ETT, endotracheal tube; End tidal pCO_2, end tidal pCO_2 before starting measurement; COMFORT scale, measurement tool to assess distress, sedation and pain in nonverbal paediatric patients; Expiratory V_T/ kg, expiratory tidal volume per kilogram body weight; PC/AC, pressure control/ assist control; PC/SIMV + SIMV, pressure control/synchronized intermittent mandatory ventilation plus pressure support ventilation; PIP, pressure above PEEP; PEEP, positive end-expiratory pressure; FiO_2, fraction of inspired oxygen; PSV, pressure support ventilation

Median percentage of patient triggered breaths was 96% [61; 99]. At the time of data recording patients received a median morphine dosage of 10 mcg/kg/h [7.7; 10.5], median midazolam dosage of 0.1 mg/kg/h [0.08; 0.2] and median fentanyl dosage of 2.0 mcg/kg/h [1.0; 2.9]. One patient received lorazepam in a dosage of 0.3 mg/kg/day. Median COMFORT score was 14 [11, 15].

Description of dEMG recordings
The recorded dEMG showed the following characteristics. Median neural inspiration was 0.86 s [0.74; 1.0], neural expiration was 0.79 s [0.57; 0.96], median baseline dEMG signal was 1.16 µV [0.76; 2.12], peak dEMG signal was 2.69 µV [1.72; 3.62], and median amplitude was 1.06 µV [0.85; 1.87]. Two patients had no detectable dEMG signal, probably caused by sedation. For all other patients during the entire breathing cycle, no loss of the dEMG signal was observed. Median trigger error (i.e. dEMG signal compared to ventilator pressurization)

for premature triggering was 0.33 s [0.24–0.46] and for delayed triggering 0.16 s [0.03–0.24]. Median cycle-off error for premature cycling was 0.11 s [0.07–0.20] and for delayed cycling 0.13 s [0.08–0.39].

dEMG-phase scale$_{AUTO}$
The automated detection algorithm and expert 1 and 2 detected 4366, 4342, 4333 NA or MV breaths, respectively. Based on the dEMG-phase scale$_{AUTO}$, the median rates of synchronous, dyssynchronous and asynchronous breaths as classified by the automated analysis were 11.0% [1.7; 32.7], 49.4% [36.0; 63.9], and 28.7% [6.3; 43.5]. Rates of synchronous, dyssynchronous and asynchronous breaths as classified by the automated analysis are displayed in Fig. 1. Median rates of complete dissociations were 40.4% [18.3; 48.7] for MV without NA, 25.9% [10.2; 48.7] for NA without MV, 4.0% [0; 25.0] multiple MV with NA and 5.8% [0; 15.4] for multiple NA with MV. Rates of complete dissociations as classified by the automated analysis are shown in Fig. 2. Examples of good and poor patient–ventilator interaction with corresponding ventilator pressure and dEMG tracings are shown in Figs. 3, 4 and 5.

Inter-rater and inter-method agreement
Results for inter-rater and inter-method are displayed in Table 2. The agreement between dEMG-phase scale$_{MANU}$ and dEMG-phase scale$_{AUTO}$ was reflected by an ICC of 1.0 95% CI [0.99–1.0].

Discussion
To our knowledge, this is the first study reporting that the interaction between infants and children and the mechanical ventilator can be quantified in a real-time non-invasive manner using transcutaneous

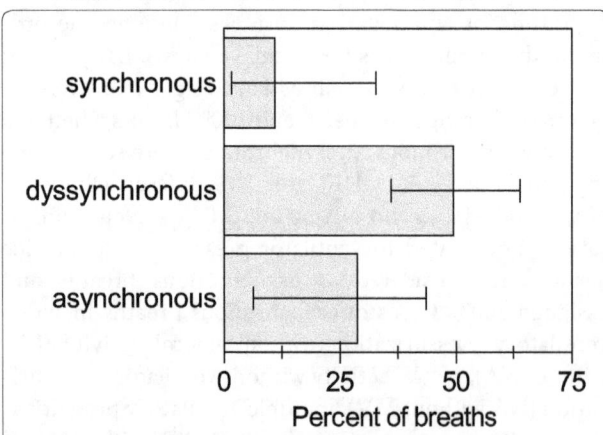

Fig. 1 Rates of synchronous, dyssynchronous and asynchronous breaths as classified by the automated analysis. Columns are median, and bars are interquartile range

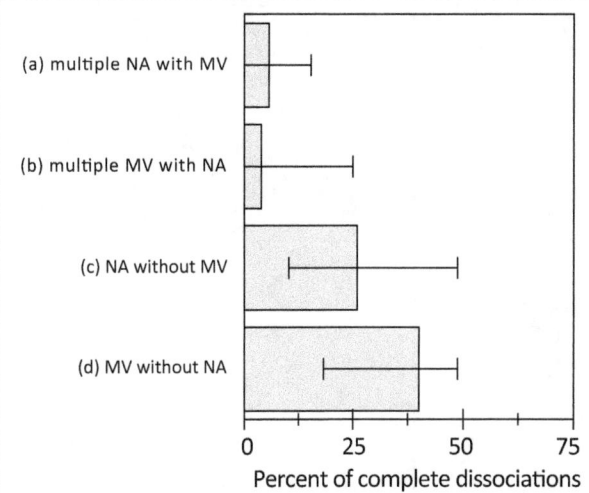

Fig. 2 Rates of multiple NA with MV (a), multiple MV with NA (b), NA without MV (c) and MV without NA (d) as classified by the automated analysis. Columns are median, and bars are interquartile range

electromyographic respiratory muscle recordings. Quantification of patient–ventilator interaction using a modification of a previously described method (dEMG-phase

scale) proved to be a feasible and reliable method, reflected by high ICCs for both trigger and cycle-off errors and the dEMG-phase scale. This method may have important implications for both clinical use and research purposes, as it is not restricted to one type of ventilator and it is a non-invasive tool implying that it can be easily implemented in the pediatric population.

To date, measuring the electrical activity of the diaphragm was only feasible using a specifically developed esophageal catheter linked to a specific brand of ventilator. Alternatively, we used surface electrodes with their own limitations. First, when measuring respiratory electrical activity by surface electrodes, also other muscle activity could be measured, a phenomenon known as cross-talk [25]. Reassuring, however, is that we noticed only minimal cross-talk in our study comparable with other studies [17, 26]. Second, electrical interference by machines commonly used in the intensive care unit may interfere with the measured electrical activity [26–29]. We therefore applied a 50 Hz notch filter and were subsequently able to use all data registrations. Third, the use of template subtraction and gating to remove heart activity from the dEMG signal could theoretically interfere with

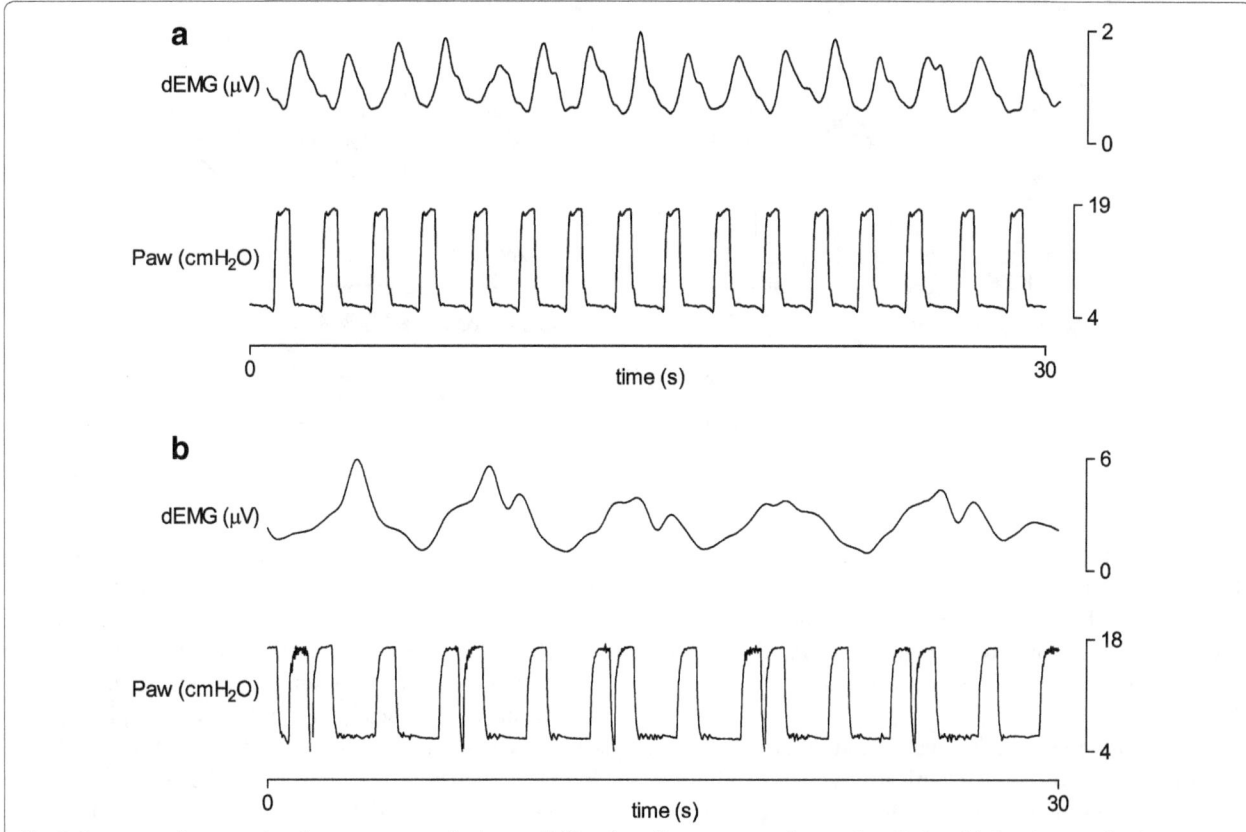

Fig. 3 Representative examples of transcutaneous diaphragm EMG and ventilator pressure–time tracings. Patient A is showing good patient–ventilator interaction. Patient B is showing poor patient–ventilator interaction with multiple ventilator pressurization within one period of neural inspiration

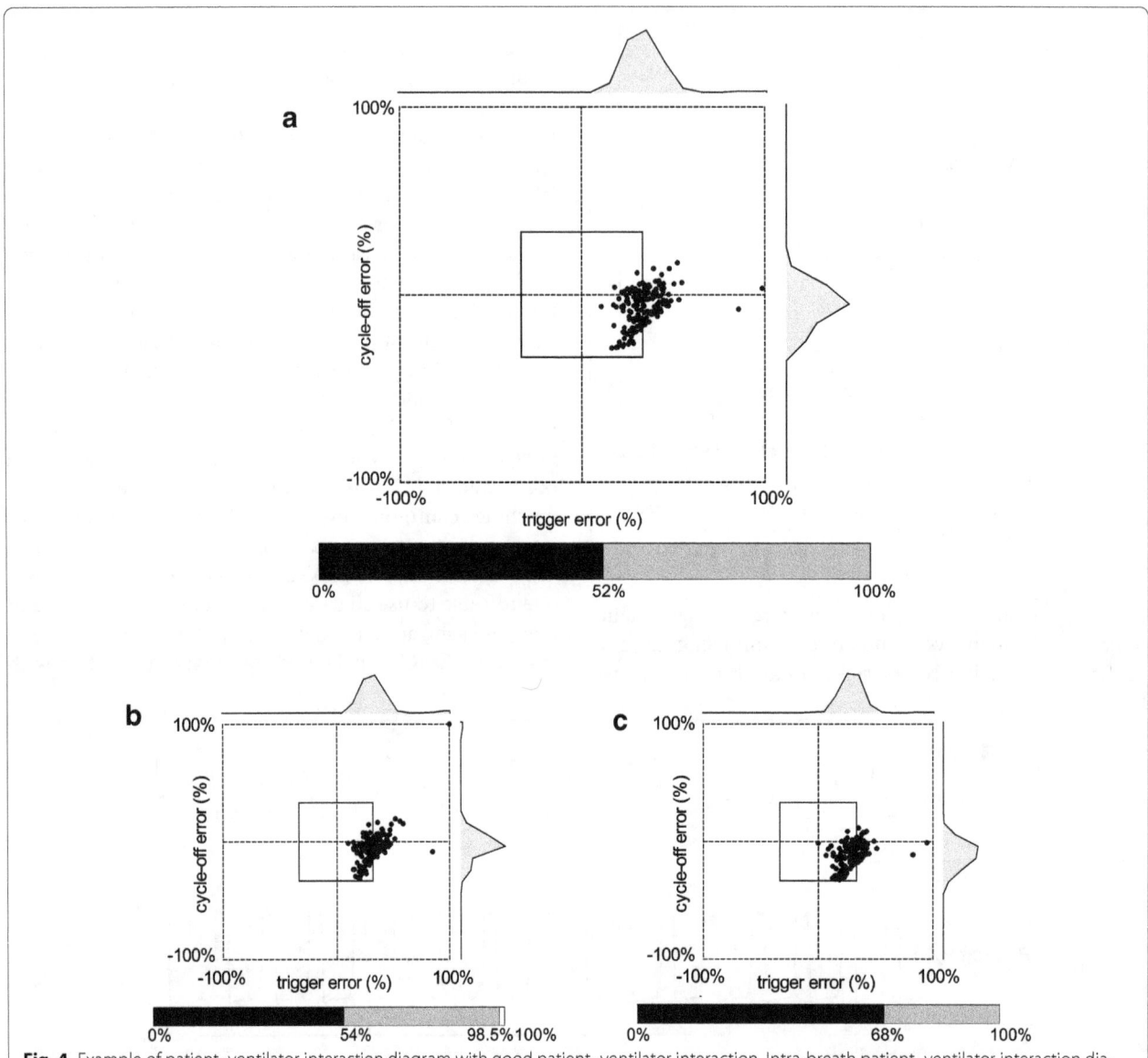

Fig. 4 Example of patient–ventilator interaction diagram with good patient–ventilator interaction. Intra-breath patient–ventilator interaction diagrams resulting from automated (**a**) and manual analysis by experts 1 (**b**) and 2 (**c**) are shown. Histograms of trigger and cycle-off errors are shown above and right of interaction diagrams. Stacked bar charts showing the relative distribution of events are depicted under the interaction diagrams. Corresponding NA and Paw tracings are shown in Fig. 3a

the exact determination of the onset and termination of the neural inspiration. Yet, Hutten et al. used a dEMG signal in which such a filter removed the ECG signal. They found that this filtered signal correlated well with tidal airflow and was fairly robust against time delays [26].

In our previous study, we found that PVA was extremely common in mechanically ventilated children and the predominant type was ineffective triggering [4]. There was some type of asynchrony in one out of every three breaths. Unlike the present study, we had detected PVA by analyzing the ventilator flow and pressure

waveforms. Such a method is prone to underreporting the true prevalence of PVA [10]. This is confirmed by the results from the present study, in which we found that only 12.2% (1.9–33.8) of breaths was synchronous. Thus, incorporating dEMG measurements and analyzing the waveforms automatically using the dEMG-phase scale is superior to manual analysis of ventilator waveforms alone. By incorporating the dEMG-phase scale, we were able to improve our definition of PVA [4]. For instance, breaths with relative timing differences > 33% were now classified as dyssynchronous instead of asynchronous, which may explain the difference in occurrence of PVA

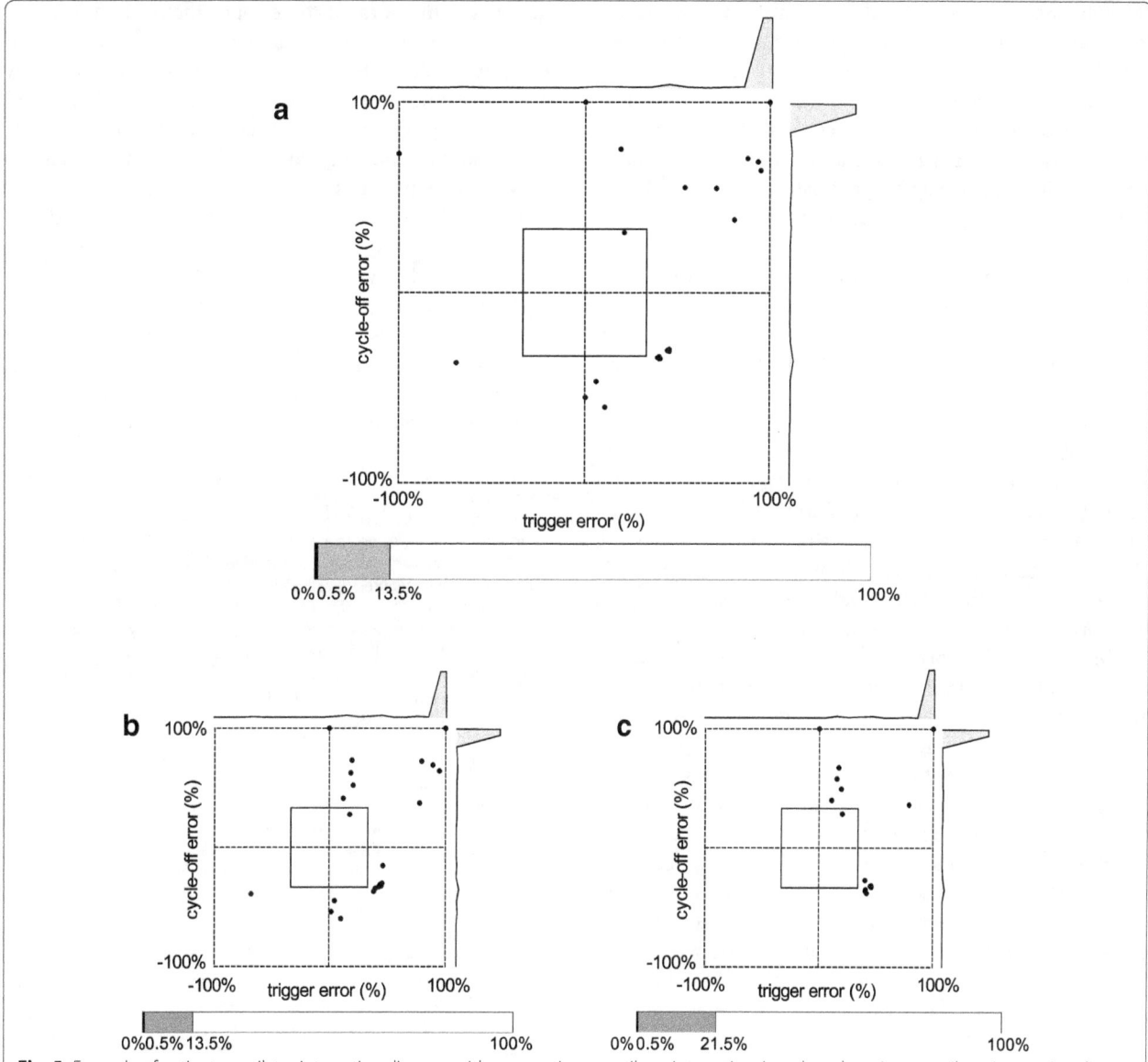

Fig. 5 Example of patient–ventilator interaction diagram with poor patient–ventilator interaction. Intra-breath patient–ventilator interaction diagrams resulting from automated (**a**) and manual analysis by experts 1 (**b**) and 2 (**c**) are shown. Histograms of trigger and cycle-off errors are shown above and right of interaction diagrams. Stacked bar charts showing the relative distribution of events are depicted under the interaction diagrams. Corresponding NA and PAW tracings are shown in Fig. 3b

Table 2 Inter-rater and inter-method agreement

	Inter-rater agreement	Inter-method agreement
Trigger error	0.92 [0.91; 0.92]	0.95 [0.94; 0.95]
Cycle-off error	0.94 [0.94; 0.95]	0.95 [0.95; 0.96]

Inter-rater and method agreements as the intra-class correlation coefficient with a 95% CI

between this and previous studies. Although the error limits were adopted from Sinderby et al., these limits were arbitrarily chosen and may not be appropriate for defining synchrony, dyssynchrony, and asynchrony in mechanically ventilated children [16]. To determine more accurate inspiration times studies comparing dEMG with the esophageal pressure versus time tracings have to be performed. In addition, in the present study we have used a different brand of ventilator (AVEA, CareFusion, Yorba Linda, CA, USA) than in our previous study (EvitaXL Draeger Medical, Lubeck, Germany). Since a poor patient–ventilator interaction is not only caused by patient but also by ventilator-related factors, it may be surmised that differences in ventilator performance may influence the observed level of asynchrony [30].

Implementing this method to quantify patient–ventilator interaction in the daily evaluation of mechanically ventilated children may be a very promising approach in individually setting the ventilator. For instance, the intra-breath patient–ventilator interaction diagram could be used to adjust the trigger sensitivity and for optimizing cycling criterion. It may be postulated that such guided individual titration may improve patient–ventilator interaction and decrease patient effort, although obviously, this assumption needs to be confirmed in clinical studies. To date, only in observational adults studies a significant association between the level of asynchrony and prolonged duration of mechanical ventilation and mortality has been shown [1, 2]. Pediatric data are lacking. However, a better understanding of patient–ventilator interaction by means of dEMG monitoring may aid in understanding the effects of dys- and asynchrony on patient outcome in ventilated children.

Some limitations of our study need to be discussed. First we used the surface EMG of the diaphragm in the same manner as the EADi signal. To our best knowledge, no correlation studies between the surface EMG and EADi have been performed. Sinderby et al. have shown in a small study population that peak EAdi signals obtained from esophageal catheter were comparable with peak costal surface EMG signal [31]. This manuscript shows that automatic algorithms for transcutaneous electromyographic respiratory muscle recordings to quantify patient–ventilator interaction in mechanically ventilated children can be developed. However, this does not mean surface EMG is equivalent to EADi measurements. More validation studies need to be performed. Secondly, we included patients in the 24 h prior to extubation. The rationale for this was the expectation that patients in the weaning phase are likely to have more interaction with the ventilator. In fact, Emeriaud et al. indeed showed a significant lower diaphragm activity during the acute phase of illness [32]. Last, it should be noted that currently to estimate a patient's respiratory center output, only dEMG was analyzed. Analyzing both dEMG and EMG of intercostal muscles simultaneously may have an added value in patients characterized by an early trigger error, because the ventilator might be triggered by inspiratory flow generated by intercostal muscle activity. Moreover, it is shown that external intercostal muscles are normally stimulated before the diaphragm as an initial stabilization of the chest wall to make diaphragmatic contraction more efficient [33].

Conclusions

The transcutaneously measured electrical activation of the diaphragm is a useful signal for evaluating and monitoring patient–ventilator interaction. The dEMG-phase scale was demonstrated to be reproducible and to be an accurate scale to quantify patient–ventilator interaction of mechanically ventilated children. This method may have important implications for both clinical use and research purposes, as it is not restricted to a type of ventilator and it is a non-invasive tool implying that it can be easily implemented in the pediatric population.

The described method could be the first step to determine the effects of patient–ventilator synchrony, dyssynchrony and asynchrony in mechanically ventilated children. Further research is needed to validate cut-off points used in this study. Finally, validation studies are needed to explore the correlation between electrical signals from the diaphragm measured transcutaneously and EADi signals obtained by an esophageal catheter.

Abbreviations

dEMG: transcuonaeous recording of the electromyographic signals of the diaphragm; ETT: endotracheal tube; FiO_2: fraction of inspired oxygen; ICC: intra-class correlation coefficient; ICU: intensive care unit; multiple MV with NA: multiple ventilatory pressurizations with one neural activity; multiple NA with MV: multiple neural activities within one ventilatory pressurization; MV without NA: ventilatory pressurization without neural activity; MV: mechanical ventilation; MV_{OFF}: end of ventilator pressurization; MV_{ON}: beginning of ventilator pressurization; NA without MV: neural activity without ventilatory pressurization; NA_{OFF}: termination of neural inspiration; NA_{ON}: onset of neural inspiration; PAP: pressure above peep; PC/AC: pressure controlled assist control; PC/SIMV + PSV: pressure controlled/synchronized intermittent mandatory ventilation + pressure support ventilation; PEEP: positive end-expiratory pressure; PICU: pediatric intensive care unit; PIM: Pediatric Index of Mortality; PIP: peak inspiratory pressure; Pmean: mean airway pressure; PRISM: Pediatric RISk of Mortality; PRVC/SIMV + PSV: pressure regulated volume controlled/synchronized intermittent mandatory ventilation + pressure support ventilation; PSV: pressure support ventilation; PVA: patient–ventilator asynchrony; RMS: root mean square; VOXP: Ventilator Open XML Protocol; V_T: expiratory tidal volume.

Authors' contributions

AAK and RGTB provided equally to the manuscript and share first authorship. AAK and RGTB collected and analyzed the data. RGTB drafted the manuscript. JB contributed to the statistical analysis and provided intellectual content to the manuscript. LvE and FdJ advised on EMG analysis and provided intellectual content to the manuscript. MK supervised the study and is responsible for the final version of the manuscript. All authors read and approved the final manuscript.

Author details

[1] Division of Paediatric Intensive Care, Department of Paediatrics, Beatrix Children's Hospital, University Medical Center Groningen, The University of Groningen, Internal Postal Code CA 62, P.O. Box 30.001, 9700 RB Groningen, The Netherlands. [2] Inbiolab B.V., Groningen, The Netherlands. [3] Faculty of Science and Technology, University of Twente, Enschede, The Netherlands. [4] Department of Epidemiology, University Medical Center Groningen, The University of Groningen, Groningen, The Netherlands. [5] Division of Paediatric Intensive Care, Department of Paediatrics, VU University Medical Center, Amsterdam, The Netherlands. [6] Critical Care, Anesthesia, Peri-operative Medicine and Emergency Medicine (CAPE), The University of Groningen, Groningen, The Netherlands.

Acknowledgements

None.

Competing interests

The authors declare that they have no competing interests.

Funding

Not applicable.

References

1. de Wit M, Miller KB, Green DA, Ostman HE, Gennings C, Epstein SK. Ineffective triggering predicts increased duration of mechanical ventilation. Crit Care Med. 2009;37(10):2740–5.
2. Blanch L, Villagra A, Sales B, Montanya J, Lucangelo U, Lujan M, Garcia-Esquirol O, Chacon E, Estruga A, Oliva JC, et al. Asynchronies during mechanical ventilation are associated with mortality. Intensive Care Med. 2015;41(4):633–41.
3. Thille AW, Rodriguez P, Cabello B, Lellouche F, Brochard L. Patient-ventilator asynchrony during assisted mechanical ventilation. Intensive Care Med. 2006;32(10):1515–22.
4. Blokpoel RG, Burgerhof JG, Markhorst DG, Kneyber MC. Patient-ventilator asynchrony during assisted ventilation in children. Pediatr Crit Care Med. 2016;17(5):e204–11.
5. Alander M, Peltoniemi O, Pokka T, Kontiokari T. Comparison of pressure-, flow-, and NAVA-triggering in pediatric and neonatal ventilatory care. Pediatr Pulmonol. 2012;47(1):76–83.
6. de la Oliva P, Schuffelmann C, Gomez-Zamora A, Villar J, Kacmarek RM. Asynchrony, neural drive, ventilatory variability and COMFORT: NAVA versus pressure support in pediatric patients. A non-randomized cross-over trial. Intensive Care Med. 2012;38(5):838–46.
7. Nilsestuen JO, Hargett KD. Using ventilator graphics to identify patient-ventilator asynchrony. Respir Care. 2005;50(2):202–34 **(discussion 232–204)**.
8. Georgopoulos D, Prinianakis G, Kondili E. Bedside waveforms interpretation as a tool to identify patient-ventilator asynchronies. Intensive Care Med. 2006;32(1):34–47.
9. de Wit M. Monitoring of patient-ventilator interaction at the bedside. Respir Care. 2011;56(1):61–72.
10. Colombo D, Cammarota G, Alemani M, Carenzo L, Barra FL, Vaschetto R, Slutsky AS, Della Corte F, Navalesi P. Efficacy of ventilator waveforms observation in detecting patient-ventilator asynchrony. Crit Care Med. 2011;39(11):2452–7.
11. Akoumianaki E, Maggiore SM, Valenza F, Bellani G, Jubran A, Loring SH, Pelosi P, Talmor D, Grasso S, Chiumello D, et al. The application of esophageal pressure measurement in patients with respiratory failure. Am J Respir Crit Care Med. 2014;189(5):520–31.
12. Mulqueeny Q, Ceriana P, Carlucci A, Fanfulla F, Delmastro M, Nava S. Automatic detection of ineffective triggering and double triggering during mechanical ventilation. Intensive Care Med. 2007;33(11):2014–8.
13. Chen CW, Lin WC, Hsu CH, Cheng KS, Lo CS. Detecting ineffective triggering in the expiratory phase in mechanically ventilated patients based on airway flow and pressure deflection: feasibility of using a computer algorithm. Crit Care Med. 2008;36(2):455–61.
14. Nguyen QT, Pastor D, L'Her E. Automatic detection of AutoPEEP during controlled mechanical ventilation. Biomed Eng Online. 2012;11:32.
15. Blanch L, Sales B, Montanya J, Lucangelo U, Garcia-Esquirol O, Villagra A, Chacon E, Estruga A, Borelli M, Burgueno MJ, et al. Validation of the Better Care® system to detect ineffective efforts during expiration in mechanically ventilated patients: a pilot study. Intensive Care Med. 2012;38(5):772–80.
16. Sinderby C, Liu S, Colombo D, Camarotta G, Slutsky AS, Navalesi P, Beck J. An automated and standardized neural index to quantify patient-ventilator interaction. Crit Care. 2013;17(5):R239.
17. Maarsingh EJ, van Eykern LA, Sprikkelman AB, Hoekstra MO, van Aalderen WM. Respiratory muscle activity measured with a noninvasive EMG technique: technical aspects and reproducibility. J Appl Physiol (1985). 2000;88(6):1955–61.
18. Kraaijenga JV, Hutten GJ, de Jongh FH, van Kaam AH. The effect of caffeine on diaphragmatic activity and tidal volume in preterm infants. J Pediatr. 2015;167(1):70–5.
19. Kraaijenga JV, Hutten GJ, de Jongh FH, van Kaam AH. Transcutaneous electromyography of the diaphragm: a cardio-respiratory monitor for preterm infants. Pediatr Pulmonol. 2015;50(9):889–95.
20. Carnevale FA, Razack S. An item analysis of the COMFORT scale in a pediatric intensive care unit. Pediatr Crit Care Med. 2002;3(2):177–80.
21. Ambuel B, Hamlett KW, Marx CM, Blumer JL. Assessing distress in pediatric intensive care environments: the COMFORT scale. J Pediatr Psychol. 1992;17(1):95–109.
22. Prechtl HF, van Eykern LA, O'Brien MJ. Respiratory muscle EMG in newborns: a non-intrusive method. Early Hum Dev. 1977;1(3):265–83.
23. Bartko JJ. The intraclass correlation coefficient as a measure of reliability. Psychol Rep. 1966;19(1):3–11.
24. Shrout PE, Fleiss JL. Intraclass correlations: uses in assessing rater reliability. Psychol Bull. 1979;86(2):420–8.
25. American Thoracic Society/European Respiratory Society. ATS/ERS Statement on respiratory muscle testing. Am J Respir Crit Care Med. 2002;166(4):518–624.
26. Hutten GJ, van Eykern LA, Latzin P, Kyburz M, van Aalderen WM, Frey U. Relative impact of respiratory muscle activity on tidal flow and end expiratory volume in healthy neonates. Pediatr Pulmonol. 2008;43(9):882–91.
27. Hutten J, van Eykern LA, Cobben JM, van Aalderen WM. Cross talk of respiratory muscles: it is possible to distinguish different muscle activity? Respir Physiol Neurobiol. 2007;158(1):1–2 **(author reply 3–4)**.
28. Winter DA, Fuglevand AJ, Archer SE. Crosstalk in surface electromyography: theoretical and practical estimates. J Electromyogr Kinesiol. 1994;4(1):15–26.
29. Ackermann KA, Brander L, Tuchscherer D, Schroder R, Jakob SM, Takala J, Z'Graggen WJ. Esophageal versus surface recording of diaphragm compound muscle action potential. Muscle Nerve. 2015;51(4):598–600.
30. Sassoon CS, Foster GT. Patient-ventilator asynchrony. Curr Opin Crit Care. 2001;7(1):28–33.
31. Sinderby C, Beck J, Spahija J, Weinberg J, Grassino A. Voluntary activation of the human diaphragm in health and disease. J Appl Physiol (1985). 1998;85(6):2146–58.
32. Emeriaud G, Larouche A, Ducharme-Crevier L, Massicotte E, Flechelles O, Pellerin-Leblanc AA, Morneau S, Beck J, Jouvet P. Evolution of inspiratory diaphragm activity in children over the course of the PICU stay. Intensive Care Med. 2014;40(11):1718–26.
33. Corda M, Eklund G, Von E. External intercostal and phrenic alpha-motor responses to changes in respiratory load. Acta Physiol Scand. 1965;63:391–400.

14

Immunohaemostasis: a new view on haemostasis during sepsis

Xavier Delabranche[1,2], Julie Helms[1,3] and Ferhat Meziani[1,2]*

Abstract

Host infection by a micro-organism triggers systemic inflammation, innate immunity and complement pathways, but also haemostasis activation. The role of thrombin and fibrin generation in host defence is now recognised, and thrombin has become a partner for survival, while it was seen only as one of the "principal suspects" of multiple organ failure and death during septic shock. This review is first focused on pathophysiology. The role of contact activation system, polyphosphates and neutrophil extracellular traps has emerged, offering new potential therapeutic targets. Interestingly, newly recognised host defence peptides (HDPs), derived from thrombin and other "coagulation" factors, are potent inhibitors of bacterial growth. Inhibition of thrombin generation could promote bacterial growth, while HDPs could become novel therapeutic agents against pathogens when resistance to conventional therapies grows. In a second part, we focused on sepsis-induced coagulopathy diagnostic challenge and stratification from "adaptive" haemostasis to "noxious" disseminated intravascular coagulation (DIC) either thrombotic or haemorrhagic. Besides usual coagulation tests, we discussed cellular haemostasis assessment including neutrophil, platelet and endothelial cell activation. Then, we examined therapeutic opportunities to prevent or to reduce "excess" thrombin generation, while preserving "adaptive" haemostasis. The fail of international randomised trials involving anticoagulants during septic shock may modify the hypothesis considering the end of haemostasis as a target to improve survival. On the one hand, patients at low risk of mortality may not be treated to preserve "immunothrombosis" as a defence when, on the other hand, patients at high risk with patent excess thrombin and fibrin generation could benefit from available (antithrombin, soluble thrombomodulin) or ongoing (FXI and FXII inhibitors) therapies. We propose to better assess coagulation response during infection by an improved knowledge of pathophysiology and systematic testing including determination of DIC scores. This is one of the clues to allocate the right treatment for the right patient at the right moment.

Keywords: Infection, Septic shock, Disseminated intravascular coagulation (DIC), Host defence peptides (HDPs), Contact phase, Neutrophil extracellular traps (NETs)

Background

The aim of this review is to describe the battle between a foreign pathogen and the host regarding thrombin generation, one of the key molecules to win or to lose the war for surviving. Thrombin is involved in thrombus formation (via fibrin network), in anticoagulation and fibrinolysis [via thrombomodulin and (activated) protein C], focalisation (via glycosaminoglycans and antithrombin), but also in vascular permeability and tone (via endothelial cell receptors and kinin pathways) [1–3].

During infection, initiation of thrombin generation may occur through different pathways [35]:

i. Bacteria initiation with endothelial invasion [4] and platelet activation (via FcγRIIa, αIIbβ3 and platelet factor 4) [5],

ii. Bacterial polyphosphate (polyP) initiation through the "contact" pathway [6],

iii. Endothelial cell expression of encrypted tissue factor (TF), vascular cell recruitment and activation by thrombin, cytokines and microparticles [1, 7, 8],

*Correspondence: ferhat.meziani@chru-strasbourg.fr
[1] Université de Strasbourg, Faculté de Médecine & Hôpitaux Universitaires de Strasbourg, Service de Réanimation, Nouvel Hôpital Civil, Strasbourg, France

iv. fibrin network, neutrophil extracellular traps (NETs) and histones [9, 10].

Haemostasis should therefore be considered as a non-specific first line of host defence—at least when localised to a unique endothelial injury—considering the growing role of platelets as immune cells [11–13]. This immune response has been called "immunothrombosis" [14]. In this line, immunohaemostasis process may help to capture pathogens, prevent tissue invasion and concentrate antimicrobial cells and peptides including thrombin-derived host defence peptides. Therefore, when regulated, a low-grade activation of thrombin generation may help survive the bacterial challenge [14]. Yet, inhibition of thrombin generation by Dabigatran promotes bacterial growth and spreading with increased mortality in experimental model of *Klebsiella pneumoniae*-induced murine pneumonia [15].

On the other hand, thrombin can become deleterious if ongoing activation of the coagulation, owing to defective natural anticoagulants, leads to excessive thrombin formation. Combined with defective fibrinolysis, thrombin results in fibrin deposits in microvessels and eventually in disseminated intravascular coagulation (DIC) [16, 17]. DIC thus represents a deregulation and/or an overwhelmed haemostasis activation response triggered by pathogens and/or host responses during septic shock [14]. DIC could be classified in "asymptomatic", "bleeding" (haemorrhagic), "thrombotic" (organ failure) and ultimately "massive bleeding" (fibrinolytic) type, according to its clinical presentation [18]. Except asymptomatic one, all types are characterised by delayed clotting times (PT and aPTT), low fibrinogen and platelets count owing to their consumption [19, 20]. Although known for many years, the role of DIC in the pathogenesis of septic shock remains a matter of debate [21–23]. Since then, coagulation was considered as a potential therapeutic target. The recognition of new targets implied in thrombosis—but not in haemostasis—opens a new window over innovative therapies.

Physiology of thrombin generation

For didactic settings, haemostasis can be separated into three phases:

i. Initiation,
ii. Propagation and regulation,
iii. Fibrinolysis.

A brief overview of haemostasis is available in Additional file 1 and Additional file 2: Figure S1 provides the different steps of thrombin generation, fibrin formation and regulation [1, 24].

Pathophysiology of thrombin and fibrin formation during infection

The contact between a prokaryote and a eukaryote can result in symbiosis or infection resulting in host or pathogen survival. To survive infection, the host initiates a complex inflammatory response including innate immunity, complement and coagulation pathways. These two cascades have a unique origin, but many refinements over the past 500 million years improved their specificities [25, 26]. In this view, coagulation is fundamental to survive and the following section will highlight the role of contact activation system (not involved in "normal" haemostasis), the interplay between pathogens, coagulation and fibrinolysis pathways, and the emerging role of antimicrobial host defence peptides generated by proteolysis of "coagulation" proteins [17, 27, 28].

Initiation: the emerging role of contact activation system (Fig. 1)
Physiology or pathophysiology?
An old view of haemostasis distinguished two initiation pathways: tissue factor ("extrinsic" pathway) and contact activation system (CAS) ("intrinsic" pathway). The latter requires a "contact" activator, prekallikrein (PK), high molecular weight kininogen (HK), factor XII (FXII) and FXI [29]. A deficit of one of these proteins results in prolonged aPTT although no haemorrhagic diathesis is evidenced in patients. CAS does not seem to be involved in "normal" haemostasis and may be restricted to pathological conditions resulting in negatively charged surfaces, including sepsis (via NETs and polyP), but also acute respiratory distress syndrome (ARDS) [30] and blood contact with artificial surfaces (intravascular catheters, extracorporeal circuits).

"Contact" activator is a negatively charged surface able to link and induce a conformational change in FXII that auto-activates FXII in α-FXIIa in the presence of Zn^{2+}. Then α-FXIIa converts PK to kallikrein (KAL) that enable a reciprocal hetero-activation of α-FXII, leading to large amount of β-FXIIa and thereafter platelet GP_{Ib}-bound FXI activation. β-FXIIa is also able to activate the classic complement system pathway via C1r and to a lesser extent C1 s linking haemostasis and complement-mediated host defence [3].

CAS and PK also activate fibrinolysis and tissue proteolysis. HK linked to urokinase-type plasminogen activator receptor (uPAR) is able to activate pro-uPA into uPA that in turn activates plasminogen into matrix-bound plasmin. Moreover, BK induces tPA release by endothelial cells when linked to B1R [2].

Besides and related to CAS, the kallikrein/kinin system (KKS) is also activated [3]. CAS and PK also activate fibrinolysis and tissue proteolysis and are regulated by

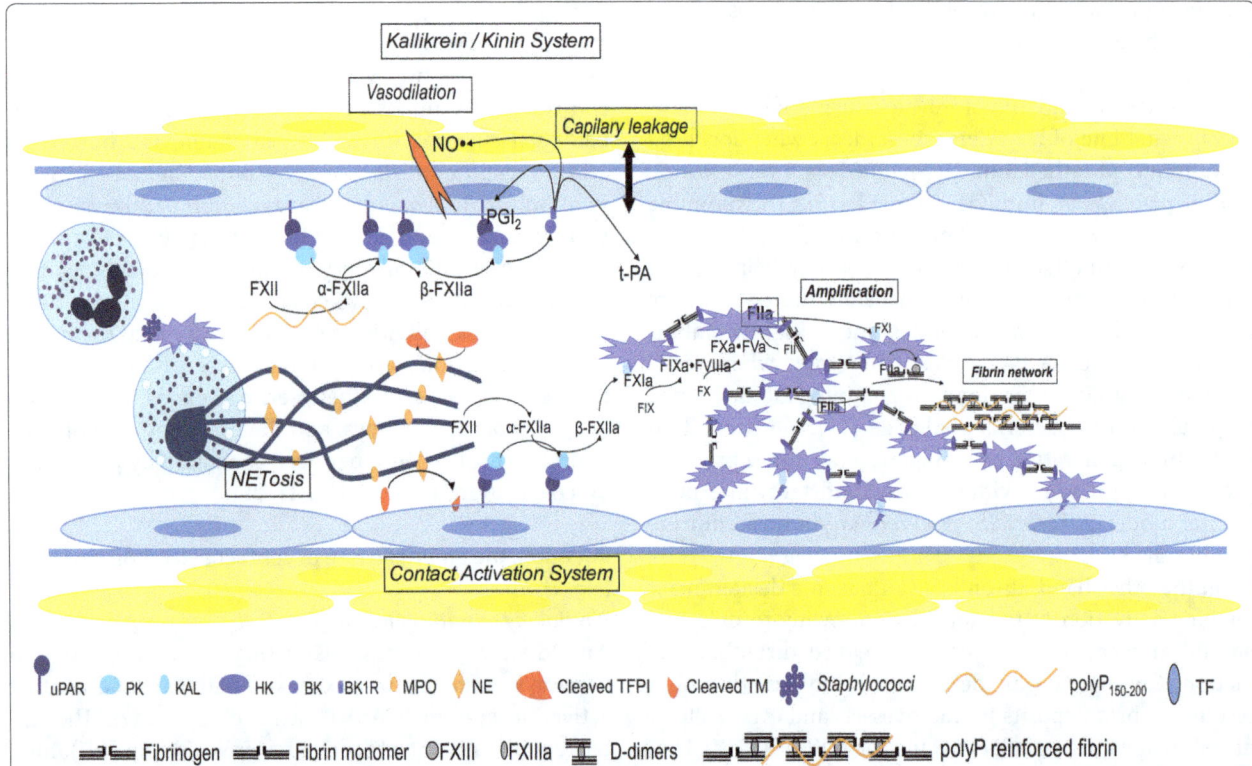

Fig. 1 Immunohaemostasis and infection. During infection, bacteria trigger platelet activation via PF4 and TLRs and can initiate neutrophil extracellular traps (NETs) release by neutrophils after chromatin decondensation and nuclear membrane disruption. Negatively charged DNA, decorated with histones, myeloperoxidase (MPO) and neutrophil elastase (NE), is a potent inducer of FXII auto-activation as well as polyphosphates (polyP$_{150-200}$) released by bacteria. Both are "contact" activators, i.e. a negatively charged surface able to link and induce a conformational change in FXII that auto-activates FXII in α-FXIIa in the presence of Zn^{2+}. Then α-FXIIa converts PK to kallikrein (KAL) that enables a reciprocal hetero-activation of α-FXII, leading to large amount of β-FXIIa and thereafter platelet GP$_{Ib}$-bound FXI activation. Large amount of FXIIa generated is able to convert platelet-bound FXI into FXIa involved in thrombin generation and fibrin generation. Interestingly, neutrophil elastase (NE) released with NETs is also able to enhance platelet adhesion and activation (inactivation of ADAMTS13) and coagulation with inhibition of tissue factor pathway inhibitor (prolonged tissue factor-induced initiation) and thrombomodulin (impaired activation of protein C). Moreover, polyP$_{150-200}$ enhances activation of platelet-bound FXI by FXIIa and can be incorporated in the fibrin network, reinforcing its structure. On the other hand the kallikrein/kinin system (KKS) is also triggered. FXIIa and KAL convert high molecular weight kininogen (HK) in biologically active bradykinin (BK). BK is not involved in thrombin generation, but mainly in inflammatory response via two G-coupled receptors, B1R and B2R. BK results in increased vascular permeability, vasodilation (mediated by both PGI$_2$ and nitric oxide after iNOS induction), oedema formation and ultimately hypotension

serpin C1 esterase inhibitor (C1-INH). A deficit (responsible for hereditary angioedema) or consumption (during septic shock but also after extracorporeal circulation) is responsible for increased permeability syndrome [31].

Polyphosphates (polyP)

PolyP are negatively charged inorganic phosphorous residue polymers, highly conserved in prokaryotes and eukaryotes. They are important source of energy, but are also involved in cell response. Half-life of polyP is very short due to their degradation by phosphatases [32, 33].

Medium-size soluble polyP$_{60-80}$ are released by activated platelets and mast cells. They are able to induce FXII activation only if large amounts are present [34, 35]. PolyP$_{60-80}$ could also bind α-FXIIa preventing further degradation, resulting in prolonged half-life. In the presence of fibrin polymers associated with polyP$_{60-80}$, α-FXIIa can activate fibrin-bound plasminogen in plasmin, resulting in "intrinsic" fibrinolytic activity overcoming antifibrinolytic properties [36, 37]. Interestingly, activated platelets could retain polyP$_{60-80}$ on their surface assembled into insoluble spherical nanoparticles with divalent metal ions (Ca^{2+}, Zn^{2+}). These nanoparticles provide higher polymer size and become able to trigger contact system activation [38, 39].

On the other hand, large-sized insoluble polyP$_{150-200}$ are released by bacteria and yeasts. PolyP$_{150-200}$ are able to support auto-activation of FXIIa and to promote thrombin generation independently of FXI activation. PolyP can bind FM resulting in clots with reduced stiffness and increased deformability [40]. Moreover, polyP$_{150-200}$ are incorporated in fibrin mesh, inhibiting fibrinolysis [34].

Neutrophil extracellular traps (NETs)

Neutrophils have long been considered as suicidal cells killing extracellular pathogens. Few years ago, biology of neutrophils has evolved for a more complex network linking innate immunity, adaptive immunity and haemostasis [41–43]. Neutrophils do not only engulf pathogens (phagocytosis) and release granules content, but also release their nuclear content, essentially histones and DNA fragments resulting in a net. These NETs support histones and other granule enzymes like myeloperoxidase (MPO) and neutrophil elastase (NE). These fragments are called NETs for neutrophils extracellular traps, and they enable to trap pathogens and blood cells, including platelets, in their meshes [44].

Two mechanisms of NETosis are described: a suicidal one [44–46] and a vital one, with functional anucleated phagocytic cell survival [47]. Finally, the plasma membrane bursts and NETs are released [48].

NETosis plays a critical role in host defence through innate immunity, but also through other procoagulant mechanisms:

i. Negatively charged DNA constitutes an activated surface for coagulation factors assembly, including contact phase;
ii. Enzymatic inhibition of tissue factor pathway inhibitor (TFPI) and thrombomodulin (TM) by neutrophil elastase;
iii. Direct recruitment and activation of platelets by histones [14].

Recent data support a direct activation by DNA and histones more than NETs themselves [49]. High levels of circulating histones have been evidenced in septic shock. Histone infusion induces intravascular coagulation with thrombocytopenia and increased D-dimers. Antihistone antibodies can prevent both lung and cardiac injuries in experimental models. C-reactive protein can bind histones and reduce histone-induced endothelial cell injury. C-reactive protein infusion rescues histone-challenged mouse [50].

Pathogen-induced modulation of blood coagulation (Table 1)

Initiation of coagulation

All bacteria can induce blood coagulation in a polyP-dependent pathway as seen above. High molecular weight kininogen (HK) can also bind bacterial surface allowing a better activation by host proteases [51]. Interestingly, some bacteria use specific pathways to induce thrombin and fibrin generation [52–58].

Degradation of fibrin clots

Fibrin formation and pathogen entrapment are key features of host defence during infection. Fibrin(ogen) is fundamental to survive infection [59]. To evade fibrin, many bacteria developed fibrinolysis activators or expressed plasminogen receptors allowing activation by host tPA or uPA [60–76].

Outer membrane proteins (omptins) are surface-exposed, transmembrane β-barrel proteases exposed by some gram-negative bacteria. They display fibrinolytic and procoagulant activities required for pathogenicity [71, 72]. *Yersinia pestis* is the agent of bubonic and pneumonic plague. Both associate haemorrhagic and thrombotic disorders and the presence of Pla, a direct activator of host plasminogen, require rough LPS. Pla is also able to promote fibrinolysis by activation of uPA, inactivation of serpins PAI-1 and α_2-antiplasmin and by cleavage of C-terminal region of TAFI with reduced activation by thrombin–thrombomodulin complex [73, 74]. Pla is also able to cleave TFPI. Interestingly, dysplasminogenemia (Ala^{601} → Thr), present in about 2% of the Chinese, Korean and Japanese populations, confers a protection against plague. Homozygous individuals have a reduced plasminogen activity about 10% with fewer thrombotic events, but enhanced survival during infection by *Y. pestis* but also by group A *streptococci* and *S. aureus* requiring plasminogen activation for pathogenicity [75].

Inactivation of fibrinolysis

Inhibition of fibrinolysis is another way to promote clot stabilisation [77, 78].

Inhibition of coagulation

Bacteria can also block contact activation pathway [79, 80] or thrombin generation [81] in order to prevent host defence.

Host defence peptides

Innate immunity is mediated by cell activation via Toll-like receptors (TLRs). Resulting cationic and amphipathic small peptides (15–30 amino acids, < 10 kDa) have many biological properties including direct bactericidal effects, but also immunomodulation and angiogenesis. They have been named "host defence peptides" (HDPs) or "antimicrobial peptides" (AMPs).

In eukaryotes, we can identify defensins (disulphide-stabilised peptides) and cathelicidins (α-helical or

Table 1 Pathogen-induced modulation of blood coagulation

Bacteria	Protein	Target	Result	References
A—initiation of coagulation				
All bacteria	PolyP	FXII → FXIIa	Contact phase activation (FXI)	[51]
S. aureus	Coagulase	FII → FIIa	Non-proteolytic activation	[52]
	von Willebrand binding protein (vWbp)	vWF (endothelium)	*S. aureus* anchorage to endothelium	[53]
		FII → FIIa	Non-proteolytic activation	[52]
		vWbp-FIIa → FXIII	Clot stabilisation	[53]
	Clumping factor A (ClfA) and fibronectin-binding protein A (FnbpA)	Fg	*S. aureus*—platelet bridging and clot formation	[54]
	Staphopains A and B (ScpA, ScpB)	HK → BK	Vascular leakage	[55, 56]
Group G *streptococci*	Fibrinogen-binding protein (FOG) and protein G (PG)	FXII → FXIIa	Contact phase complex assembly and activation (FXI) at bacterial surface	[57]
B. anthracis	Zinc metalloprotease InhA1	FX → FXa/FII → FIIa	Fibrin deposition	[57, 58]
		ADAMTS13 inhibition	Platelet adhesion/activation by UL-vWF	[58]
B—degradation of fibrin clot				
B. burgdorferi	Outer surface proteins (OspA and OspC) and Erp proteins (ErpA, ErpC and ErpP)	Plasmin(ogen)	Plasminogen activation by tPA/uPA	[62]
H. influenzae	Surface protein E (PE)	Plasmin(ogen)	Plasminogen activation by tPA/uPA	[63]
Streptococci spp.	α-Enolase	Plasmin(ogen)	Plasminogen activation by tPA/uPA	[64–67]
B. anthracis	α-Enolase and elongation factor tu	Plasmin(ogen)	Plasminogen activation by tPA/uPA	[66]
S. pyogenes	Plasminogen-binding M-like protein (PAM) and streptokinase (SK)	Plasminogen	Direct non-enzymatic activation	[51]
			Metalloprotease activation and tissue invasion by PAM-bound SK·PM	[68, 69]
S. agalactiae	Skizzle (SkzL)	tPA/uPA	Enhanced plasminogen activation	[70]
Y. pestis	Omptin Pla	Plasminogen	Direct activation in presence of LPS	[71]
		PAI-1/TAFI/α₂-AP	Inactivation of serpins	[72–74]
S. enterica	Omptin PgtE	PAI-1/α₂-AP	Inactivation of serpins	[76]
C—inactivation of fibrinolysis				
Group A *streptococci*	Collagen-like proteins (SclA and SclB)	TAFI and FIIa	TAFI → TAFIa	[77, 78]
D—Inhibition of coagulation				
Group A *streptococci*	Streptococcal inhibitor of complement (SIC)	HK	Inhibition of HK binding and contact phase activation	[79, 80]
S. aureus	Staphylococcal superantigen-like protein 10 (SSLP-10)	FII	Inhibition of platelet binding and activation	[81]

extended peptides). HDPs can be classified into three categories regarding their target on prokaryotes:

i. Plasma membrane-active peptides disrupting membrane integrity,
ii. Intracellular inhibitors of transcription or translational factors and
iii. Cell wall-active peptides interfering with cell wall synthesis and bacterial replication [82].

Limited proteolysis of many proteins involved in blood coagulation (activators as well as inhibitors) is now recognised as HDPs and may participate to host defence. Interestingly, the development of synthetic HDPs is a new therapeutic anti-infectious strategy regarding resistance of pathogens to (conventional) antibiotics [83].

Serine protease-derived peptides
Human serine proteases (including vitamin K-dependent blood coagulation factors and kallikrein system peptides) can be cleaved by proteases to generate C-terminal peptides with direct antimicrobial activities [84]. GKY25 is released from FIIa, FXa and FXIa after cleavage by neutrophil elastase [85]. This peptide is able to slightly reduce *P. aeruginosa* growth but also to significantly reduce both inflammatory response and mortality [86]. Bacteria are also able, mainly by unknown mechanisms, to generate HDPs from fibrinogen (GHR28) and high molecular weight kininogen (HKH20 and NAT26).

Serpin-derived peptides
Serpins (or serine protease inhibitors) can also generate HDPs. Heparin cofactor II (HCII) can be cleaved

by neutrophil elastase after binding to glycosaminogly-can [87], and KYE28 displays antimicrobial properties against gram-negative and gram-positive bacteria but also against fungus [87]. Moreover, KYE28 can bind LPS dampening inflammatory response [88]. FFF21 derived from antithrombin also shares antimicrobial activity after permeabilisation of bacterial membrane [89]. Protein C inhibitor-derived SEK20 peptide displays antimicrobial activity [90]. Interestingly, platelets can bind PCI under activation resulting in high concentration of PCI at site of platelet recruitment as observed during infection [91].

Diagnosis

Activation of the coagulation cascade is a physiologic, innate and adaptive response during infection. This response can be overwhelmed, becoming hazardous and referred to as DIC meaning disseminated intravascular coagulation, as well as "death is coming" [92]. For many years, only two conditions were distinguished: "no DIC" and "DIC". This "schizophrenic" view of haemostasis needs to be reissued, as proposed by Dutt and Toh [93]: "The Ying-Yang of thrombin and protein C". There is indeed a *continuum* from adaptive to noxious thrombin generation. Moreover, DIC remains a medical paradigm for critical care physicians: clinical diagnosis is often (too) late and biological diagnosis (too) frequent in the absence of clinical signs or therapeutic opportunities [94].

Clinical diagnosis

Most patients with sepsis and septic shock do not present any clinical sign of "coagulopathy", while routine laboratory tests are disturbed. Clinical examination should focus on purpura, symmetric ischaemic limb gangrene (with pulses) [95] and diffuse oozing. A very specific sign is "retiform purpura", which is a netlike purpura reminiscent of livedo. However, unlike classic livedo, in which meshes are erythematous, meshes are here purpuric. The absence of induced bleeding on retrieval when the skin is punctured to a depth of 3 to 4 mm within a livid or purpuric area is a good indication of thrombotic microangiopathy [96].

Laboratory criteria

A single test will never be able to diagnose and stratify sepsis-induced coagulopathy. Only a combination of the presence of underlying disease associated with evidence of cellular activation in the vascular compartment (including endothelial cells, leucocytes and platelets), procoagulant activation, fibrinolytic activation, inhibitor consumption and end-organ damage or failure will allow such diagnosis.

Underlying disease

In sepsis and septic shock, vascular injury is central and prompted by different actors with overlapping kinetics, leading to difficulties in deciphering a sequential order [97].

Acute kidney injury (AKI) is present in about half patients, one-third of non-DIC patients *versus* four-fifth in DIC patients. This association between AKI and low platelets may be symptomatic of thrombotic microangiopathy (TMA) all the more that Ono et al. [98] reported low ADAMTS13 activity and high UL-vWF in septic shock-induced DIC. Nevertheless, there are two important differences: the presence of schizocytes and the absence of prolonged clotting times in TMAs [99, 100].

Hepatic injury is frequent, but remains mild to moderate, with a slight increase in liver enzymes and bilirubin and decrease in PT. On the other hand, severe hepatic ischaemia may lead to fulminant hypoxic hepatitis with very low PT, but also inhibitors AT and PC mimicking DIC with ischaemic limb gangrene with pulses [101].

Cellular activation

Only indirect markers of cellular activation are available; most of them are not routinely assessed. These markers could be soluble molecules (released by shedding or by proteolytic cleavage) or cell-derived microvesicles, including microparticles (MPs). The role of MPs in septic shock and infection has been discussed elsewhere [102–104].

Endothelial cells E-selectin (CD62E), or endothelial-leucocyte adhesion molecule-1 (ELAM-1), is only expressed by endothelial cells after cytokine stimulation. CD62E is involved in leucocyte recruitment at site of injury and could be released in the blood stream as free, soluble molecule (sCD62E) or membrane bound after MP shedding (CD62$^+$-MPs). sCD62E is dramatically increased during septic shock, especially in DIC patients [8], but was not associated with DIC diagnosis in one study [105, 106]. Interestingly, CD62$^+$-MPs were not increased in septic shock due to proteolysis [8].

Endoglin (CD105, Eng) is a membrane protein expressed mainly by endothelial cells in the vascular repair and angiogenesis during inflammation [107]. It contains an arginine-glycine-aspartic acid (RGD) tripeptide sequence that enables cellular adhesion, through the binding of integrins or other RGD binding receptors that are present in the extracellular matrix. Membrane-bound CD105 is involved in leucocyte α5β1 activation, resulting in leucocyte recruitment and extravasation on the one hand and in angiogenesis on the other hand, whereas MMP-14-cleaved soluble (s)CD105 abolishes extravasation and inhibits angiogenesis [107]. CD105 plays a pivotal role in endothelial cell adhesion to mural cells [108]. Soluble CD105 overexpression is actually linked to other typical systemic and vascular inflammation states, as pre-eclampsia and HELLP syndrome, that are also characterised by a haemostatic activation/deregulation [109] and podocyturia [108]. We evidenced the presence of CD105$^+$-MPs during septic shock, especially in DIC patients [8, 110].

Endothelial cells also release soluble and microparticle-bound EPCR. sEPCR is a marker of endothelial injury and severity [111], while EPCR$^+$-MPs can display an anticoagulant and cytoprotective pattern in the bloodstream [112, 113].

Leucocytes Neutrophils and monocytes play a major role in sepsis-induced coagulopathy. After stimulation by thrombin and cytokines, monocytes could express TF and promote thrombin generation after cell membrane remodelling and phosphatidylserine (PhtdSer) exposition. Moreover, TF$^+$-MPs of monocyte origin have been identified and could disseminate a procoagulant potential [7].

The role of neutrophils is more complex, involving both TF expression (fusion of TF$^+$-MPs) [114] and NETs [115]. Direct evidence of the presence of NETs in bloodstream is lacking, but histones (or nucleosomes), free DNA and myeloperoxidase could be detected in plasma and are significantly increased in septic shock-induced DIC [116]. Recently, our group showed cytological modification of neutrophils in blood smears of patients with DIC [117]. Moreover, we evidenced neutrophil chromatin decondensation assessed by measuring neutrophil fluorescence (NEUT-SFL) using a routine automated flow cytometer Sysmex^{TM} XN20 [118].

Platelets Inflammation resulting in systemic inflammatory response syndrome (SIRS) is a potent inducer of both fibrinogen synthesis and platelet circulating pool mobilisation. Platelet count can reach 700–800 G/L, but thrombocytopenia can occur during sepsis. A "normal" value—that is to say in the normal range—may be interpreted cautiously and represent patent consumption. Moreover, enumeration is not function. During sepsis-induced coagulopathy, platelet activation follows thrombin generation and does not support the propagation phase of haemostasis with impaired P-selectin, ADP, Ca^{2+} and cFXIII local supply.

Erythrocytes Schizocytes are fragmented erythrocytes and are the cornerstone of TMA diagnosis. They are frequently observed on blood smears during DIC and remain of poor value for DIC diagnosis [119].

Procoagulant activation

Routine coagulation tests evidence a prolongation of both prothrombin time (PT) and activated partial thromboplastin time (aPTT). Nevertheless, PT is the more accurate. aPTT is only slightly elevated during DIC due to inflammatory response and very high level of FVIII released by injured endothelial cells.

Evidence of thrombin generation can be evaluated by quantification of prothrombin fragment 1 + 2 (F1 + 2) and/or thrombin–antithrombin (TAT) complexes. These tests are not routinely available. Moreover, we evidenced the lack of discrimination of F1 + 2 between DIC and non-DIC patients despite significant differences [8].

Fibrin formation is quantified by fibrinopeptide A (FpA) (with a 2:1 ratio), not available in routine [120]. Soluble fibrin monomers (FM) can be routinely quantified. They do not represent fibrin formation, but resting fibrin monomers not yet polymerised by FXIIIa. High FM can evidence increased production and/or defective polymerisation [121, 122]. The accuracy of this biomarker is still matter of debate (see below) [123, 124].

Fibrinolytic activation

Fibrin(ogen) degradation products (FDPs) are heterogeneous small molecules generated by the action of plasmin on both fibrin network (secondary fibrinolysis) and fibrinogen (primary fibrinogenolysis). D-dimers (D-domain of two fibrin molecules stabilised by FXIIIa) are specific of fibrinolysis and must be preferred when available [125–127]. D-dimers sign thrombin generation, fibrin formation and polymerisation then fibrinolysis, while the absence of D-dimers could represent defective fibrinolysis despite the presence of fibrin. Other markers could be useful but are not available in routine laboratories: PAP (plasmin–antiplasmin complexes), tPA and PAI-1 [128, 129]. Both tPA and PAI-1 are dramatically increased during septic shock, regardless of DIC diagnosis. Early inhibition of fibrinolysis during sepsis-induced coagulopathy may cause diagnostic delay regarding the importance of FDPs in DIC diagnosis.

Inhibitors consumption

Sustained thrombin generation leads to activation, then consumption, of regulatory mechanisms. TFPI is decreased during DIC [130]. Antithrombin can be—and should be—routinely assessed during sepsis-induced coagulopathy. The absence of low AT level challenges the diagnosis of DIC [131]. Concerning the TM-APC pathway, assessment is complex. PC is decreased by consumption, but APC is increased, at least at the beginning of sepsis. Moreover, soluble forms of EPCR (sEPCR) [111] and TM (sTM) [132] can be found in plasma of septic patients and are correlated to vascular injury.

Global assessment of haemostasis

Thromboelastography (TEG) and rotational thromboelastometry (ROTEM™) are routinely used in operative theatres to monitor blood coagulation and "assess global haemostasis" [133]. Interestingly, they can also evaluate fibrinolysis at 30 and 60 min. Nevertheless, a recent Cochrane review concluded that there was little or no evidence of the accuracy of such devices, strongly suggesting that they should only be used for research [99, 100]. Few data are available regarding septic shock-induced coagulation/coagulopathy. A prospective study comparing septic shock patients, surgical patients and healthy volunteers evidences a hypocoagulability during DIC [134]. In this study, we may hypothesise that DIC patients were in "fibrinolytic" phase.

Scoring systems

Different scoring systems have been developed to ensure DIC diagnosis and are discussed in supplementary data (Additional file 1, Additional file 3: Table S1).

New therapeutic opportunities?

A syllogism precludes anticoagulant therapy during severe sepsis and septic shock: "more severe is the infection, more thrombin is generated", "more thrombin is generated, more organ failure and death supervene", so "more you prevent thrombin generation, more you will improve your patient with severe infection". This view forgets that haemostasis is mandatory to survive sepsis via many pathways, including newly recognised immunothrombosis and HDPs. In fact, "anticoagulant" treatments disrupt a tight equilibrium between pathogen and adaptive host response and may lead to more deaths in a group of patients (adaptive haemostasis) and to fewer deaths in another group (noxious haemostasis). Recognition of "noxious haemostasis" remains a medical paradigm for critical care physicians. Negative therapeutic interventions [135, 136], drotrecogin alfa withdrawal [137], but also emerging concept of immunothrombosis [14] could argue for a radical "tabula rasa" regarding coagulation during septic shock. The debate is still open and can be summarised in one question: "Should all patients with sepsis receive anticoagulation?" [138, 139]. Finally, whether immunohaemostasis/DIC clinical assessment is reliable remains a major issue (Fig. 2).

A mini-review of current (and past) therapies is provided in supplementary data (Additional file 1, Additional file 4: Table S2, Additional file 5: Table S3 and Additional file 6: Figure S2) regarding:

i. limitation of thrombin and fibrin generation,
ii. DIC with thrombotic/multiple organ failure pattern,
iii. DIC with haemorrhagic pattern.

In the following section, we will present an overview of therapies focused on immunohaemostasis activation.

Inhibition of contact pathway

Contact pathway is not necessary for "normal" haemostasis. FXII(a) and FXI(a) are new targets to develop "safe" antithrombotic drugs without antihaemostatic effects [140–142]. Moreover, these drugs could improve hypotension targeting bradykinin release.

C1-inhibitor

C1-inhibitor regulates both complement activation and FXII and could improve both capillary leakage and hypotension on the one hand and contact phase-induced thrombin generation on the other. As other serpins, C1-inhibitor is dramatically reduced in septic shock and C1-inhibitor supplementation could improve patients or renal function in short randomised trials [143–145]. Nevertheless, no large randomised trial can support its use. Interestingly, bradykinin receptor antagonist icatibant had no effect on a porcine model of septic shock [146].

FXII blockade

In a baboon model challenged with a lethal dose of *E. coli*, the monoclonal antibody C6B7 directed against FXIIa improved survival with higher blood pressure. In the treated group, the inflammatory response was reduced with lower IL-6 and neutrophil elastase release as well as complement activation. Inhibition of FXIIa was obvious with reduced BK released and fibrinolysis. Nevertheless, both groups experiment DIC with low platelet count, low fibrinogen and low FV [147]. Another FXIIa monoclonal blocking antibody is 3F7. This antibody seems to be safe as an anticoagulant in experimental extracorporeal membrane oxygenation model, with reduced bleeding compared to heparin, but no data are yet available regarding septic shock [148].

FXI blockade

14E11 is an anti-FXI monoclonal antibody that blocks FXI activation by FXIIa but not by FIIa. 14E11 displays antithrombotic properties. This molecule was used in mouse polymicrobial sepsis. Inflammation and coagulopathy were improved as well as survival after 14E11 treatment up to 12 h after bowel perforation onset. Clotting time was not modified, and no bleeding could be evidenced in this model [149].

Interestingly, FXI KO mice (FXI$^{-/-}$) evidence increased inflammatory response with impaired neutrophil functions—but not haemorrhage in lungs—in a model of *Klebsiella pneumoniae* and *Streptococcus pneumoniae* pneumonia resulting in an increased mortality. Inhibition

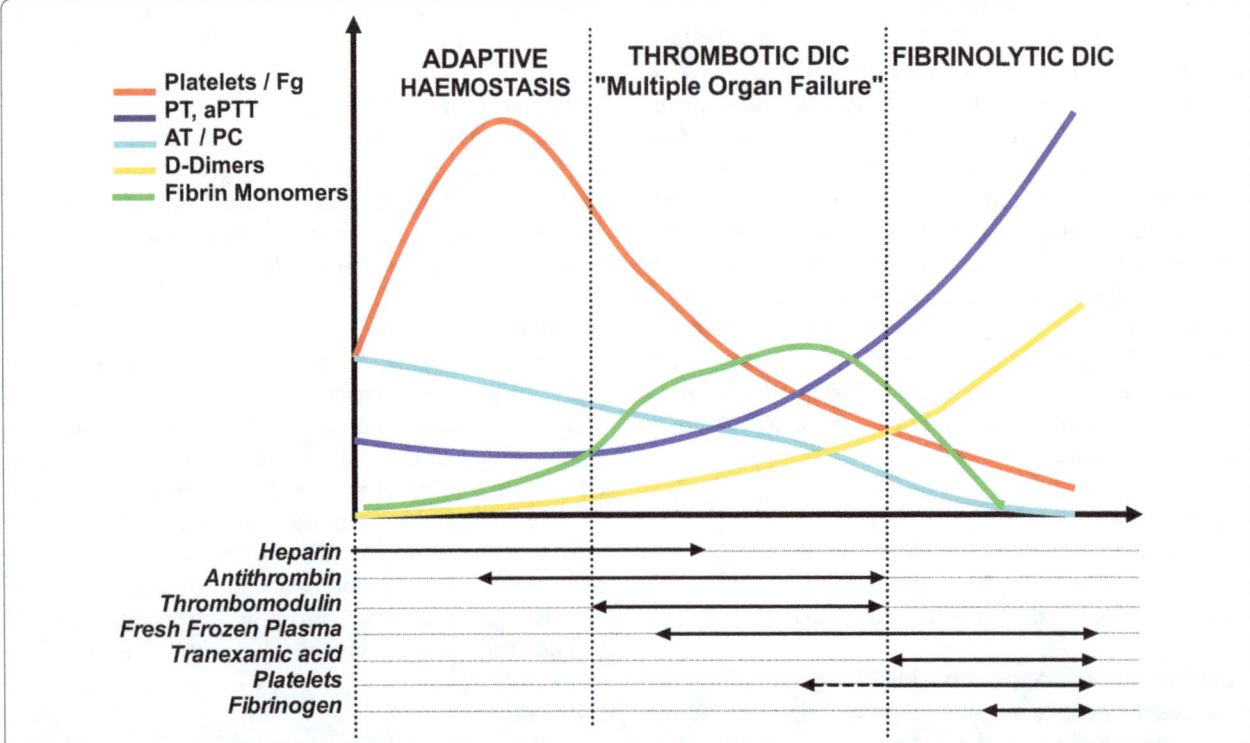

Fig. 2 Natural history of coagulation during infection and potential therapeutics. The first step is "adaptive haemostasis" associated with the systemic inflammatory syndrome. Platelet count increases and fibrinogen production is dramatically increased (red curve). Thrombin generation is initiated with slight shortening of PT and aPTT (dark blue curve) resulting in fibrin monomers generation (green curve). Natural anticoagulants, antithrombin and protein C are decreased by consumption and downregulation (light blue curve). Inhibition of fibrinolysis by PAI-1 results in low D-dimers (yellow curve). Only low-dose heparin (unfractionated or low molecular weight) could be recommended to prevent thrombosis (inferior part of the graph). Reduction of anticoagulants and continuous thrombin generation results in prolonged clotting times (PT and aPTT) and platelet and fibrinogen consumption that remain in the high normal range. Fibrin monomers increased due to sustained fibrin formation and defective polymerisation by FXIIIa. D-dimers are moderately increased. This step can be called "thrombotic/multiple organ failure DIC" step and could be treated by natural anticoagulant infusion (antithrombin or soluble thrombomodulin) or fresh-frozen plasma. Later in the natural evolution of coagulation, consumption of all factors and platelets results in very low levels of fibrinogen, AT and PC, prolonged PT and aPTT and massive fibrinolysis with very high D-dimers. This "fibrinolytic DIC" step is characterised by oozing and massive bleeding, and supportive therapy associates fresh-frozen plasma and platelet transfusions, fibrinogen supply and tranexamic acid to prevent fibrinolysis

of FXI activation by FXIIa does not reproduce this pattern [150].

A genetically engineered fusion protein (MR1007) containing anti-CD14 antibody (to block LPS receptor) and the modified second domain of bikunin (with anti-FXIa activity) improves survival in a rabbit model of sepsis without increasing spontaneous bleeding [151].

Inhibition of platelet functions in thrombus formation
Platelets are important immune cells, and thrombocytopenia is associated with an increased mortality in septic shock [152, 153]. Few data support a benefit of previous aspirin treatment in community-onset pneumonia with [154] or without septic shock [155]. In a retrospective study of patients with septic shock, chronic antiplatelet treatment was not associated with reduced mortality [156]. There are no data to support introduction

of antiplatelet therapy or to transfuse platelets in the absence of obvious thrombocytopenia with bleeding.

Inhibition of polyP
Targeting polyP is a new opportunity in the treatment of contact phase-induced thrombosis, including immunothrombosis, but some of them are toxic in vivo and cannot be used in humans (polymyxin B, polyethylenimine and polyamidoamine dendrimers) [157].

Universal heparin reversal agents (UHRAs)
UHRAs have been developed to reverse heparin effects but also displayed anticoagulant effects. UHRA-9 and UHRA-10 specifically inhibit polyP and prove antithrombotic effects without increasing bleeding in a mouse model of arterial thrombosis [158]. Nevertheless, these agents have not been used in experimental septic shock to date.

Phosphatases

Platelet-derived polyP are rapidly degraded by phosphatases. During septic shock, alkaline phosphatase activity is dramatically decreased and could enhance polyP activity. A recombinant human alkaline phosphatase (RecAP) is able to improve renal function due to acute kidney injury during septic shock [159–161]. Moreover, RecAP inhibits platelet activation ex vivo by converting ADP in adenosine and reverse hyperactivity of septic shock-derived platelets [162]. Effects on polyP were not specifically studied in this experimental study but cannot be excluded.

Dabrafenib

Dabrafenib is a B-Raf kinase inhibitor indicated in unresectable or metastatic melanoma with BRAF V600E mutation. This molecule has anti-inflammatory effects on polyP-mediated vascular disruption and cytokine production. In a mouse model of CLP-induced septic shock, administration of Dabrafenib 12 and 50 h after ligation improves survival [163].

Inhibition of NETs/histones

Deoxyribonuclease 1 (DNase 1)

Deoxyribonuclease 1 or dornase alfa (Pulmozyme®) is an inhaled potent inhibitor of bacterial DNA used in patients with cystic fibrosis. Few experimental data are available regarding NETs. In a mouse model of thrombosis, DNase 1 infusion disassembles NETs and prevents thrombus formation [164]. Interestingly, in a CLP model of sepsis, DNase 1 delayed—but not early—infusion reduces organ failure and improves outcome [165]. More recently, DNase 1 infusion in mice challenged with LPS, *E. coli* or *S. aureus* reduces thrombin generation and platelet aggregation and improves microvascular perfusion [166] and survival [167].

Interferon-λ1/IL-29

IFN-λ1/IL-29 is a potent antiviral cytokine able to prevent NETs release induced by septic shock sera or platelet-derived polyP after phosphorylation of mammalian target of rapamycin (mTOR) to downregulate autophagy. Moreover, IFN-λ1/IL-29 does not alter neutrophil viability and ROS production preserving phagocytosis. IFN-λ1/IL-29 has a strong antithrombotic activity in experimental arterial thrombosis but could also regulate immunohaemostasis [168].

Conclusion: evidence-based versus pragmatic medicine

Up to date, it is not possible to propose a unique strategy to diagnose and treat coagulation disorders during infection and septic shock. On the one hand, an "old view" consid-ered activation of blood coagulation as one of the principal ways to die and thrombin as the principal suspect. This view was the rationale for anticoagulation during septic shock, with many experimental data supporting it. Nevertheless, all clinical trials—with the exception of PROWESS trial—failed to improve survival in unselected septic shock patients. On the other hand, recent experimental and clinical data support a beneficial role of blood coagulation to survive sepsis, including immunohaemostasis. The first step to improve patients' care is to stratify the "coagulopathy". A combination of biological tests must be used daily, eventually combined in scores. We believe that JAAM 2006 and JAAM-DIC scores, taking into account the inflammatory syndrome and evolution, are the most appropriate. New markers of cell activation may be of interest. The second step is the choice of therapeutic intervention. Treatment of both infection and shock without delay is mandatory. Then, anticoagulation may be considered. To date, no recommendation can be made according to international guidelines with a high level of proof. Nevertheless, three different patterns could be recognised (Fig. 2):

i. Absence of obvious coagulopathy with high platelet count, low D-dimers, subnormal PT and AT requiring only prevention of thrombosis by unfractionated or low molecular weight heparins.

ii. Thrombotic/multiple organ failure coagulopathy (also referred as thrombotic DIC) with "low normal" platelet count, prolonged PT, decreased AT and mild to moderate D-dimers level; clinical presentation may combine organ failure and cutaneous signs like symmetric limb gangrene with pulses and retiform purpura. Antithrombin and recombinant soluble thrombomodulin must be considered. New treatments targeting FXIIa, FXIa, polyP and NETs preventing thrombosis are in development and improve survival in experimental sepsis or septic shock. They have not yet been tested in humans.

iii. Haemorrhagic/fibrinolytic coagulopathy with very low platelets, fibrinogen and AT, prolonged coagulation times and clinical oozing. Massive transfusion of fresh-frozen plasma, platelets and fibrinogen is required, with antifibrinolytic drugs.

New clinical trials are necessary to support this view and to improve patients' care.

Abbreviations

ADAMTS13: a disintegrin and metalloprotease with thrombospondin type 1 motif; CAS: contact activation system; DIC: disseminated intravascular coagulation; FDPs: fibrin(ogen) degradation products; HDPs: host defence peptides; HK: high molecular weight kallikrein; ISTH: International Society for Thrombosis and Haemostasis; JAAM: Japanese Association for Acute Medicine; KAL: kallikrein; KKS: kallikrein/kinin system; MPO: myeloperoxidase; MPs: microparticles; NE: neutrophil elastase; NETs: neutrophil extracellular traps; PCI: protein C inhibitor; Pg: plasminogen; polyP: polyphosphates; SK: streptokinase; TAFI: thrombin-activatable fibrinolysis inhibitor; TMAs: thrombotic microangiopathies; UL-vWF: ultralarge von Willebrand factor.

Authors' contributions

XD was the primary author responsible for literature search and review. XD, JH and FM were involved in the generation of the first version of the manuscript and then in critical revision, editing and generation of revised manuscript. All authors read and approved the final manuscript.

Authors' information

XD (MD, Ph.D.), consultant, JH (MD, Ph.D.), consultant and lecturer and FM (MD, Ph.D.), consultant, professor and head, all in critical care medicine—service de réanimation médicale, Nouvel Hôpital Civil—Hôpitaux Universitaires de Strasbourg, Strasbourg (France).

Author details

[1] Université de Strasbourg, Faculté de Médecine & Hôpitaux Universitaires de Strasbourg, Service de Réanimation, Nouvel Hôpital Civil, Strasbourg, France. [2] INSERM (French National Institute of Health and Medical Research), UMR 1260, Regenerative Nanomedicine (RNM), FMTS, Université de Strasbourg, Strasbourg, France. [3] INSERM, EFS Grand Est, BPPS UMR-S 949, Université de Strasbourg, Strasbourg, France.

Acknowledgements

We want to thank Asaël BERGER (MD) for literature search.

Competing interests

The authors declare that they have no competing interests.

Funding

No funding was obtained for the creation of this review.

References

1. Lane DA, Philippou H, Huntington JA. Directing thrombin. Blood. 2005;106(8):2605–12.
2. Schmaier AH. The contact activation and kallikrein/kinin systems: pathophysiologic and physiologic activities. J Thromb Haemost. 2016;14(1):28–39.
3. Long AT, Kenne E, Jung R, Fuchs TA, Renne T. Contact system revisited: an interface between inflammation, coagulation, and innate immunity. J Thromb Haemost. 2016;14(3):427–37.
4. Lerolle N, Carlotti A, Melican K, et al. Assessment of the interplay between blood and skin vascular abnormalities in adult purpura fulminans. Am J Respir Crit Care Med. 2013;188(6):684–92.
5. Arman M, Krauel K, Tilley DO, et al. Amplification of bacteria-induced platelet activation is triggered by FcγRIIA, integrin αIIbβ3, and platelet factor 4. Blood. 2014;123(20):3166–74.
6. Morrissey JH. Polyphosphate: a link between platelets, coagulation and inflammation. Int J Hematol. 2012;95(4):346–52.
7. Nieuwland R, Berckmans RJ, McGregor S, et al. Cellular origin and procoagulant properties of microparticles in meningococcal sepsis. Blood. 2000;95(3):930–5.
8. Delabranche X, Boisrame-Helms J, Asfar P, et al. Microparticles are new biomarkers of septic shock-induced disseminated intravascular coagulopathy. Intensive Care Med. 2013;39(10):1695–703.
9. Xu J, Zhang X, Pelayo R, et al. Extracellular histones are major mediators of death in sepsis. Nat Med. 2009;15(11):1318–21.
10. Kambas K, Mitroulis I, Ritis K. The emerging role of neutrophils in thrombosis-the journey of TF through NETs. Front Immunol. 2012;3:385.
11. Marshall JC. Why have clinical trials in sepsis failed? Trends Mol Med. 2014;20(4):195–203.
12. Dellinger RP, Levy MM, Rhodes A, et al. Surviving sepsis campaign: international guidelines for management of severe sepsis and septic shock: 2012. Crit Care Med. 2013;41(2):580–637.
13. Iba T, Gando S, Thachil J. Anticoagulant therapy for sepsis-associated disseminated intravascular coagulation: the view from Japan. J Thromb Haemost. 2014;12(7):1010–9.
14. Engelmann B, Massberg S. Thrombosis as an intravascular effector of innate immunity. Nat Rev Immunol. 2013;13(1):34–45.
15. Claushuis TA, de Stoppelaar SF, Stroo I, et al. Thrombin contributes to protective immunity in pneumonia-derived sepsis via fibrin polymerization and platelet-neutrophil interactions. J Thromb Haemost. 2017;15(4):744–57.
16. Angus DC, van der Poll T. Severe sepsis and septic shock. N Engl J Med. 2013;369(9):840–51.
17. van der Poll T, Herwald H. The coagulation system and its function in early immune defense. Thromb Haemost. 2014;112(4):640–8.
18. Wada H, Matsumoto T, Yamashita Y. Diagnosis and treatment of disseminated intravascular coagulation (DIC) according to four DIC guidelines. J Intensive Care. 2014;2(1):15.
19. Gando S, Wada H, Thachil J. Scientific and Standardization Committee on DIC of the International Society on Thrombosis and Haemostasis (ISTH). Differentiating disseminated intravascular coagulation (DIC) with the fibrinolytic phenotype from coagulopathy of trauma and acute coagulopathy of trauma-shock (COT/ACOTS). J Thromb Haemost. 2013;11(5):826–35.
20. Gando S, Otomo Y. Local hemostasis, immunothrombosis, and systemic disseminated intravascular coagulation in trauma and traumatic shock. Crit Care. 2015;19:72.
21. Fourrier F. Severe sepsis, coagulation, and fibrinolysis: dead end or one way? Crit Care Med. 2012;40(9):2704–8.
22. Levi M. The coagulant response in sepsis and inflammation. Hamostaseologie 2010; 30(1): 10–2, 4–6.
23. Levi M, van der Poll T. Endothelial injury in sepsis. Intensive Care Med. 2013;39(10):1839–42.
24. Versteeg HH, Heemskerk JW, Levi M, Reitsma PH. New fundamentals in hemostasis. Physiol Rev. 2013;93(1):327–58.
25. Krem MM, Rose T, Di Cera E. Sequence determinants of function and evolution in serine proteases. Trends Cardiovasc Med. 2000;10(4):171–6.
26. Davidson CJ, Tuddenham EG, McVey JH. 450 million years of hemostasis. J Thromb Haemost. 2003;1(7):1487–94.
27. Oikonomopoulou K, Ricklin D, Ward PA, Lambris JD. Interactions between coagulation and complement–their role in inflammation. Semin Immunopathol. 2012;34(1):151–65.
28. Berends ET, Kuipers A, Ravesloot MM, Urbanus RT, Rooijakkers SH. Bacteria under stress by complement and coagulation. FEMS Microbiol Rev. 2014;38(6):1146–71.
29. White GC 2nd. The partial thromboplastin time: defining an era in coagulation. J Thromb Haemost. 2003;1(11):2267–70.
30. Evans CE, Zhao YY. Impact of thrombosis on pulmonary endothelial injury and repair following sepsis. Am J Physiol Lung Cell Mol Physiol. 2017;312(4):L441–51.
31. Frick IM, Bjorck L, Herwald H. The dual role of the contact system in bacterial infectious disease. Thromb Haemost. 2007;98(3):497–502.

32. Brown MR, Kornberg A. Inorganic polyphosphate in the origin and survival of species. Proc Natl Acad Sci USA. 2004;101(46):16085–7.

33. Kornberg A, Rao NN, Ault-Riche D. Inorganic polyphosphate: a molecule of many functions. Annu Rev Biochem. 1999;68:89–125.

34. Smith SA, Choi SH, Davis-Harrison R, et al. Polyphosphate exerts differential effects on blood clotting, depending on polymer size. Blood. 2010;116(20):4353–9.

35. Semeraro N, Ammollo CT, Semeraro F, Colucci M. Sepsis, thrombosis and organ dysfunction. Thromb Res. 2012;129(3):290–5.

36. Mitchell JL, Lionikiene AS, Georgiev G, et al. Polyphosphate colocalizes with factor XII on platelet-bound fibrin and augments its plasminogen activator activity. Blood. 2016;128(24):2834–45.

37. Maas C. Polyphosphate strikes back. Blood. 2016;128(24):2754–6.

38. Verhoef JJ, Barendrecht AD, Nickel KF, et al. Polyphosphate nanoparticles on the platelet surface trigger contact system activation. Blood. 2017;129(12):1707–17.

39. Weitz JI, Fredenburgh JC. Platelet polyphosphate: the long and the short of it. Blood. 2017;129(12):1574–5.

40. Whyte CS, Chernysh IN, Domingues MM, et al. Polyphosphate delays fibrin polymerisation and alters the mechanical properties of the fibrin network. Thromb Haemost. 2016;116(5):897–903.

41. Mocsai A. Diverse novel functions of neutrophils in immunity, inflammation, and beyond. J Exp Med. 2013;210(7):1283–99.

42. Amulic B, Cazalet C, Hayes GL, Metzler KD, Zychlinsky A. Neutrophil function: from mechanisms to disease. Annu Rev Immunol. 2012;30:459–89.

43. Stiel L, Meziani F, Helms J. Neutrophil activation during septic shock. Shock. 2017. https://doi.org/10.1097/SHK.0000000000000980.

44. Brinkmann V, Reichard U, Goosmann C, et al. Neutrophil extracellular traps kill bacteria. Science. 2004;303(5663):1532–5.

45. Fuchs TA, Abed U, Goosmann C, et al. Novel cell death program leads to neutrophil extracellular traps. J Cell Biol. 2007;176(2):231–41.

46. Papayannopoulos V, Metzler KD, Hakkim A, Zychlinsky A. Neutrophil elastase and myeloperoxidase regulate the formation of neutrophil extracellular traps. J Cell Biol. 2010;191(3):677–91.

47. Pilsczek FH, Salina D, Poon KK, et al. A novel mechanism of rapid nuclear neutrophil extracellular trap formation in response to Staphylococcus aureus. J Immunol. 2010;185(12):7413–25.

48. Phillipson M, Kubes P. The neutrophil in vascular inflammation. Nat Med. 2011;17(11):1381–90.

49. Noubouossie DF, Whelihan MF, Yu YB, et al. In vitro activation of coagulation by human neutrophil DNA and histone proteins but not neutrophil extracellular traps. Blood. 2017;129(8):1021–9.

50. Abrams ST, Zhang N, Dart C, et al. Human CRP defends against the toxicity of circulating histones. J Immunol. 2013;191(5):2495–502.

51. Smeesters PR, McMillan DJ, Sriprakash KS. The streptococcal M protein: a highly versatile molecule. Trends Microbiol. 2010;18(6):275–82.

52. McAdow M, Missiakas DM, Schneewind O. Staphylococcus aureus secretes coagulase and von Willebrand factor binding protein to modify the coagulation cascade and establish host infections. J Innate Immun. 2012;4(2):141–8.

53. Thomer L, Schneewind O, Missiakas D. Multiple ligands of von Willebrand factor-binding protein (vWbp) promote Staphylococcus aureus clot formation in human plasma. J Biol Chem. 2013;288(39):28283–92.

54. Fitzgerald JR, Loughman A, Keane F, et al. Fibronectin-binding proteins of Staphylococcus aureus mediate activation of human platelets via fibrinogen and fibronectin bridges to integrin GPIIb/IIIa and IgG binding to the FcγRIIa receptor. Mol Microbiol. 2006;59(1):212–30.

55. Imamura T, Tanase S, Szmyd G, Kozik A, Travis J, Potempa J. Induction of vascular leakage through release of bradykinin and a novel kinin by cysteine proteinases from Staphylococcus aureus. J Exp Med. 2005;201(10):1669–76.

56. Wollein Waldetoft K, Svensson L, Morgelin M, et al. Streptococcal surface proteins activate the contact system and control its antibacterial activity. J Biol Chem. 2012;287(30):25010–8.

57. Chung MC, Popova TG, Jorgensen SC, et al. Degradation of circulating von Willebrand factor and its regulator ADAMTS13 implicates secreted Bacillus anthracis metalloproteases in anthrax consumptive coagulopathy. J Biol Chem. 2008;283(15):9531–42.

58. Kastrup CJ, Boedicker JQ, Pomerantsev AP, et al. Spatial localization of bacteria controls coagulation of human blood by 'quorum acting'. Nat Chem Biol. 2008;4(12):742–50.

59. Sun H, Wang X, Degen JL, Ginsburg D. Reduced thrombin generation increases host susceptibility to group A streptococcal infection. Blood. 2009;113(6):1358–64.

60. Rivera J, Vannakambadi G, Hook M, Speziale P. Fibrinogen-binding proteins of Gram-positive bacteria. Thromb Haemost. 2007;98(3):503–11.

61. Degen JL, Bugge TH, Goguen JD. Fibrin and fibrinolysis in infection and host defense. J Thromb Haemost. 2007;5(Suppl 1):24–31.

62. Brissette CA, Haupt K, Barthel D, et al. Borrelia burgdorferi infection-associated surface proteins ErpP, ErpA, and ErpC bind human plasminogen. Infect Immun. 2009;77(1):300–6.

63. Barthel D, Singh B, Riesbeck K, Zipfel PF. Haemophilus influenzae uses the surface protein E to acquire human plasminogen and to evade innate immunity. J Immunol. 2012;188(1):379–85.

64. Pancholi V, Fischetti VA. alpha-enolase, a novel strong plasmin(ogen) binding protein on the surface of pathogenic streptococci. J Biol Chem. 1998;273(23):14503–15.

65. Bergmann S, Rohde M, Chhatwal GS, Hammerschmidt S. Alpha-enolase of Streptococcus pneumoniae is a plasmin(ogen)-binding protein displayed on the bacterial cell surface. Mol Microbiol. 2001;40(6):1273–87.

66. Chung MC, Tonry JH, Narayanan A, et al. Bacillus anthracis interacts with plasmin(ogen) to evade C3b-dependent innate immunity. PLoS ONE. 2011;6(3):0018119.

67. Floden AM, Watt JA, Brissette CA. Borrelia burgdorferi enolase is a surface-exposed plasminogen binding protein. PLoS ONE. 2011;6(11):8.

68. Bisno AL, Brito MO, Collins CM. Molecular basis of group A streptococcal virulence. Lancet Infect Dis. 2003;3(4):191–200.

69. Verhamme IM, Panizzi PR, Bock PE. Pathogen activators of plasminogen. J Thromb Haemost. 2015;13(1):12939.

70. Wiles KG, Panizzi P, Kroh HK, Bock PE. Skizzle is a novel plasminogen- and plasmin-binding protein from Streptococcus agalactiae that targets proteins of human fibrinolysis to promote plasmin generation. J Biol Chem. 2010;285(27):21153–64.

71. Stathopoulos C. Structural features, physiological roles, and biotechnological applications of the membrane proteases of the OmpT bacterial endopeptidase family: a micro-review. Membr Cell Biol. 1998;12(1):1–8.

72. Haiko J, Suomalainen M, Ojala T, Lahteenmaki K, Korhonen TK. Invited review: breaking barriers—attack on innate immune defences by omptin surface proteases of enterobacterial pathogens. Innate Immun. 2009;15(2):67–80.

73. Korhonen TK, Haiko J, Laakkonen L, Jarvinen HM, Westerlund-Wikstrom B. Fibrinolytic and coagulative activities of Yersinia pestis. Front Cell Infect Microbiol. 2013;3:35.

74. Korhonen TK. Fibrinolytic and procoagulant activities of Yersinia pestis and Salmonella enterica. J Thromb Haemost. 2015;13(1):12932.

75. Ooe A, Kida M, Yamazaki T, et al. Common mutation of plasminogen detected in three Asian populations by an amplification refractory mutation system and rapid automated capillary electrophoresis. Thromb Haemost. 1999;82(4):1342–6.

76. Thomassin JL, Brannon JR, Gibbs BF, Gruenheid S, Le Moual H. OmpT outer membrane proteases of enterohemorrhagic and enteropathogenic Escherichia coli contribute differently to the degradation of human LL-37. Infect Immun. 2012;80(2):483–92.

77. Bengtson SH, Sanden C, Morgelin M, et al. Activation of TAFI on the surface of Streptococcus pyogenes evokes inflammatory reactions by modulating the kallikrein/kinin system. J Innate Immun. 2009;1(1):18–28.

78. Mook-Kanamori BB, Valls Seron M, Geldhoff M, et al. Thrombin-activatable fibrinolysis inhibitor influences disease severity in humans and mice with pneumococcal meningitis. J Thromb Haemost. 2015;13(11):2076–86.

79. Akesson P, Herwald H, Rasmussen M, et al. Streptococcal inhibitor of complement-mediated lysis (SIC): an anti-inflammatory virulence determinant. Microbiology. 2010;156(Pt 12):3660–8.

80. Frick IM, Shannon O, Akesson P, et al. Antibacterial activity of the contact and complement systems is blocked by SIC, a protein secreted by Streptococcus pyogenes. J Biol Chem. 2011;286(2):1331–40.

81. Itoh S, Yokoyama R, Kamoshida G, et al. Staphylococcal superantigen-like protein 10 (SSL10) inhibits blood coagulation by binding to prothrombin and factor Xa via their gamma-carboxyglutamic acid (Gla) domain. J Biol Chem. 2013;288(30):21569–80.

82. Yount NY, Yeaman MR. Peptide antimicrobials: cell wall as a bacterial target. Ann N Y Acad Sci. 2013;1277:127–38.

83. Yount NY, Yeaman MR. Emerging themes and therapeutic prospects for anti-infective peptides. Annu Rev Pharmacol Toxicol. 2012;52:337–60.

84. Kasetty G, Papareddy P, Kalle M, et al. The C-terminal sequence of several human serine proteases encodes host defense functions. J Innate Immun. 2011;3(5):471–82.

85. Papareddy P, Rydengard V, Pasupuleti M, et al. Proteolysis of human thrombin generates novel host defense peptides. PLoS Pathog. 2010;6(4):1000857.

86. Kalle M, Papareddy P, Kasetty G, et al. Host defense peptides of thrombin modulate inflammation and coagulation in endotoxin-mediated shock and *Pseudomonas aeruginosa* sepsis. PLoS ONE. 2012;7(12):13.

87. Kalle M, Papareddy P, Kasetty G, et al. Proteolytic activation transforms heparin cofactor II into a host defense molecule. J Immunol. 2013;190(12):6303–10.

88. Kalle M, Papareddy P, Kasetty G, et al. A peptide of heparin cofactor II inhibits endotoxin-mediated shock and invasive *Pseudomonas aeruginosa* infection. PLoS ONE. 2014;9(7):e102577.

89. Papareddy P, Kalle M, Bhongir RK, Morgelin M, Malmsten M, Schmidtchen A. Antimicrobial effects of helix D-derived peptides of human antithrombin III. J Biol Chem. 2014;289(43):29790–800.

90. Malmstrom E, Morgelin M, Malmsten M, et al. Protein C inhibitor–a novel antimicrobial agent. PLoS Pathog. 2009;5(12):18.

91. Rieger D, Assinger A, Einfinger K, Sokolikova B, Geiger M. Protein C inhibitor (PCI) binds to phosphatidylserine exposing cells with implications in the phagocytosis of apoptotic cells and activated platelets. PLoS ONE. 2014;9(7):e101794.

92. Spero JA, Lewis JH, Hasiba U. Disseminated intravascular coagulation. Findings in 346 patients. Thromb Haemost. 1980;43(1):28–33.

93. Dutt T, Toh CH. The Yin-Yang of thrombin and activated protein C. Br J Haematol. 2008;140(5):505–15.

94. Wada H, Thachil J, Di Nisio M, et al. Guidance for diagnosis and treatment of DIC from harmonization of the recommendations from three guidelines. J Thromb Haemost. 2013;4(10):12155.

95. Warkentin TE. Ischemic Limb Gangrene with Pulses. N Engl J Med. 2015;373(7):642–55.

96. Lipsker D. Ischemic limb gangrene with pulses [Correspondance]. N Engl J Med. 2015;373(24):2385–6.

97. Shapiro NI, Schuetz P, Yano K, et al. The association of endothelial cell signaling, severity of illness, and organ dysfunction in sepsis. Crit Care. 2010;14(5):R182.

98. Ono T, Mimuro J, Madoiwa S, et al. Severe secondary deficiency of von Willebrand factor-cleaving protease (ADAMTS13) in patients with sepsis-induced disseminated intravascular coagulation: its correlation with development of renal failure. Blood. 2006;107(2):528–34.

99. George JN, Nester CM. Syndromes of thrombotic microangiopathy. N Engl J Med. 2014;371(7):654–66.

100. Hunt BJ. Bleeding and coagulopathies in critical care. N Engl J Med. 2014;370(9):847–59.

101. Warkentin TE, Pai M. Shock, acute disseminated intravascular coagulation, and microvascular thrombosis: is 'shock liver' the unrecognized provocateur of ischemic limb necrosis? J Thromb Haemost. 2016;14(2):231–5.

102. Delabranche X, Berger A, Boisrame-Helms J, Meziani F. Microparticles and infectious diseases. Med Mal Infect. 2012;42(8):335–43.

103. Meziani F, Delabranche X, Asfar P, Toti F. Bench-to-bedside review: circulating microparticles—a new player in sepsis? Crit Care. 2010;14(5):236.

104. Reid VL, Webster NR. Role of microparticles in sepsis. Br J Anaesth. 2012;109(4):503–13.

105. Okajima K, Uchiba M, Murakami K, Okabe H, Takatsuki K. Plasma levels of soluble E-selectin in patients with disseminated intravascular coagulation. Am J Hematol. 1997;54(3):219–24.

106. Koyama K, Madoiwa S, Nunomiya S, et al. Combination of thrombin-antithrombin complex, plasminogen activator inhibitor-1, and protein C activity for early identification of severe coagulopathy in initial phase of sepsis: a prospective observational study. Crit Care. 2014;18(1):R13.

107. Rossi E, Sanz-Rodriguez F, Eleno N, et al. Endothelial endoglin is involved in inflammation: role in leukocyte adhesion and transmigration. Blood. 2012;16:16.

108. Rossi E, Smadja DM, Boscolo E, et al. Endoglin regulates mural cell adhesion in the circulatory system. Cell Mol Life Sci. 2016;73(8):1715–39.

109. Ramma W, Ahmed A. Is inflammation the cause of pre-eclampsia? Biochem Soc Trans. 2011;39(6):1619–27.

110. Delabranche X, Quenot JP, Lavigne T, et al. Early detection of disseminated intravascular coagulation during septic shock: a multicentre prospective study. Crit Care Med. 2016;17:17.

111. Guitton C, Gerard N, Sebille V, et al. Early rise in circulating endothelial protein C receptor correlates with poor outcome in severe sepsis. Intensive Care Med. 2011;37(6):950–6.

112. Perez-Casal M, Downey C, Fukudome K, Marx G, Toh CH. Activated protein C induces the release of microparticle-associated endothelial protein C receptor. Blood. 2005;105(4):1515–22.

113. Perez-Casal M, Thompson V, Downey C, et al. The clinical and functional relevance of microparticles induced by activated protein C treatment in sepsis. Crit Care. 2011;15(4):R195.

114. Osterud B. Tissue factor expression in blood cells. Thromb Res. 2010;125(1):10.

115. Stakos DA, Kambas K, Konstantinidis T, et al. Expression of functional tissue factor by neutrophil extracellular traps in culprit artery of acute myocardial infarction. Eur Heart J. 2015;36(22):1405–14.

116. Gould TJ, Lysov Z, Liaw PC. Extracellular DNA and histones: double-edged swords in immunothrombosis. JJ Thromb Haemost. 2015;13(Suppl 1):S82–91.

117. Delabranche X, Stiel L, Severac F, et al. Evidence of netosis in septic shock-induced disseminated intravascular coagulation. Shock. 2017;47(3):313–7.

118. Stiel L, Delabranche X, Galoisy AC, et al. Neutrophil fluorescence: a new indicator of cell activation during septic shock-induced disseminated intravascular coagulation. Crit Care Med. 2016;44(11):e1132–6.

119. Lesesve JF, Martin M, Banasiak C, et al. Schistocytes in disseminated intravascular coagulation. Int J Lab Hematol. 2014;36(4):439–43.

120. Pfitzner SA, Dempfle CE, Matsuda M, Heene DL. Fibrin detected in plasma of patients with disseminated intravascular coagulation by fibrin-specific antibodies consists primarily of high molecular weight factor XIIIa-crosslinked and plasmin-modified complexes partially containing fibrinopeptide A. Thromb Haemost. 1997;78(3):1069–78.

121. Cauchie P, Cauchie C, Boudjeltia KZ, et al. Diagnosis and prognosis of overt disseminated intravascular coagulation in a general hospital—meaning of the ISTH score system, fibrin monomers, and lipoprotein-C-reactive protein complex formation. Am J Hematol. 2006;81(6):414–9.

122. Dickneite G, Czech J, Keuper H. Formation of fibrin monomers in experimental disseminated intravascular coagulation and its inhibition by recombinant hirudin. Circ Shock. 1994;42(4):183–9.

123. Gris JC, Faillie JL, Cochery-Nouvellon E, Lissalde-Lavigne G, Lefrant JY. ISTH overt disseminated intravascular coagulation score in patients with septic shock: automated immunoturbidimetric soluble fibrin assay vs. D-dimer assay. J Thromb Haemost. 2011;9(6):1252–5.

124. Gris JC, Bouvier S, Cochery-Nouvellon E, Faillie JL, Lissalde-Lavigne G, Lefrant JY. Fibrin-related markers in patients with septic shock: individual comparison of D-dimers and fibrin monomers impacts on prognosis. Thromb Haemost. 2011;106(6):1228–30.

125. Greenberg CS, Devine DV, McCrae KM. Measurement of plasma fibrin D-dimer levels with the use of a monoclonal antibody coupled to latex beads. Am J Clin Pathol. 1987;87(1):94–100.

126. Wilde JT, Kitchen S, Kinsey S, Greaves M, Preston FE. Plasma D-dimer levels and their relationship to serum fibrinogen/fibrin degradation products in hypercoagulable states. Br J Haematol. 1989;71(1):65–70.

127. Carr JM, McKinney M, McDonagh J. Diagnosis of disseminated intravascular coagulation. Role of D-dimer. Am J Clin Pathol. 1989;91(3):280–7.

128. Boisclair MD, Ireland H, Lane DA. Assessment of hypercoagulable states by measurement of activation fragments and peptides. Blood Rev. 1990;4(1):25–40.

129. Boisclair MD, Lane DA, Wilde JT, Ireland H, Preston FE, Ofosu FA. A comparative evaluation of assays for markers of activated coagulation and/or fibrinolysis: thrombin-antithrombin complex, D-dimer and fibrinogen/fibrin fragment E antigen. Br J Haematol. 1990;74(4):471–9.

130. Fourrier F, Jourdain M, Tournois A, Caron C, Goudemand J, Chopin C. Coagulation inhibitor substitution during sepsis. Intensive Care Med. 1995;21(2):S264–8.

131. Fourrier F, Chopin C, Goudemand J, et al. Septic shock, multiple organ failure, and disseminated intravascular coagulation. Compared patterns of antithrombin III, protein C, and protein S deficiencies. Chest. 1992;101(3):816–23.

132. Gando S, Kameue T, Matsuda N, Hayakawa M, Hoshino H, Kato H. Serial changes in neutrophil-endothelial activation markers during the course of sepsis associated with disseminated intravascular coagulation. Thromb Res. 2005;116(2):91–100.

133. Hans GA, Besser MW. The place of viscoelastic testing in clinical practice. Br J Haematol. 2016;173(1):37–48.

134. Brenner T, Schmidt K, Delang M, et al. Viscoelastic and aggregometric point-of-care testing in patients with septic shock—cross-links between inflammation and haemostasis. Acta Anaesthesiol Scand. 2012;56(10):1277–90.

135. Abraham E, Reinhart K, Opal S, et al. Efficacy and safety of tifacogin (recombinant tissue factor pathway inhibitor) in severe sepsis: a randomized controlled trial. JAMA. 2003;290(2):238–47.

136. Warren BL, Eid A, Singer P, et al. Caring for the critically ill patient. High-dose antithrombin III in severe sepsis: a randomized controlled trial. JAMA. 2001;286(15):1869–78.

137. Ranieri VM, Thompson BT, Barie PS, et al. Drotrecogin alfa (activated) in adults with septic shock. N Engl J Med. 2012;366(22):2055–64.

138. Meziani F, Vincent JL, Gando S. Should all patients with sepsis receive anticoagulation? Yes. Intensive Care Med. 2017;43:452–4.

139. van der Poll T, Opal SM. Should all septic patients be given systemic anticoagulation? No. Intensive Care Med. 2017;43(3):455–7.

140. Kenne E, Renne T. Factor XII: a drug target for safe interference with thrombosis and inflammation. Drug Discov Today. 2014;19(9):1459–64.

141. Chen Z, Seiffert D, Hawes B. Inhibition of Factor XI activity as a promising antithrombotic strategy. Drug Discov Today. 2014;19(9):1435–9.

142. Labberton L, Kenne E, Renne T. New agents for thromboprotection. A role for factor XII and XIIa inhibition. Hamostaseologie. 2015;35(4):338–50.

143. Caliezi C, Zeerleder S, Redondo M, et al. C1-inhibitor in patients with severe sepsis and septic shock: beneficial effect on renal dysfunction. Crit Care Med. 2002;30(8):1722–8.

144. Zeerleder S, Caliezi C, van Mierlo G, et al. Administration of C1 inhibitor reduces neutrophil activation in patients with sepsis. Clin Diag Lab Immunol. 2003;10(4):529–35.

145. Igonin AA, Protsenko DN, Galstyan GM, et al. C1-esterase inhibitor infusion increases survival rates for patients with sepsis. Crit Care Med. 2012;40(3):770–7.

146. Barratt-Due A, Johansen HT, Sokolov A, et al. The role of bradykinin and the effect of the bradykinin receptor antagonist icatibant in porcine sepsis. Shock. 2011;36(5):517–23.

147. Pixley RA, De La Cadena R, Page JD, et al. The contact system contributes to hypotension but not disseminated intravascular coagulation in lethal bacteremia. In vivo use of a monoclonal anti-factor XII antibody to block contact activation in baboons. J Clin Invest. 1993;91(1):61–8.

148. Worm M, Kohler EC, Panda R, et al. The factor XIIa blocking antibody 3F7: a safe anticoagulant with anti-inflammatory activities. Ann Transl Med. 2015;3(17):2305–5839.

149. Tucker EI, Verbout NG, Leung PY, et al. Inhibition of factor XI activation attenuates inflammation and coagulopathy while improving the survival of mouse polymicrobial sepsis. Blood. 2012;119(20):4762–8.

150. Stroo I, Zeerleder S, Ding C, et al. Coagulation factor XI improves host defence during murine pneumonia-derived sepsis independent of factor XII activation. Thromb Haemost. 2017;117(8):1601–14.

151. Nakamura M, Takeuchi T, Kawahara T, et al. Simultaneous targeting of CD14 and factor XIa by a fusion protein consisting of an anti-CD14 antibody and the modified second domain of bikunin improves survival in rabbit sepsis models. Eur J Pharmacol. 2017;802:60–8.

152. Thiery-Antier N, Binquet C, Vinault S, et al. Is thrombocytopenia an early prognostic marker in septic shock? Crit Care Med. 2016;44(4):764–72.

153. Tsirigotis P, Chondropoulos S, Frantzeskaki F, et al. Thrombocytopenia in critically ill patients with severe sepsis/septic shock: prognostic value and association with a distinct serum cytokine profile. J Crit Care. 2016;32:9–15.

154. Falcone M, Russo A, Farcomeni A, et al. Septic shock from community-onset pneumonia: is there a role for aspirin plus macrolides combination? Intensive Care Med. 2016;42(2):301–2.

155. Falcone M, Russo A, Cangemi R, et al. Lower mortality rate in elderly patients with community-onset pneumonia on treatment with aspirin. J Am Heart Assoc. 2015;4(1):e001595.

156. Valerio-Rojas JC, Jaffer IJ, Kor DJ, Gajic O, Cartin-Ceba R. Outcomes of severe sepsis and septic shock patients on chronic antiplatelet treatment: a historical cohort study. Crit Care Res Pract. 2013;2013:782573.

157. Smith SA, Choi SH, Collins JN, Travers RJ, Cooley BC, Morrissey JH. Inhibition of polyphosphate as a novel strategy for preventing thrombosis and inflammation. Blood. 2012;120(26):5103–10.

158. Travers RJ, Shenoi RA, Kalathottukaren MT, Kizhakkedathu JN, Morrissey JH. Nontoxic polyphosphate inhibitors reduce thrombosis while sparing hemostasis. Blood. 2014;124(22):3183–90.

159. Heemskerk S, Masereeuw R, Moesker O, et al. Alkaline phosphatase treatment improves renal function in severe sepsis or septic shock patients. Critical care medicine. 2009;37(2):417–23.

160. Pickkers P, Heemskerk S, Schouten J, et al. Alkaline phosphatase for treatment of sepsis-induced acute kidney injury: a prospective randomized double-blind placebo-controlled trial. Crit Care. 2012;16(1):R14.

161. Su F, Brands R, Wang Z, et al. Beneficial effects of alkaline phosphatase in septic shock. Crit Care Med. 2006;34(8):2182–7.

162. Tunjungputri RN, Peters E, van der Ven A, de Groot PG, de Mast Q, Pickkers P. Human recombinant alkaline phosphatase inhibits ex vivo platelet activation in humans. Thromb Haemost. 2016;116(6):1111–21.

163. Lee S, Ku SK, Bae JS. Anti-inflammatory effects of dabrafenib on polyphosphate-mediated vascular disruption. Chem Biol Interact. 2016;256:266–73.

164. Brill A, Fuchs TA, Savchenko AS, et al. Neutrophil extracellular traps promote deep vein thrombosis in mice. Journal of thrombosis and haemostasis: JTH. 2012;10(1):136–44.

165. Mai SH, Khan M, Dwivedi DJ, et al. Delayed but not early treatment with DNase reduces organ damage and improves outcome in a murine model of sepsis. Shock. 2015;44(2):166–72.

166. McDonald B, Davis RP, Kim SJ, et al. Platelets and neutrophil extracellular traps collaborate to promote intravascular coagulation during sepsis in mice. Blood. 2017;129(10):1357–67.

167. Laukova L, Konecna B, Babickova J, et al. Exogenous deoxyribonuclease has a protective effect in a mouse model of sepsis. Biomed Pharmacother. 2017;93:8–16.

168. Chrysanthopoulou A, Kambas K, Stakos D, et al. Interferon lambda1/IL-29 and inorganic polyphosphate are novel regulators of neutrophil-driven thromboinflammation. J Pathol. 2017;243(1):111–22.

15

Quality of life and life satisfaction are severely impaired in patients with long-term invasive ventilation following ICU treatment and unsuccessful weaning

Sophie Emilia Huttmann[1], Friederike Sophie Magnet[1], Christian Karagiannidis[1], Jan Hendrik Storre[2,3] and Wolfram Windisch[1*]

Abstract

Background: Health-related quality of life (HRQL), life satisfaction, living conditions, patients' attitudes towards life and death, expectations, beliefs and unmet needs are all poorly understood aspects associated with patients receiving invasive home mechanical ventilation (HMV) following ICU treatment and unsuccessful weaning. Therefore, the present study aimed to assess (1) HRQL, (2) life satisfaction and (3) patients' perspectives on life and death associated with invasive HMV as the consequence of unsuccessful weaning.

Results: Patients undergoing invasive HMV with full technical supply and maximal patient care were screened over a 1-year period and assessed in their home environment. The study comprised the following: (1) detailed information on specific aspects of daily life, (2) self-evaluation of 23 specific daily life aspects, (3) HRQL assessment using the Severe Respiratory Insufficiency Questionnaire, (4) open interviews about the patient's living situation, HRQL, unsolved problems, treatment options, dying and the concept of an afterlife. Out of 112 patients admitted to a specialized weaning centre, 50 were discharged with invasive HMV and 25 out of these (14 COPD and 11 neuromuscular patients) were ultimately enrolled. HRQL and life satisfaction were severely impaired, despite maximal patient care and full supply of technical aids. The most important areas of dissatisfaction identified were mobility, communication, social contact and care dependency. Importantly, 32% of patients would have elected to die in hindsight rather than receive invasive HMV.

Conclusions: Despite maximal patient care and a full supply of technical aids, both HRQL and life satisfaction are severely impaired in many invasive HMV patients who have failed prolonged weaning. These findings raise ethical concerns about the use of long-term invasive HMV following unsuccessful weaning.

Keywords: Health-related quality of life, Home mechanical ventilation, ICU outcome, Respiratory failure, Tracheostomy, End of life

Background

Long-term home mechanical ventilation (HMV) is an increasingly used treatment option for patients with chronic respiratory failure [1, 2]. For this purpose, HMV

*Correspondence: windischw@kliniken-koeln.de
[1] Department of Pneumology, Cologne-Merheim Hospital, Kliniken der Stadt Köln gGmbH, Witten/Herdecke University Hospital, Ostmerheimer Strasse 200, 51109 Cologne, Germany

can be performed either invasively following tracheotomy, or noninvasively using face masks, the latter being the preferred mode [1]. Invasive HMV is only chosen in cases where noninvasive HMV is no longer feasible or sufficient [3]. Here, particularly in patients with neuromuscular disorders (NMDs), invasive HMV should only be electively established after detailed, fully informed consent is given for the procedures involved and their potential consequences [3].

In addition, intubation of ICU patients suffering from acute respiratory failure is often accompanied by tracheotomy if mechanical ventilation (MV) has to be applied for a longer period, or if there are foreseeable difficulties with weaning [4]. Even though many patients can eventually be liberated from invasive MV once the acute respiratory failure has been successfully treated, some still require prolonged weaning [4]. In the event that this fails, invasive HMV must once again be implemented [5].

Such patients do not usually have the opportunity during stable phases of their disease to decide whether or not they wish to become tracheotomized. While there is increasing evidence that outcome and health-related quality of life (HRQL) are improved in many patients receiving noninvasive HMV [2, 6], the impact of invasive HMV remains especially unclear in patients receiving invasive HMV after an unsuccessful attempt at weaning.

According to the Severe Respiratory Insufficiency Questionnaire (SRI), a specific HRQL measuring tool [6–8] (https://www.pneumologie.de/service/patienteninformation/patienten-fragebogen-zur-befindlichkeit-bei-schwerer-respiratorischer-insuffizienz/), we found that HRQL differed substantially among patients undergoing invasive HMV primarily following weaning failure, with scores ranging from very good to very poor [9]. Older patients with chronic obstructive pulmonary disease (COPD) and more co-morbidities showed a higher tendency for reduced HRQL than patients with NMD. In addition, some patients verbally expressed the severe limitations they faced in daily life [9]. Therefore, it appears that even the most specific questionnaires cannot fully assess the specific and complex living conditions of patients with invasive HMV.

The present study therefore aimed to assess (1) HRQL, (2) life satisfaction and (3) patients' perspectives on life and death associated with invasive HMV following unsuccessful weaning in patients with intubation and subsequent tracheostomy that have become necessary to treat acute-on-chronic respiratory failure by carrying out detailed assessments of the specific living conditions experienced by patients in their respective home environments. The purpose of this was to identify specific problems and undiscovered needs of these patients, as well as the reasons for reduced HRQL and life satisfaction following a new study different from the authors' previous one [9].

Methods

The study protocol was approved by the local ethics committee (Ethikkommission der Ärztekammer Nordrhein, Germany) and performed in accordance with the ethical standards laid down in the Declaration of Helsinki. The study was registered under the German Clinical Trials Register (DRKS00006524) with the Universal Trial Number (UTN): U1111-1159-5354. Informed written consent was obtained from all subjects or legal guardians.

Subjects

The study was performed in adult tracheotomized patients undergoing long-term invasive HMV. All patients were treated on a specialized weaning unit for prolonged weaning (Department of Pneumology, Cologne-Merheim Hospital, University Witten/Herdecke, Germany) following the need for intubation and tracheotomy due to acute respiratory failure prior to the study. Specifically, the weaning unit was accredited by the German Society of Pneumology and Mechanical Ventilation (DGP) and aims for tracheotomized patients who are ready to wean, but who still fit with the category of prolonged weaning according to international criteria while decannulation has not become successful in the external referring hospital [5].

For the purpose of the study, we screened all patients who underwent prolonged weaning (as defined by international and national guidelines [5, 10]) and were treated on the specialized weaning unit between January and December 2014. Eligible patients who died during the recruitment period, as well as those who were successfully weaned from invasive ventilation, with or without the adjunct of NIV, were not included in the final study. Thus, only patients who were discharged to an outpatient environment to continue invasive HMV following unsuccessful weaning were included in the study. A prerequisite for the study was that patients had to be acclimatized to their home environment; therefore, only patients who underwent invasive HMV for at least 2 months were included. Since the patient's ability to perceive his or her own situation was mandatory for the study, severe mental retardation served as an exclusion criterion.

Study design

All patients were visited in their home environment by a physician experienced with ICU medicine and prolonged weaning (first author) who was also experienced in performing interviews in these patients in the home environment according to previous research [9]. Four consecutive steps were performed for each patient:

1. Detailed information about sociodemographics, medical history, living situation, nursing care, medical care, MV, supply of technical aids, treatments (physiotherapy, occupational therapy and speech therapy), nursing dependency and daily living activities, social contacts, daily routine, legal guardianship, and religion/faith was collected. Information from medical documents was also recorded, and inspec-

tion of the home environment as well as interviews with patients, caregivers and relatives was carried out.

2. Based on the collated information, 23 important aspects of living with invasive HMV were defined following discussion and final agreement within the expert panel (all authors). Here, patients were required to indicate whether or not they were satisfied with each of these conditions (yes/no). Care was taken to ensure that the patients' opinion was exclusively assessed, whereby relatives, caregivers or other people were not allowed to answer these questions.

3. Patients completed the original German version of the SRI, an instrument specifically designed to measure HRQL in patients with severe respiratory insufficiency [6–8]. The SRI Questionnaire contains 49 items with seven subscales measuring different aspects of HRQL (Respiratory Complaints, Physical Functioning, Attendant Symptoms and Sleep, Social Relationships, Anxiety, Psychological Well-being, Social Functioning). Each subscale produces a score (0–100), with lower scores indicating poorer health status. The scales can be aggregated to one Summary Score. Answers are given on a 5-point Likert scale ranging from "completely untrue" to "always true". Again, relatives and caregivers were excluded from answering questions.

4. An open interview was performed by posing questions about (1) the living situation, (2) quality of life, (3) unsolved problems regarding the underlying disease, (4) treatment options, (5) dying, and (6) the concept of an afterlife. Again, the six topics for the open interview were determined within the expert group.

Statistical analysis

Demographics, numeric data and SRI values were subjected to normality testing using the Shapiro–Wilk test. All normally distributed data are presented as mean ± standard deviation. Non-normally distributed data (Shapiro–Wilk with P value < 0.05) are provided as median values with minimum and maximum values. Binary data are presented with absolute numbers and percentages [n (%)].

Group comparison of SRI results was performed with respect to (1) the underlying disease (NMD vs. COPD) and (2) the individual's attitude towards tracheostomy and invasive HMV (no regret vs. regret). Therefore, paired t tests were used for normally distributed data. A nonparametric test (Wilcoxon–Mann–Whitney rank-sum test) was used on non-normally distributed data. Group effects were estimated with 95% confidence intervals and tested with a 2-sided level of 0.05.

Results

A flow chart of the study cohort is displayed in Fig. 1.

A total of 25 patients (10 females, median age 64 years, min/max 20;82 years, 14 primarily with COPD, 11 with NMD) were visited in their home environment and intensively studied as outlined in Methods section. Further demographic data, disease classifications, co-morbidities, but also patients' marital statuses and education are listed in Additional file 1: Tables S1 and S2, respectively. Self-evaluation of the relevant daily life aspects is illustrated in Fig. 2.

Overall, 23 different topics were rated by the patients. Data are also provided according to disease categories, showing that COPD patients are more frequently unsatisfied than neuromuscular patients with regard to the 23 listed aspects (Additional file 1: Table S3). Adding to this, detailed information on the underlying circumstances for each of the 23 topics is listed in Additional file 1: Table S4.

As an example, two of the 23 topics (No. 10, Fig. 3 and No. 1, Fig. 4) are illustrated according to the underlying disease.

To this end, the topic most frequently reported as being unsatisfactory was mobility. In particular, a much larger proportion of COPD patients (85.7%) were unsatisfied with their mobility compared to NMD patients (45.5%) (Additional file 1: Table S3). Only one patient (4%) was able to get out of bed without help, 23 patients (92%) were dependent on technical aids and/or personal help and one patient (4%) could not leave the bed at all. However, all patients had individually prescribed technical aids for mobility such as wheel chairs, rollators and lifters (Additional file 1: Table S4). Furthermore, leaving the house with or without help was only possible for 16 patients (64%). Excursions and travelling were possible for 13 (52%) and two patients (8%), respectively.

Regarding the question about "choosing tracheostomy again, in hindsight", 42.9% of COPD patients ($N=6$) and 18.2% of NMD patients ($N=2$; one with amyotrophic lateral sclerosis, one with spinal cord injury) indicated that they would have refused to have a tracheotomy if they had to choose again. Importantly, this question was raised under the assumption that the alternative to tracheotomy was death, as communicated to all patients during the interview. Unfortunately, it remains unclear whether some of these patients eventually asked for withdrawing of mechanical ventilation. Of note, tracheotomy dated back to a median of 23 months (min 6; max 145 months), with no difference between patients who refused and those who didn't. Seven out of eight and 8/8 patients who would have refused a tracheotomy indicated dissatisfaction with MV and mobility, respectively. Finally, 18 patients (72%) had had unplanned hospital

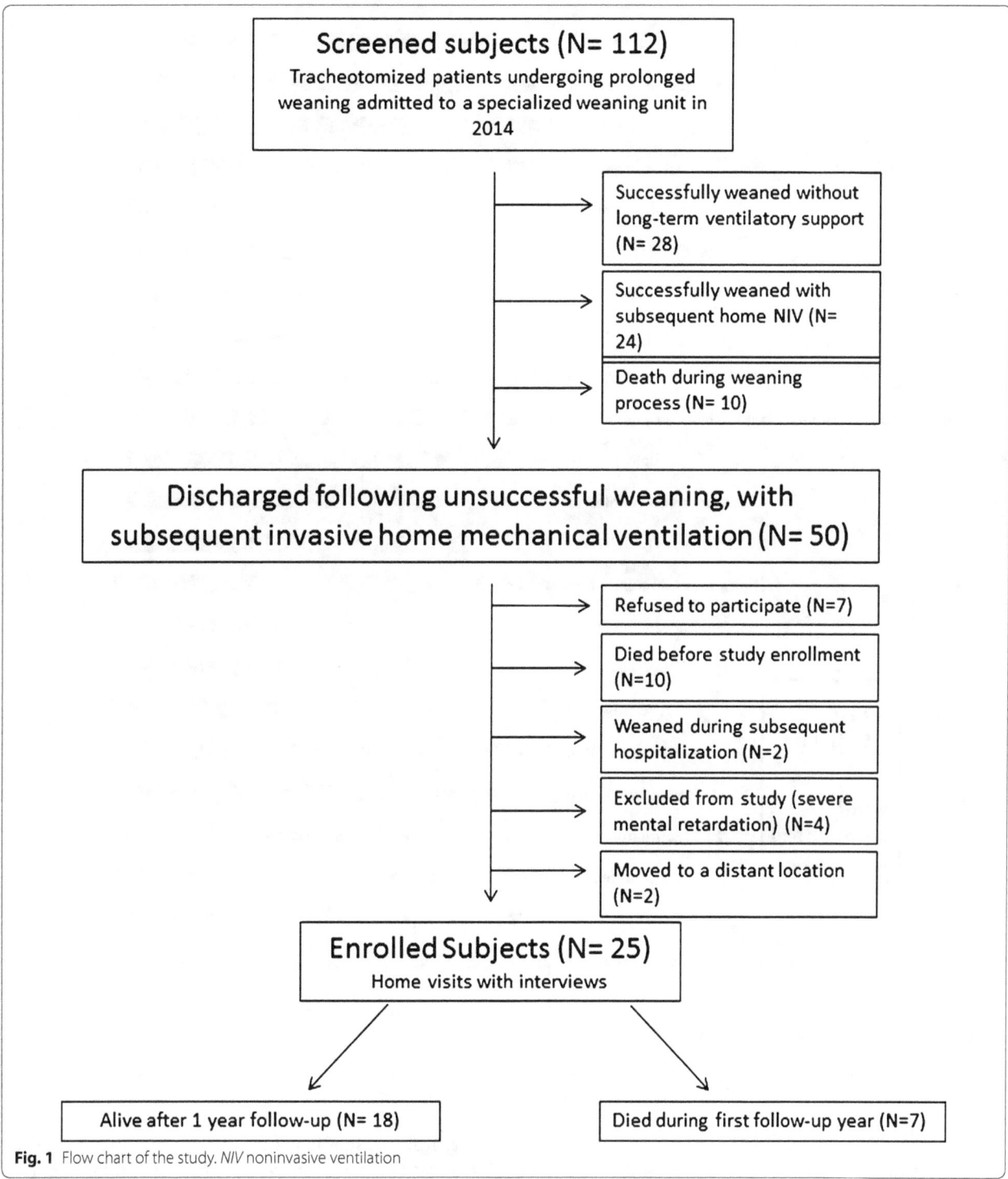

Fig. 1 Flow chart of the study. *NIV* noninvasive ventilation

admissions for the management of acute deteriorations prior to the study.

Another important issue addressed in the interview was communication. In order to communicate, 21 (84%) patients required technical aids (Additional file 1: Table S4). Despite this, the ability to speak was impaired in 48% of patients, to write by hand in 24%, and to write using a computer in 48%. Remarkably, three NMD patients could only communicate with eye movements.

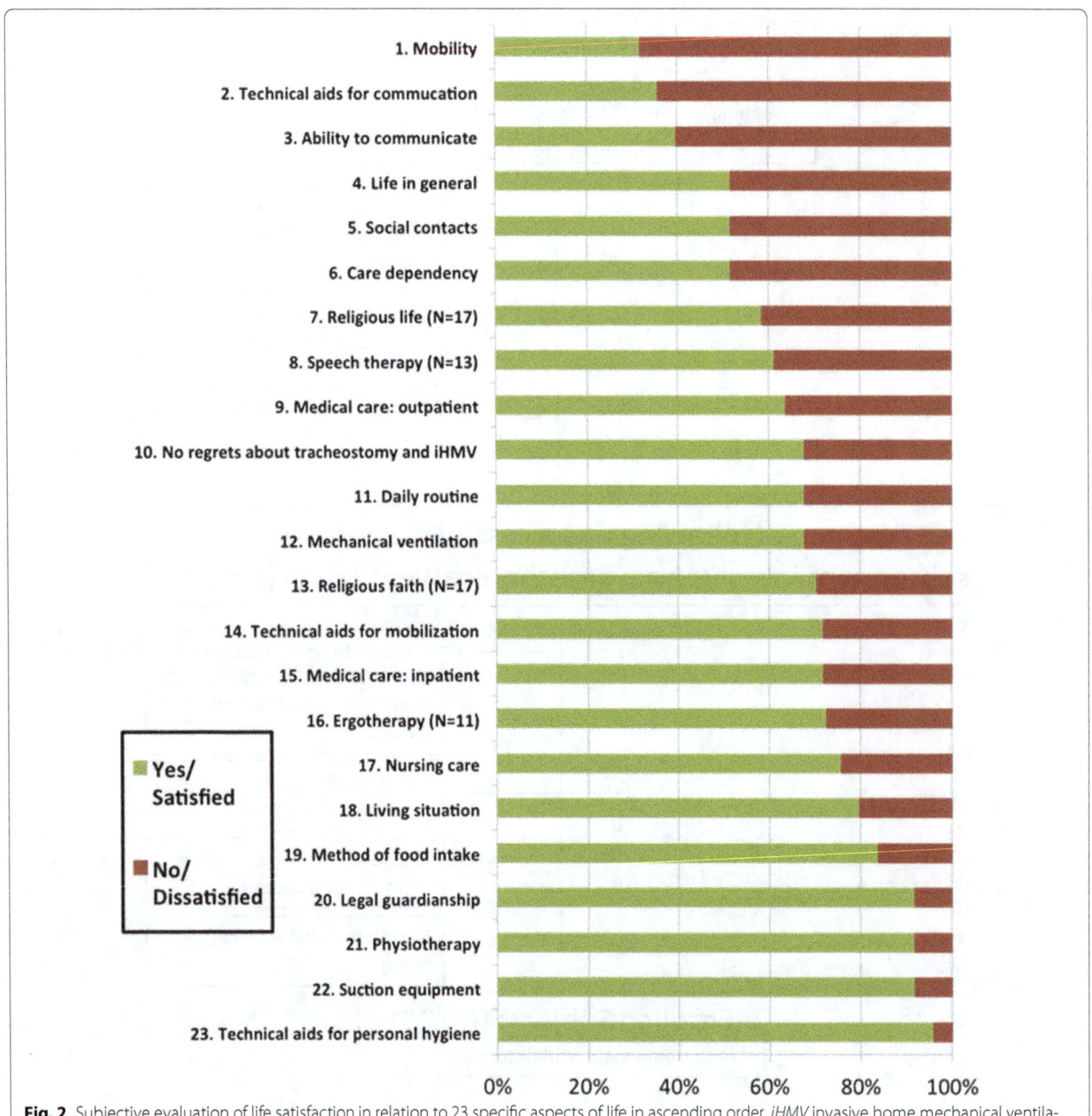

Fig. 2 Subjective evaluation of life satisfaction in relation to 23 specific aspects of life in ascending order. *iHMV* invasive home mechanical ventilation

Most of the patients had family members and/or close friends (Additional file 1: Table S4). Fifteen patients (60%) lived with family members. In contrast, after invasive HMV was established, six (24%) and 14 patients (56%) lost contact with close family members and close friends, respectively. Patients were also highly dependent on nursing care: bathing (100%), dressing (96%), use of the toilet (92%), grooming (76%), feeding (44%).

Regarding outpatient care, 23 patients (92%) received home visits from a general practitioner and four patients (16%) were visited by a specialized respiratory physician. Nevertheless, all patients were assigned to a specialized ventilation centre with a median (min/max) distance of 15 km (0.1/104 km). Outpatient nursing care was provided in 92% of patients. In addition, family members were involved in the nursing care of 48% of patients: primarily in basic care and to a lesser extent in respiratory

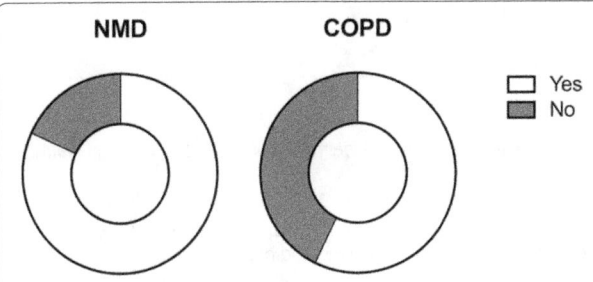

Fig. 3 Degree of satisfaction with history of tracheostomy according to underlying disease—question: In hindsight, would you choose tracheostomy for long-term invasive HMV again? *NMD* neuromuscular disease, *COPD* chronic obstructive pulmonary disease, *HMW* home mechanical ventilation

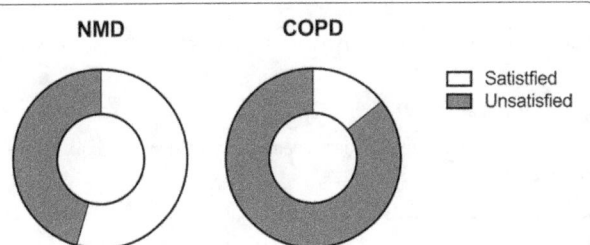

Fig. 4 Degree of satisfaction with mobilization according to underlying disease—question: Are you satisfied with your level of mobility? *NMD* neuromuscular disease, *COPD* chronic obstructive pulmonary disease

care. Eighteen patients (72%) lived in a private home and seven patients (28%) in a nursing facility (Additional file 1: Table S4). Nutrition was provided via percutaneous endoscopic gastrostomy in nine patients (36%).

The daily routine of the 25 patients who underwent invasive HMV is illustrated in Additional file 1: Figure S1 and Table S4. Importantly, patients spent most of their time watching television when they were not asleep (8 h per day). Eleven patients (44%) received continuous ventilation for 24 h per day. In contrast, 14 patients (66%) were intermittently able to breathe spontaneously, with a mean spontaneous breathing period of 8.5 ± 5.7 h per day.

Information on the Subscales and Summary Scale of the SRI is provided in Table 1, with emphasis on the differences between the two patient groups, as well as between those who regretted their tracheostomy and those who didn't. To this end, patients who regretted their tracheostomy had significantly lower SRI results for both the Subscale Anxiety and the Summary Scale, while most of the remaining scales also tended to be lower.

The results of the open interview on the topics of life and death and afterlife are summarized in Table 2. Since the interview was too exhausting for one patient suffering from both COPD and obesity hypoventilation syndrome, detailed interviews are available for 24 patients. With regard to these results, 21 patients (84%) had a religious affiliation: Catholic ($N=13$), Protestant ($N=5$), Muslim ($N=2$) and Hindu ($N=1$). However, only 17 of these patients (68%) reported having an active faith.

Discussion

This is the first study to provide a detailed description of patient characteristics, living conditions, specific aspects of HRQL and attitudes towards life, dying and death in patients with long-term invasive HMV following ICU treatment and unsuccessful weaning. The main finding was that HRQL and life satisfaction are massively impaired in many of these patients, despite maximal patient care and full supply of technical aids. Importantly, one-third of patients indicated that they would not have chosen to have a tracheostomy inserted if they had the chance to decide again, with this decision being based on

Table 1 Sub- and summary scales of the SRI according to underlying disease (NMD vs. COPD) and individual attitudes towards tracheostomy and invasive HMV

$N=25$	Underlying disease			Attitude towards tracheostomy and invasive HMV		
	NMD ($N=11$)	COPD ($N=14$)	*P* value	No regrets ($N=17$)	Regrets ($N=8$)	*P* value
Respiratory complaints	52 ± 27	54 ± 27	0.912	56.7 ± 24.9	36.3 ± 21.5	0.059
Physical functioning	27 ± 23	13 (0;58)	0.267	16.7 (0;58,3)	22.9 ± 22.8	0.617
Attendant symptoms and sleep	58 ± 18	66 ± 26	0.393	63.0 ± 21.7	45.1 ± 26.9	0.087
Social relationships	64 ± 19	54 ± 27	0.278	63.9 ± 23.8	47.8 ± 14.5	0.136
Anxiety	58 ± 23	53 ± 35	0.693	58.2 ± 30.3	34.4 ± 24.0	0.063
Psychological well-being	51 ± 26	46 ± 27	0.267	54.9 ± 21.0	34.0 ± 24.6	0.038
Social functioning	33 ± 20	42 ± 23	0.320	40.9 ± 24.8	31.0 ± 22.3	0.350
Summary scale	49 ± 16	47 ± 20	0.814	51.2 ± 18.3	35.9 ± 13.3	0.046

Data are presented as mean ± standard deviation. For non-normally distributed data, median values with minimum and maximum ranges are given

NMD neuromuscular disorders; *HMV* home mechanical ventilation; *SRI* Severe Respiratory Insufficiency Questionnaire

Table 2 Summary of open interview (*N* = 24)

Questions 1–6

1. How is your current living situation?
Three patients said that they are able to cope with their respective living conditions
Twenty-one patients felt lousy, stressed and massively impaired. Emotions such as anxiety and sadness, and feelings of being dependent and waiting for death were frequently reported

2. How would you assess your quality of life? What makes your life worth living?
Seventeen patients emphasized that despite their reduced quality of life, the deep relationship with family members and (to a lesser extent) friends, nevertheless, made life worth living. Among these patients, two had the hope of eventually becoming weaned and healed, respectively
Seven patients reported a severely reduced quality of life with nothing available to make it worth living again

3. What are your wishes regarding the treatment of your disease. What are the unresolved problems?
Fourteen patients had wishes that related to their treatment: better ability to speak (*N* = 1), less pain (*N* = 2), no further disease progression (*N* = 1), lung transplantation (*N* = 1), definitive weaning (*N* = 2), more awareness (*N* = 2), technical advances aimed at healing (*N* = 5)
Ten patients had no wishes relating to their treatment

4. What are your wishes regarding your ventilation therapy? How could this potentially be improved?
Fourteen patients had wishes that related to potential improvements in ventilation therapy: Switching to NIV (*N* = 1), less dyspnoea (*N* = 1), no further admissions to hospital (*N* = 2), longer periods of spontaneous breathing (*N* = 5), definitive weaning (*N* = 5)
Ten patients had no wishes relating to potential improvements in ventilation therapy

5. What do you think about dying and death?
Seventeen patients did think about dying and their own death: two patients expressed the wish to die, seven patients had a fear of dying/suffering during dying, and eight patients had no fear of dying
Seven patients thought neither about dying, nor their own death

6. Do you believe in an afterlife? What do you think is going to happen after you die?
Eleven patients believed in an afterlife: two patients had no idea how life after death would be, and nine patients had hopes (being with family members, being free, an eternal life, transmigration of souls, resurrection, being a spirit)
Thirteen patients did not believe in an afterlife

the understanding that refusing a tracheostomy would have led to death. Importantly, based on the SRI scores and interview findings, these patients had the worst HRQL.

Overall, these findings raise ethical concerns about the use of long-term invasive HMV following unsuccessful weaning. In addition, the prognosis of patients with prolonged weaning in the present study was severely impaired. Some patients had already died during the weaning process, others died shortly after they were assigned to invasive HMV prior to study inclusion, and some died in the year following study inclusion. This is in line with recent research that also reported severely impaired prognoses of patients who failed the weaning process [11–13]. In addition, there is increasing evidence to suggest that weaning success rates and patient outcome steadily deteriorate over time, an effect attributed to the observation that more severely ill patients are admitted to weaning centres [12]. This is presumably due to the fact that greater numbers of chronically critical patients are surviving catastrophic illnesses as a result of modern ICU medicine [12]. However, despite the increased success of modern medicine in saving lives, the flipside is that surviving ICU treatment—but remaining dependent on invasive ventilation—is associated with a high risk of extremely poor quality of life. Moreover, there are reportedly many problems and individually raised discomforts and dissatisfactions voiced by HMV

patients in their final months of life [14]. In addition, it has been emphasized that we need to increase our level of consideration for how patients with HMV die [15]. Therefore, ICU medicine should not simply focus on how to best preserve life; it should also consider the long-term living conditions of patients who remain dependent on long-term invasive ventilation. Finally, it remains unclear how many patients regretting getting tracheotomized would eventually asked for withdrawing of mechanical ventilation and how this can be brought to the clinician's attention.

The outcome of the present study is somewhat in contrast to the findings reported by Marchese et al. [13], whereby 90% of patients undergoing invasive HMV would have chosen a tracheostomy again. However, the tracheotomies in the latter study were performed electively, and the patients were younger and had a promising median survival of 49 months. Furthermore, they were cared for primarily by family members, in contrast to our study population, whose primary care was provided by specialized nurses. In addition, the proportion of patients with pulmonary diseases was considerably lower in the Marchese study than the present one [13]. Of note, HRQL and life satisfaction in the present trial were particularly impaired in patients with COPD, in line with the previous observations [9]. Finally, patients in the current study had significant co-morbidities. Therefore, in the light of the evidence presented here and elsewhere, it is most likely that COPD patients in whom weaning has failed after ICU treatment may no longer have a life worth living.

The strength of the present study is that the comprehensive, detailed interview process that took place in the home environment provided meticulous details on how HMV patients live, feel and think. Of note, the two conditions that were associated with the most dissatisfaction were impaired mobility and communication. To this end, 36% of patients could not leave the house and 48% were unable to speak (Additional file 1: Table S3). This is remarkable, especially since aids for mobility and communication were thoroughly provided. Thus, in most cases it is the nature of the maximally advanced disease state that impairs life satisfaction, and this cannot be fully compensated by technical aids and patient care.

Social contact and care dependency were two additional aspects with which patients were dissatisfied. Importantly, patients spent most of their time watching television (median 8 h) during waking hours, with only a median social contact time of 1.5 h. In addition, many patients had lost contact with family members and close friends after the establishment of invasive HMV. However, 71% of the patients emphasized that they had a meaningful relationship with family members, and most were satisfied with their living conditions. To this end, 72% of patients lived in their own private home, and 60% of all patients lived with family members. Based on this finding, it is remarkable that nearly 50% of patients were not satisfied with their social situation. Finally, all patients were extremely dependent on nursing care, and the family members of 48% of patients were involved in patient care, indicating the close interlink between living situation, family contact and patient care. Of note, while there is no information available about how family members would evaluate their level of life satisfaction if a close relative become ventilator dependent in the home environment, previous research has indicated that family members were less satisfied with a relative having a tracheostomy than the patient him/herself [13].

Finally, there was a broad heterogeneity among patients regarding religious life, faith and belief in an afterlife. This was also dependent on different religious affiliations. Some patients had detailed thoughts about their deaths, ranging between positive and negative, and some even verbally expressed their wish to die. In contrast, other patients had no definitive thoughts on this subject and avoided thinking about death. The impact of religious life on HRQL and life satisfaction, however, needs to be further elucidated in future.

As a limitation of the current study and as the prize for the individually detailed investigation, the number of patients was low. In addition, this was a monocentric study. Therefore, it cannot be excluded that patients may respond differently under different conditions, particularly in other countries. Therefore, further studies in different countries are needed to verify the current findings.

Conclusions

In conclusion, despite maximal patient care and a full supply of technical aids, both HRQL and life satisfaction are severely impaired in many invasive HMV patients who have failed prolonged weaning. The most important areas of dissatisfaction are mobility, communication, social contacts and care dependency. Importantly, one-third of patients would have preferred to die rather than receive invasive HMV. This raises ethical concerns about the practice of long-term MV following unsuccessful weaning, even though it still should be taken into account that some patients clearly benefit from long-term invasive HMV. Therefore, to avoid unethical prolongation of life, the disciplines of ICU medicine, prolonged weaning care and long-term outpatient care need to move closer together in order to improve individual decision-making processes that incorporate patients' beliefs, expectations and circumstances.

Abbreviations
COPD: chronic obstructive pulmonary disease; HMV: home mechanical ventilation; iHMV: invasive home mechanical ventilation; MV: mechanical ventilation; HRQL: health-related quality of life; NMD: neuromuscular disorders; SRI: Severe Respiratory Insufficiency Questionnaire.

Authors' contributions
SEH takes responsibility for (is the guarantor of) the content of the manuscript, including the data and analysis. All other authors contributed substantially to the study design, data analysis and interpretation, and the writing of the manuscript, with special contributions as follows: FSM assisted in the collection of data and writing of the manuscript. CK assisted in designing the study and writing the manuscript. JHS assisted in designing the study, collection of data as well as writing the manuscript. WW assisted in designing the study, the collection of the data and writing the manuscript. All authors read and approved the final manuscript.

Author details
[1] Department of Pneumology, Cologne-Merheim Hospital, Kliniken der Stadt Köln gGmbH, Witten/Herdecke University Hospital, Ostmerheimer Strasse 200, 51109 Cologne, Germany. [2] Department of Pneumology, University Medical Hospital, Freiburg, Germany. [3] Department of Intensive Care, Sleep Medicine and Mechanical Ventilation, Asklepios Fachkliniken Munich-Gauting, Gauting, Germany.

Acknowledgements
We acknowledge all participants for the effort they devoted to this study and Dr. Sandra Dieni for proofreading the manuscript prior to submission.

Competing interests
SEH, FSM, CK, JHS and WW received speaking fees from companies dealing with mechanical ventilation outside the presented work.

Funding

All authors state that none of the discussed issues in the present article were dependent on or influenced by financial support or funding. The study was supported by Weinmann Geräte für Medizin GmbH & Co. KG and VIVISOL Deutschland GmbH.

References

1. Lloyd-Owen SJ, Donaldson GC, Ambrosino N, Escarabill J, Farre R, Fauroux B, Robert D, Schoenhofer B, Simonds AK, Wedzicha JA. Patterns of home mechanical ventilation use in Europe: results from the Eurovent survey. Eur Respir J. 2005;25:1025–31.

2. Windisch W. Home mechanical ventilation. In: Tobin MJ, editor. Principles and practice of mechanical ventilation, 3rd edn. p. 683–697. Nex Yoek: Mc Graw Hill Medical; 2012.

3. Windisch W, Walterspacher S, Siemon K, Geiseler J, Sitter H. Guidelines for non-invasive and invasive mechanical ventilation for treatment of chronic respiratory failure. Published by the German Society for Pneumology (DGP). Pneumologie. 2010;64:640–52.

4. Beduneau G, Pham T, Schortgen F, Piquilloud L, Zogheib E, Jonas M, Grelon F, Runge I, Nicolas T, Grange S, et al. Epidemiology of weaning outcome according to a new definition. The WIND study. Am J Respir Crit Care Med. 2017;195:772–83.

5. Boles JM, Bion J, Connors A, Herridge M, Marsh B, Melot C, Pearl R, Silverman H, Stanchina M, Vieillard-Baron A, et al. Weaning from mechanical ventilation. Eur Respir J. 2007;29:1033–56.

6. Windisch W. Quality of life in home mechanical ventilation study g: impact of home mechanical ventilation on health-related quality of life. Eur Respir J. 2008;32:1328–36.

7. Windisch W, Freidel K, Schucher B, Baumann H, Wiebel M, Matthys H, Petermann F. The Severe Respiratory Insufficiency (SRI) Questionnaire: a specific measure of health-related quality of life in patients receiving home mechanical ventilation. J Clin Epidemiol. 2003;56:752–9.

8. Windisch W, Budweiser S, Heinemann F, Pfeifer M, Rzehak P. The Severe Respiratory Insufficiency Questionnaire was valid for COPD patients with severe chronic respiratory failure. J Clin Epidemiol. 2008;61:848–53.

9. Huttmann SE, Windisch W, Storre JH. Invasive home mechanical ventilation: living conditions and health-related quality of life. Respiration. 2015;89:312–21.

10. Schönhofer B, Geiseler J, Dellweg D, Moerer O, Barchfeld T, Fuchs H, Karg O, Rosseau S, Sitter H, Weber-Carstens S, et al. S2k-guideline "prolonged weaning". Pneumologie. 2015;69:595–607.

11. Schönhofer B, Euteneuer S, Nava S, Suchi S, Kohler D. Survival of mechanically ventilated patients admitted to a specialised weaning centre. Intensive Care Med. 2002;28:908–16.

12. Polverino E, Nava S, Ferrer M, Ceriana P, Clini E, Spada E, Zanotti E, Trianni L, Barbano L, Fracchia C, et al. Patients' characterization, hospital course and clinical outcomes in five Italian respiratory intensive care units. Intensive Care Med. 2010;36:137–42.

13. Marchese S, Lo Coco D, Lo Coco A. Outcome and attitudes toward home tracheostomy ventilation of consecutive patients: a 10-year experience. Respir Med. 2008;102:430–6.

14. Vitacca M, Grassi M, Barbano L, Galavotti G, Sturani C, Vianello A, Zanotti E, Ballerin L, Potena A, Scala R, et al. Last 3 months of life in home-ventilated patients: the family perception. Eur Respir J. 2010;35:1064–71.

15. Windisch W. Home mechanical ventilation: who cares about how patients die? Eur Respir J. 2010;35:955–7.

16

Risks of bleeding and thrombosis in intensive care unit patients with haematological malignancies

Lene Russell[1,2]* ⓘ, Lars Broksø Holst[1], Lars Kjeldsen[3], Jakob Stensballe[4,5] and Anders Perner[1]

Abstract

Background: Patients with malignant haematological disease and especially those who require intensive care have an increased risk of bleeding and thrombosis, but none of these data were obtained in ICU patients only. We assessed the incidence of bleeding and thrombotic complications, use of blood products and risk factors for bleeding in an adult population of ICU patients with haematological malignancies.

Methods: We screened all patients with acute leukaemia and myelodysplastic syndrome admitted to a university hospital ICU during 2008–2012. Bleeding in ICU was scored according to the WHO grading system, and risk factors were evaluated using unadjusted and adjusted analyses.

Results: In total, 116 of 129 ICU patients were included; their median length of stay was 7 (IQR 2–16) days. Of these, 66 patients (57%) had at least one bleeding episode in ICU; they bled for 3 (2–6) days and most often from lower and upper airways and upper GI tract. Thirty-nine (59%) of the 66 patients had severe or debilitating (WHO grade 3 or 4) bleeding. The median platelet count on the day of grade 3 or 4 bleeding was 23×10^9 per litre (IQR 13–39). Nine patients (8%) died in ICU following a bleeding episode; five of these had intra-cerebral haemorrhage. Platelet count on admission was associated with subsequent bleeding (adjusted odds ratio 1.18 (95% CI 1.03–1.35) for every 10×10^9 per litre drop in platelet count, $p = 0.016$). Eleven of the 116 patients (9%) developed a clinically significant thrombosis in ICU, which was the cause of death in four patients. The median platelet count was 20×10^9 per litre (15–48) at the time of thrombosis. The patients received a median of 6 units of red blood cells, 1 unit of fresh frozen plasma and 8 units of platelet concentrates in ICU.

Conclusions: Severe and debilitating bleeding complications were frequent in our ICU patients with haematological malignancies, but thrombosis also occurred in spite of low platelet counts. Platelet count on ICU admission was associated with subsequent bleeding.

Keywords: Bleeding, ICU, Intensive care, Haematology, Leukaemia, Myelodysplastic syndrome, Thrombosis, Sepsis, Transfusion

Background

Acute leukaemia and myelodysplastic syndrome are devastating diseases that, in worst cases, involve life-threatening complications such as bleeding, sepsis, respiratory failure and renal failure, often caused by disease or treatment-related pancytopenia [1–4]. Some patients will require admission to the intensive care unit (ICU), and although the mortality for these patients appears to have declined over the last two decades, it continues to be very high [4–6].

Patients with malignant haematological disease and especially those who require intensive care have an increased risk of bleeding and thrombosis [7–11], but none of the studies were in ICU patients only. The prevention of haemorrhage and thrombosis is a challenging task as the risk of both complications is likely to increase

*Correspondence: lene.russell@mail.dk
[1] Department of Intensive Care 4131, Copenhagen University Hospital, Rigshospitalet, Blegdamsvej 9, 2100 Copenhagen, Denmark
Full list of author information is available at the end of the article

in patients with sepsis [12–14], which is very frequent in ICU patients with malignant haematological disease [2, 5]. Thrombocytopenia increases risk of bleeding complications [11], and platelet transfusions remain the cornerstone in treatment and prevention of bleeding [15, 16]. Large multicentre studies on prophylactic platelet transfusions in thrombocytopenic non-ICU patients have shown that a restrictive prophylactic platelet transfusion strategy is likely to be safe [9], although the degree of restrictiveness is still controversial [10]. The vast majority of patients with malignant haematological disease are receiving blood products [17] so complications secondary to transfusions are also likely [14].

Because of these complexities and the lack of ICU data, we aimed to assess the following: incidence of bleeding, time to onset, risk factors for bleeding, transfusion requirements, risk of thrombotic complications and association with death in an ICU population of patients with haematological malignancies.

Methods

All patients with acute myeloid leukaemia (AML), acute lymphoblastic leukaemia (ALL) and myelodysplastic syndrome (MDS) admitted to the general ICU at Copenhagen University Hospital, Rigshospitalet, between 1 January 2008 and 3 December 2012 were identified through the local electronic ICU database (CIS, Daintel, Copenhagen). All electronic files including computed tomography (CT) reports, ultrasound scan reports and autopsy reports, when available, were reviewed. Use of pro-coagulant and anti-thrombotic medications was collected from the electronic medication charges and blood transfusion usage from the Blood Bank database.

Bleeding and thrombosis data were reviewed every single day of the ICU admission. The electronic patient chart system has a pre-defined section for coagulation issues, prompting the physician to prospectively fill out data on coagulation/bleeding/thrombosis status on a daily basis. Bleeding was graded retrospectively according to the WHO criteria [18]. The WHO grading system, which is the most common method for categorising bleeding severity in platelet transfusion trials [10, 19, 20], categorises bleeding episodes as grade 1 (mild), grade 2 (moderate), grade 3 (severe, requiring red blood cell (RBC) transfusion within 24 h) or grade 4 (debilitating or life-threatening). Details of grading system are presented in Additional file 1: Table S1.

The blood transfusion products used were standard pre-storage leuko-reduced RBC suspended in saline–adenine–glucose and mannitol, fresh frozen separated donor plasma (with 70% of coagulation factors preserved) and platelet concentrates from four donors. All transfusions were type/cross-match compatible. One unit RBC = 245 ml, one unit fresh frozen plasma (FFP) = 275 ml, and one unit platelet concentrates = 350 ml.

Daily platelet counts were done with an automated haematology analyser (Sysmex XE-500, Denmark). Thrombocytopenic patients with bleeding had platelet counts analysed twice a day. Platelet counts of less than 10×10^9 per litre were manually counted.

Simplified Acute Physiology Score (SAPS) II and the Sequential Organ Failure Assessment (SOFA) score were calculated using the worst value for that variable during the first 24 h of ICU admission [21, 22].

Statistical analysis

Qualitative data were analysed using Mann–Whitney test for nonparametric data. For categorical data, the Chi-square test was used, and in the few cases when expected values were less than 5, Fisher's exact test was used. The odds ratio (OR) was calculated where appropriate and expressed together with 95% confidence interval (CI). Risk factors for bleeding with a p value of less than 0.10 in unadjusted analyses were included in a multiple logistic regression analysis. Survival analysis of bleeding within the first 3 days in the ICU was conducted using the Kaplan–Meier method, and log-rank test was used to compare the survival curves. The linear assumptions for qualitative data included in the regression models were tested with linear splines with knot points at the quartiles. We used SAS version 9.4 (USA) and GraphPad Prism 6.00 for OS (USA) for the analyses and considered any differences statistically significant if the two-sided p value was less than 0.05.

Results

Clinical and general characteristics

One hundred and twenty-nine consecutive patients with ALL, AML or MDS were admitted during 2008–2012 and screened for inclusion; 13 patients were excluded from the study due to post-procedural observation ($n = 11$) and observation less than 24-h due to allergic reactions ($n = 2$). Thus, 116 patients were included (Table 1).

The primary reasons for ICU admission were respiratory failure and severe sepsis/septic shock; 109 (94%) of the patients fulfilled the criteria for sepsis, severe sepsis and septic shock according to the International Sepsis Definitions of 2003 [23], and 82 patients (71%) had shock on admission. The median admission SAPS II and SOFA scores were 58 (interquartile range (IQR) 50–75) and 12 (9–14), respectively.

Bleeding and platelets

In total, 66 patients (57%) had one or more bleeding episodes during the ICU stay (WHO grade 1–4).

Table 1 Characteristics of the study population (N = 116)

Baseline characteristics		
Age	60	(48–66)
Female	52	(45)
Diagnosis		
ALL	15	(13)
AML	75	(65)
MDS	26	(22)
Time from leukaemia diagnosis to ICU admission		
Less than 3 months	35	(30)
3–6 months	12	(10)
6–12 months	20	(17)
More than 12 months	50	(43)
Chemotherapy within 6 weeks prior to admission	76	(66)
Haematopoietic Stem Cell Transplantation (HSCT)	43	(37)
Graft-versus-host reaction	20	(17)
Relapse after having received treatment	20	(17)
Transformation from other haematological malignancy	18	(16)
From MDS to AML	10	(9)
From CML to AML	2	(2)
From CMML to AML	2	(2)
From Mb. Waldenstrom to AML	1	(1)
Respiratory or systemic fungal infection	19	(16)
Primary reason for ICU admission		
Respiratory failure	59	(51)
Septic shock/severe sepsis	39	(34)
Bleeding	3	(3)
Severe graft-versus-host reaction	3	(3)
Other	13	(11)
WBC count at admission ($\times 10^9$ per litre)	3	(0.2–11)
ICU characteristics		
Sepsis[a]	109	(94)
Sepsis	9	(8)
Severe sepsis	18	(15)
Septic shock	82	(71)
Mechanical ventilation in ICU	101	(87)
Vasopressor in ICU	95	(82)
Renal replacement therapy in ICU	42	(37)
Emergency surgery immediately before or during ICU stay	3	(3)
SAPS II	58	(50–75)
SOFA (admission)	12	(9–14)
SOFA (admission) without platelet score[b]	8	(6–11)
SOFA (maximum)	14	(11–17)
Length of ICU stay, days	7	(2–16)

Values are number (%) or median (IQR)

AML acute myeloid leukaemia, *ALL* acute lymphoblastic leukaemia, *MDS* myelodysplastic syndrome, *CML* chronic myeloid leukaemia, *CMML* chronic myelomonocytic leukaemia, *SAPS II* Simplified Acute Physiology Score, *SOFA* Sequential Organ Failure Assessment score, *WBC* white blood cell

[a] According to the International Sepsis Definitions 2003 [23]

[b] SOFA score at admission minus score values given for platelets count ($\times 10^9$ per litre): ≥ 150: score = 0; ≥ 150: score = 0; < 150: score = 1; < 100: score = 2; < 50: score = 3; < 20: score = 4

The median number of days with bleeding was 3 (IQR 2–6). One-third ($n = 38$, 33%) of the patients had a bleeding episode during the first 24 h in ICU, and 49 patients (42%) had an episode during the first 5 days. The 116 included patients spent a total of 1728 days in the ICU and of these, 333 (19%) were days when bleeding occurred.

The majority of the patients bled from more than one location; only 17/66 (26%) bled from one location only (Table 2). The most common locations were lower/upper airways and upper gastrointestinal (GI) tract. Respiratory tract bleedings were more common among mechanically ventilated patients [49/101 (49%) vs. 1/15 (7%)]; however, three patients were intubated and mechanically ventilated due to bleedings in the airways. Six patients developed intracranial bleeding (ICH). One of the patients with ICH had severe leukocytosis (WBC > 100×10^9 per litre) with predominance of myeloblasts, known to be associated with increased risk of intracranial haemorrhage [24].

More than half of the patients with bleeding had a severe (WHO grade 3) or debilitating (WHO grade 4) bleeding episode (39 patients, 59%). There was no significant difference in the number of bleeding complications when stratifying for ALL, AML and MDS patients ($p = 0.67$), and haematopoietic stem cell transplantation (HSCT) patients had similar numbers of bleeding complications to non-HSCT patients ($p = 0.86$) (Fig. 1).

Patients' median platelet count at ICU admission was 29×10^9 per litre (IQR 18–48), and the majority (88 patients, 76%) were severely thrombocytopenic at admission with platelet counts < 50×10^9 per litre.

The platelet count on admission was the only variable associated with subsequent bleeding (Fig. 2, Table 3). The adjusted OR for bleeding within the first 5 days in the ICU was 1.15 (95% CI 1.00–1.33) for every drop in platelet count by 10×10^9 per litre, $p = 0.058$ and 1.18 (1.03–1.35), $p = 0.016$ for bleeding in the ICU. The median platelet count on the first bleeding day was 21×10^9 per litre (IQR 15–31), and the median platelet count on the day of having a severe or debilitating bleeding episode (WHO grade 3 or 4) was 23×10^9 per litre (13–39). In patients with subsequent bleeding in the ICU, we found that the individual differences in platelet counts on the first day of bleeding compared to at admission were minor [median difference 0 (IQR 0–0), mean $- 3.8 \times 10^9$(min–max: $- 98 - (+ 28)$).].

Mortality

Within the first week in ICU, 33 of the 116 patients (28%) had died and in total 64 (55%) of the patients died in the ICU. The 30-day, 90-day and 1-year mortality was 60, 72 and 86%, respectively.

Table 2 Anatomical site of bleeding

Intracranial bleeding	6	(5)
Upper airway bleeding[a]	23	(20)
Lower airway bleeding	41	(35)
Upper gastrointestinal bleeding	22	(19)
Lower gastrointestinal bleeding	14	(12)
Skin bleedings[b]	17	(15)
Bleeding from sites of vascular catheters	13	(11)
Urinary tract	10	(9)
Eyes[c]	1	(1)
Post-biopsy[d]	4	(3)
Post-surgical bleeding	3	(3)
Eyes[c]	1	(1)
Other sites[e]	7	(6)

All values are number (%)

Many patients bled from more than one site: 17 (26%) bled from one site only; 25 (38%) bled from two sites; 12 (18%) bled from three sites; 12 (18%) bled from four or more sites

[a] Upper airway bleeding included bleedings from the nose, mouth, pharynx and larynx

[b] Skin bleedings included petechia, purpura and ecchymosis

[c] Subconjunctival bleeding

[d] The biopsy sites were: liver (N = 2), skin and bone marrow (pelvis)

[e] Other sites included vaginal (non-menstrual) bleedings, pelvic bleedings, a pericardial bleedings and a bleeding from spontaneous spleen rupture

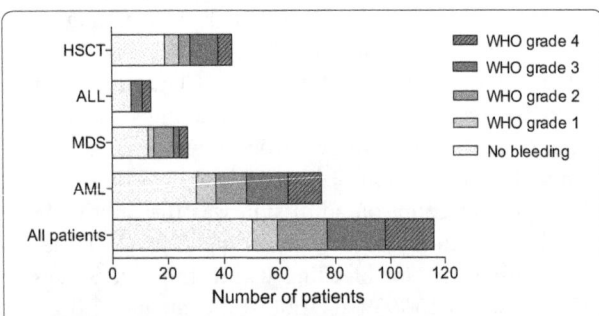

Fig. 1 Bleeding complications during ICU stay. No significant difference was seen in number of bleedings complications between the different diagnoses or in patients with haematopoietic stem cell transplantation (HSCT). *ALL* acute lymphoblastic leukaemia, *MDS* myelodysplastic syndrome, *AML* acute myeloid leukaemia

Nine patients (8%) died in ICU following an acute bleeding episode; five of these had ICH, three had pulmonary bleeding and one a large post-operative bleeding after acute hemi-colectomy for bowel ischaemia. The unadjusted 30-day and 1-year mortality was higher in bleeding vs. non-bleeding patients (68 vs. 50%, $p = 0.047$ and 92 vs. 78%, $p = 0.022$), but the Kaplan–Meier survival analysis curve stratified by bleeding or not within the first 3 ICU days did not indicate any difference between the two groups (Fig. 3). Including age and SOFA

score at admission in the survival analysis, the HR for death in bleeding versus non-bleeding patients was 1.28 (95% CI 0.79–2.1, $p = 0.31$).

Transfusions

Due to lack of Danish national identification numbers, four patients did not have their transfusion data registered in the Blood Bank database. Of the remaining 112 patients, 100 patients (89%) received one or more transfusions of RBC, FFP or platelets concentrates during their ICU stay. The 112 patients received a total of 3561 units of blood products, and half of the units (1749 units, 49%) were given within the first week in ICU. Only four patients with bleeding did not receive any transfusions at all; two patients had large intracranial bleedings that was the immediate cause of death, and two had minor bleedings not requiring transfusions. The amount of transfusions increased on the days leading up to a grade 3 or 4 bleeding episode (Fig. 4).

Red blood cell transfusions

Ninety patients (80%) had at least one RBC transfusion during their ICU stay and received median 6 (IQR 1–13) units; 32/90 (36%) did not have any signs of clinical bleeding during the ICU stay.

Bleeding patients received a median of 10 (4–20) units of RBC during ICU stay as compared with 2 (0–7) units in non-bleeding patients ($p = < 0.0001$) or 0.78 unit/ICU day for bleeding patients versus 0.30 unit/ICU day for non-bleeding patients ($p = 0.0003$).

Fresh frozen plasma transfusions

Sixty of the 112 patients (54%) received a median 1 unit of FFP during ICU stay (IQR 0–4 units). The median amount of FFP administered to bleeding patients was 4 (0–12) units while in ICU or 0.28 units/ICU day. Twenty-seven per cent of the patients who received FFP did not have any signs of clinical bleeding during the ICU stay.

Platelet transfusions

Ninety of the 112 patients (80%) received a median 8 (IQR 2–23) units of platelets during ICU stay equalling a median of 2800 (700–8050) ml of platelets; 32 (36%) did not have any signs of clinical bleeding during the ICU stay. Patients with platelets $< 50 \times 10^9$ per litre received a median of 10 (4–28) units during ICU or 1.7 (0.8–2.3) units/day.

Bleeding patients received a median of 22 (8–39) units of platelets during ICU stay as compared with 2 (0–7) units for non-bleeding patients ($p < 0.0001$) or 1.8 unit/ day for bleeding patients versus 0.5 unit/day for non-bleeding patients ($p < 0.0001$).

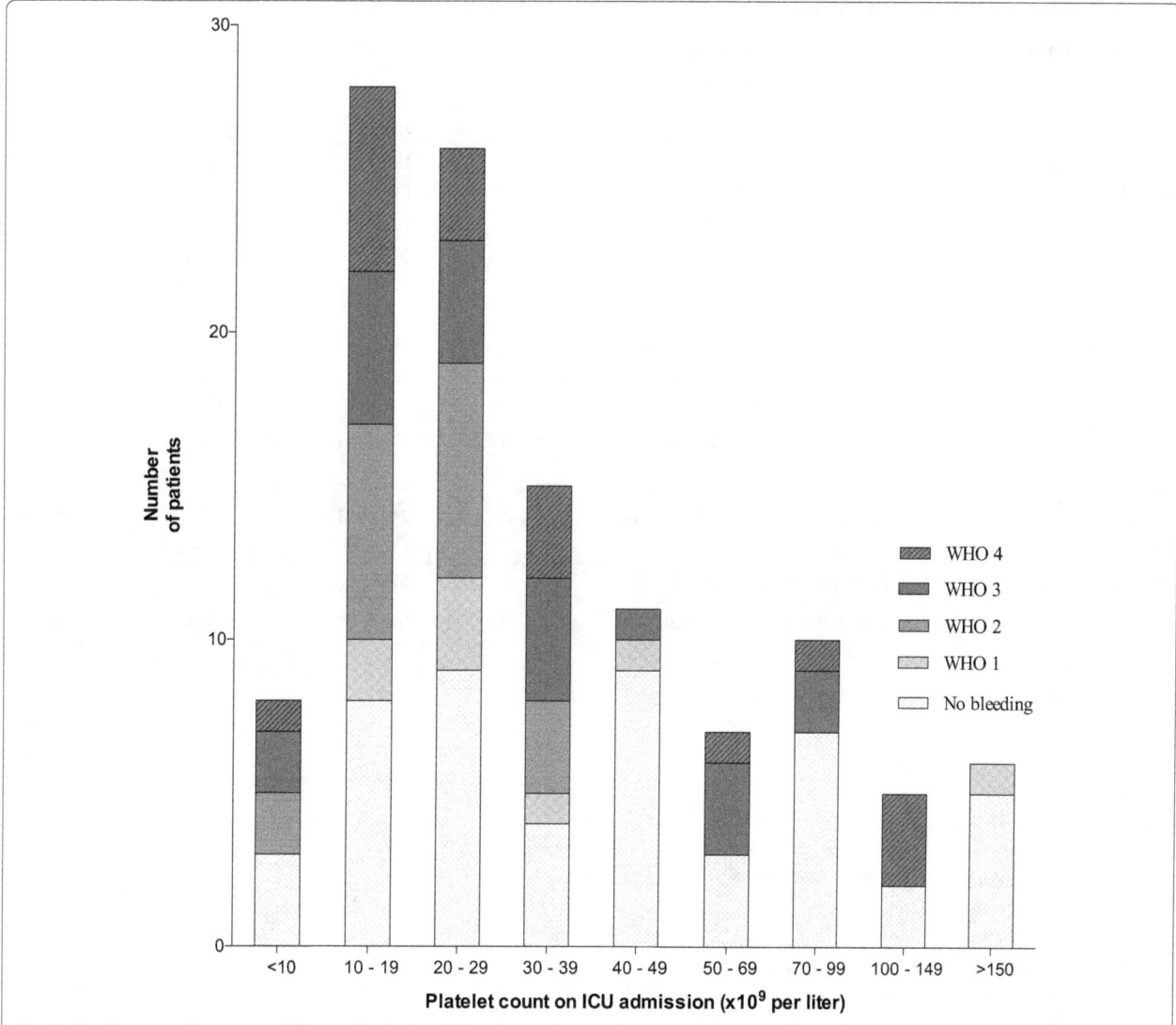

Fig. 2 Bleeding complications at different platelet levels. This figure shows the range of platelet level at ICU admission across our patient population and frequency of bleeding complications in ICU graded according to WHO, in which bleeding episodes are categorised as grade 1 (mild), grade 2 (moderate), grade 3 (severe; requiring red blood cell (RBC) transfusion within 24-h) or grade 4 (debilitating or life-threatening)

Thrombosis

Eleven of the 116 patients (9%) developed a clinically significant thrombotic event (Table 4), which was the cause of death in four patients. The median platelet count was 20×10^9 per litre (IQR $15 - 48 \times 10^9$ per litre) at the time of thrombosis. Six of the 11 patients with thrombosis also had bleeding episodes during their ICU stay. Patients with thrombosis had the same amount of RBC and slightly more platelets/day than patients without thrombosis. Nine (82%) of the patients with thrombosis had received plasma transfusion as compared with 50/101 (50%) of the patients without thrombosis ($p = 0.06$) and those with thrombosis received more units of FFP per ICU day than patients without thrombosis (0.5 unit/day (0.1–1.5) vs. 0.02 (0–0.62) unit/day, $p = 0.053$).

Thrombosis prophylaxis

Forty-seven patients (41%) received the low molecular weight heparin (LMWH) enoxaparin in prophylactic doses during the ICU stay. There was no difference in bleeding complications between patients receiving LMWH and those who did not ($p = 0.39$). None of the patients received anti-platelet treatments when admitted to the ICU or during the ICU stay.

Among the 88 patients with platelet levels less than 50×10^9 per litre on admission, 30 patients (34%) received LMWH and 58 (66%) did not. No difference in bleeding complications was seen between these groups of patients either ($p = 0.13$). Four of the 11 patients with thrombotic events had received prophylactic LMWH at the time of the event.

Table 3 Risk factors at ICU admission for bleeding in unadjusted and adjusted analyses

Unadjusted analyses	Bleeding within 5 days of admission			Bleeding in ICU[a]		
	No. (%)	OR (95% CI)	p value	No. (%)	OR (95% CI)	p value
Acute lymphatic leukaemia	5 (36)	1.37 (0.43–4.36)	0.60	7 (50)	1.37 (0.44–4.20)	0.58
Acute myeloid leukaemia	33 (44)	0.82 (0.38–1.77)	0.82	45 (60)	0.70 (0.33–1.51)	0.36
Myelodysplastic syndrome	11 (40)	1.08 (0.45–2.60)	0.85	14 (52)	1.31 (0.55–3.10)	0.55
Recent chemotherapy[b]	39 (51)	**3.16 (1.36–7.36)**	**0.006**	49 (64)	**2.45 (1.12–5.37)**	**0.02**
HSCT	15 (35)	0.61 (0.28–1.33)	0.22	24 (56)	0.93 (0.44–2.00)	0.86
Leukopenia at admission[c]	31 (56)	**3.09 (1.43–6.64)**	**0.004**	35 (64)	1.69 (0.80–3.56)	0.16
Fungal infection[d]	10 (48)	1.31 (0.51–3.37)	0.58	14 (67)	1.65 (0.61–4.47)	0.32
Renal replacement therapy	11 (48)	1.33 (0.53–3.32)	0.54	13 (57)	0.98 (0.39–2.46)	0.97
Mechanical ventilation[e]	28 (41)	0.90 (0.43–1.90)	0.78	39 (57)	1.05 (0.50–2.21)	0.91
Use of LMWH[f]	9 (29)	0.49 (0.19–1.19)	0.11	16 (52)	0.81 (0.35–1.86)	0.62
	Median (IQR)	OR (95% CI)	p value	Median (IQR)	OR (95% CI)	p value
Age	58 (48–65)	1.00 (0.97–1.03)	0.73	59 (45–66)	1.00 (0.95–1.03)	0.97
Platelet count at admission	**22 (15–31)**	**1.16 (1.03–1.32)[f]**	**0.001**	**24 (15–35)**	**1.14 (1.03–1.26)[f]**	**0.004**
SOFA-score at admission	12 (9–14)	1.05 (0.96–1.15)	0.14	12(9–14)	1.03 (0.95–1.13)	0.34
Adjusted analyses[g]	**Bleeding within 5 days**			**Bleeding in ICU**		
	Median(IQR)	OR (95%CI)	p value	Median(IQR)	OR (95% CI)	p value
Recent chemotherapy	n/a	2.27 (0.93–5.56)	0.07	n/a	1.70 (0.70–3.95)	0.24
White blood cell count	2.8 (0.2–11)	1.01 (0.99–1.02)	0.39	1.2 (0.1–8.5)	1.02 (1.00–1.04)	0.07
Platelet count[h]	22 (15–31)	1.15 (1.00–1.33)	0.058	**24 (15–35)**	**1.18 (1.03–1.35)**	**0.016**

Bold indicates significant results ($p < 0.05$)

n/a not applicable

[a] One patient lost at 1-year follow up

[b] Chemotherapy within 6 weeks of ICU-admission

[c] Leukopenia at ICU admission defined as white blood cell (WBC) count < 2 (missing data = 1)

[d] Confirmed systemic or respiratory fungal infection

[e] Mechanical ventilation on day one in ICU

[f] Low molecular weight heparin (enoxaparin 20–40 mg daily)

[g] Logistic regression analysis with bleeding as outcome and chemotherapy, WBC count and platelet count as co-variates

[h] Platelet count OR for every decrease in platelet count by 10×10^9 (at admission)

Pro-coagulant drugs and vitamin K

Pro-coagulant drugs were administered to 11 patients (9%); 8 patients had vitamin K administered (7%), and 2 had so without prior bleeding. Both these patients developed large thrombi, which were the immediate cause of death. Nine patients received tranexamic acid.

Discussion

This study confirmed that a high percentage of ICU patients with acute leukaemia and myelodysplastic syndrome are subject to bleeding. Low platelet count at ICU admission was associated with bleeding. Despite bleeding being the cause of death in some patients, bleeding was not associated with time to death after adjustments for known risk factors. The patients were transfused with a large amount of blood products compared to haematological non-ICU patients [9, 10]. This is not surprising, given the inherent bone marrow failure of either the disease itself or its treatment with chemotherapy, which 66% of patients had received less than 6 weeks prior to ICU admission. Thrombotic events also occurred in some patients despite low platelet counts.

It is well known that patients with haematological cancer receiving chemotherapy or undergoing HSCT have an increased risk of bleeding. The number of bleeding events has been studied as primary end-point in several large, multicentre platelet transfusion trials performed outside the ICU. In the PLADO (Platelet Dose) trial, including 1272 patients undergoing chemotherapy or HSCT, 67% had a bleeding episode before leaving the hospital or within 30 days [9]. In the TOPPS study (Trial

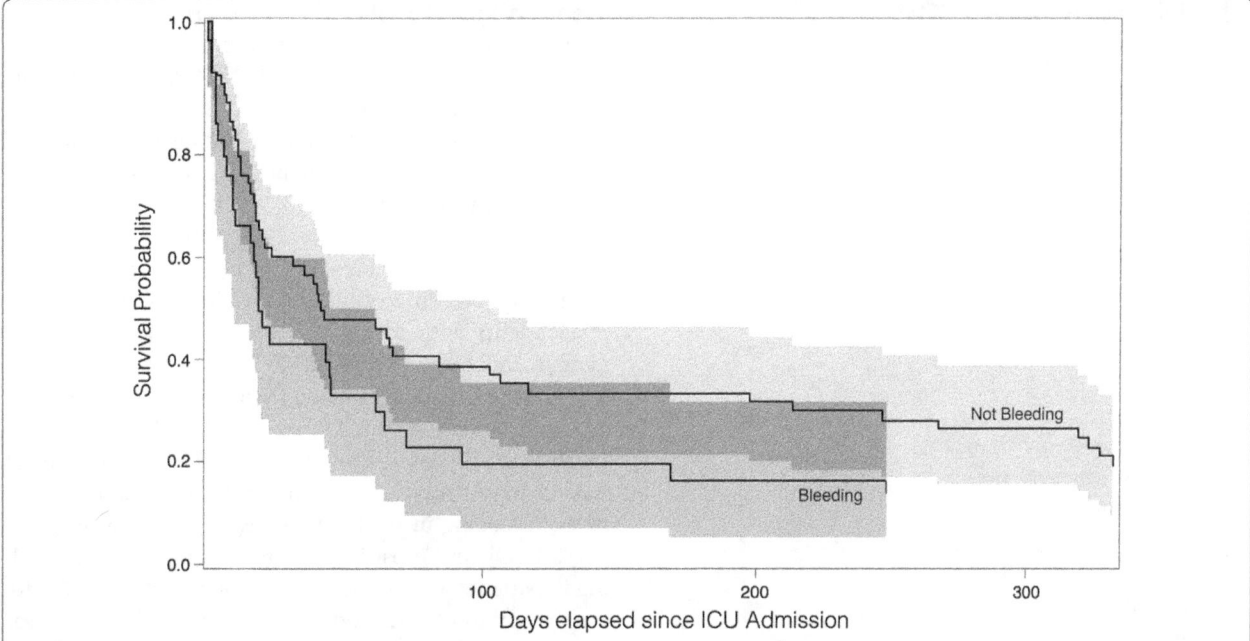

Fig. 3 Time to death showed as Kaplan–Meier survival curves in bleeding and non-bleeding patients. The log-rank score for bleeding was 1.74 ($p = 0.19$) and the hazard ratio (HR) for patients with bleeding as compared to non-bleeders was 1.37 (95% CI 0.86–2.19). Survival curves are presented with 95% confidential intervals

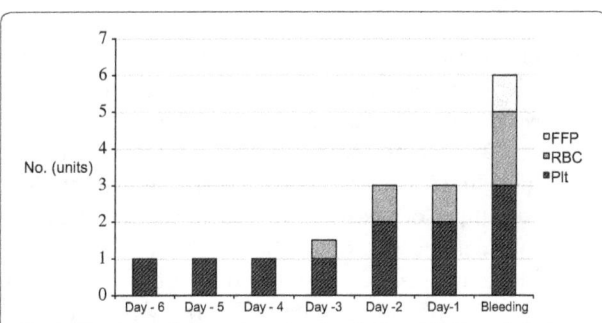

Fig. 4 Blood transfusions given the days *before* a WHO grade 3–4 bleeding episode. This figure shows the median amount of blood products given during the days leading up to a major bleeding. *FFP* fresh frozen plasma, *RBC* red blood cells, *Plt* platelet concentrate

of Prophylactic Platelets), including 598 patients undergoing chemotherapy for haematological cancer or HSCT, 47% of the 598 patients bleed within 30 days [10]. Both studies had low platelet levels as one of the inclusion criteria.

Likewise, in a German platelet dose study, 391 patients undergoing HSCT or intensive chemotherapy for AML were randomised to receive platelets either when bleeding or when platelet counts were less than 10×10^9 per litre. Patients were only followed as long as platelet counts were less than 20×10^9 per litre. In the HSCT group, grade 3 bleedings were rare and grade 4 bleedings

non-existent. In the leukaemia group, 15 patients had non-fatal haemorrhages, including six with minor cerebral bleeds. Two fatal intracranial bleeds were registered, both in the group receiving platelets when bleeding [16].

Our study population was small compared to the three trials described above, but overall we found the same number of bleeding complications. In other words, despite our patients having considerably shorter observation periods the same incidence of bleeding was found. We also found that our patients had longer bleeding episodes. The median number of days with bleeding in the PLADO study was one day, whereas our patients bled for 3 days. Importantly, in our study population, more than half of the bleedings were severe or debilitating and 8% had fatal bleedings. In contrast, in PLADO 10% of the patients had WHO grade 3 or 4 bleedings and only one patient died from bleeding. In TOPPS, 1% (7 patients) had grade 3 or 4 bleeding episodes and none died from bleeding.

Patients with lower platelet levels did have a higher frequency of bleeding complications. Most patients received prophylactic platelet transfusions when platelet levels fell below 20×10^9 per litre, although the platelet levels at which the individual patient was transfused was at the clinicians' discretion. The proportion of severe and debilitating bleedings (WHO grade 3–4) did not decrease as might have been expected at increasing platelet levels, which probably explains why platelet levels did not

Table 4 Thrombotic events in ICU

No. of thrombotic events—no (%)	11	(9)
Site of thrombosis		
Brain	5	
Arm, fingers, toes	2	
Liver veins	2	
Spleen (post-mortem finding)	1	
Inferior vena cava	1	
Haematological diagnosis		
AML	10	
ALL	1	
MDS	0	
Severe sepsis/septic shock—no (%)	11	(100)
Death directly related to thrombosis—no	4	
Bleeding prior to thrombotic event	3	
Bleeding after thrombotic event	3	
LMWH[a]	4	
Drugs given prior to thrombotic event		
Tranexamic acid	2	[b]
Vitamin K	2	[c]

Data are in number (%)

AML acute myeloid leukaemia, *ALL* acute lymphoblastic leukaemia, *MDS* myelodysplastic syndrome, *LMWH* low molecular weight heparin

[a] Enoxaparin 20–40 mg daily in ICU before thrombotic event

[b] Site of thrombi: 1. spleen (post-mortem finding); 2. thalamus (MRI finding)

[c] Site of thrombi: 1. inferior vena cava; 2. brain (multiple sites)

influence survival in our population. However, use of platelet and RBC transfusions was increasing in the days leading up to a severe bleeding, which might indicate that increasing platelet dependency and minor bleedings could be warning signs of severe/debilitating bleeding.

We also analysed biochemical coagulation parameters and calculated the disseminated intravascular coagulation (DIC) scores according to the definition by the International Society of Thrombosis and Haemostasis (ISTH) [25]. Among these other markers of coagulation (International normalised ratio (INR), activated pro-thrombin time (APTT), anti-thrombin, D-dimer and fibrinogen) only INR was weakly associated with subsequent bleeding (odds ratio 2.91 for bleeding within 24 h, 95% CI 1.01–8.43, $p = 0.048$). The DIC score was neither associated with bleeding nor thrombosis. None of the biochemical parameters had any predictive value with regard to bleeding in these patients as described elsewhere [26].

The majority of bleedings in our ICU started within the first 5 days. Several bleedings were severe and in nine patients (8%) the direct cause of death, thereby contributing to the high mortality. More than half of the patients died in ICU, and the 30-day mortality was 60%. This is similar to the mortality rates described by Pène et al. in critically ill HSCT patients [27], but higher than

described in some other studies of critically ill haematology patients. However, our population differs from some of the previous studies [3, 5, 28–31] in that the vast majority were mechanically ventilated (87%) and received vasopressor (82%). In most other studies, the ratio of mechanically ventilated patients has been considerably lower, in some less than 50% [3, 30–32].

So why are our patients bleeding more? Sepsis-induced coagulopathy causes bleeding in ICU patients [33], so the risk of bleeding is likely to be increased in leukaemia patients with sepsis and a large proportion of our patients indeed had sepsis at ICU admission. A low platelet count has been associated with adverse outcome in a general population of ICU patients [32, 34–37] although thrombocytopenia as a determinant of severe bleeding in ICU remains unclear. Several studies have assessed the risk of bleeding in ICU patients with thrombocytopenia [34, 37–39], and most have found a higher risk of bleeding in patients with lower platelet counts [36, 38, 40] with the exception of one study, which found that sepsis was the single variable associated with bleeding in multivariate analysis [41]. However, none of these studies were in haematological patients only.

Although the incidence of bleeding in medical ICU patients without haematological malignancies is lower, the exact numbers are not certain, as haematological patients often are included in the general ICU populations. The prospective multicentre Scandinavian Starch for Severe Sepsis/Septic Shock (6S) trial [42], which included 798 general ICU patients with severe sepsis, had severe bleeding (defined as clinical bleeding that required 3 or more units of packed red cells within 24 h) as one of the pre-defined outcomes. In 6S, 19% of the patients had a bleeding episode and 8% had severe bleeding [43]. However, 35% of the patients had surgery prior to ICU admission. Among the patients without prior surgery, only 16% had a bleeding episode and 6% had severe bleeding. Haematological patients were included in this study, constituting 9% of the total study population.

Some of our patients also had thrombotic events in spite of low platelet counts, which was the cause of death in four patients. The patients with thrombosis also had low platelet counts on the day of the thrombus, and several of them had one or more bleeding episodes before the thrombotic episode. All except one of the thrombotic events in our study were in patients with AML. Patients with acute leukaemia have an increased risk of thrombosis that may be as high, or even higher than in patients with solid tumours [44, 45]. There are several reasons why thrombocytopenic leukaemia patients still have an increased risk of thrombosis [8, 46, 47]: Leukaemic cells express pro-coagulant mediators including tissue factor [48, 49], produce pro-inflammatory and pro-coagulant cytokines [50, 51], release leukaemia cell derived micro-particles into the blood stream which are expressing tissue factor on the surface [52] and directly activate platelets [53, 54]. The rapid cell death induced by chemotherapy further increases the release of pro-coagulant factors into the blood stream [50]. Furthermore, all our patients had central venous catheters which is a likely risk factor for thrombosis in patients with acute leukaemia, although the incidence has varied in different studies and no studies have been in ICU patients only [55–57].

Preventing thromboembolic complications in thrombocytopenic patients with haematological malignancy is indeed complicated due to the high risk of bleeding. There are no available guidelines for prevention of thrombosis in acute leukaemia patients outside the ICU setting, and in ICU the risk is likely to be even more increased due to immobilisation, use of vasopressors and sepsis [58, 59]. To our knowledge, no randomised trials on thrombosis prophylaxis in leukaemia patients have been made. A prospective multicentre study on the incidence of thrombosis in non-ICU haematological patients with central venous catheters found no increase in bleeding in the 14% of patients receiving thrombosis prophylaxis [55]. However, even though thrombosis prophylaxis was not found to increase the number of bleeding episodes, the incidence of thrombosis was not reduced. Similar results were found in a retrospective study of central venous catheters in AML patients [57] as well as in a study of low-dose warfarin prophylaxis in oncology patients [60]. In our study, 47 patients (41%) received enoxaparin as thrombosis prophylaxis during the ICU stay. No increase in bleeding events was observed among these patients.

Our patients received large amounts of blood products. Severely thrombocytopenic patients would be expected to bleed more and therefore receive more RBC transfusions, but this was not the case. Bleeding patients did, for obvious reasons, receive more blood products than non-bleeding patients, but it is worth noticing that 36% of the patients who received RBC transfusion and 27% of the patients who received fresh frozen plasma did not have any signs of clinical bleeding.

This study has several limitations. Due to its retrospective nature, there is a risk of underestimating the occurrence of minor bleedings. Furthermore, this is a single-centre study and it may be that the results are different in other centres. Most importantly, we cannot make any inferences about cause and effect because of the observational design, in particular as the time at risk of bleeding for any patient is related to the time spent in ICU, and as such it is difficult to analyse any associations to mortality.

The strength of this study is the high availability of data achieved by using three separate databases linked using the patients' unique identification number. We also included a relatively homogenous group of patients with only three acute haematological diagnoses, and where the majority had sepsis, required mechanical ventilation and had received chemotherapy within 6 weeks of ICU admission. We had few exclusions and full follow-up of all included patients.

Conclusions

ICU patients with acute leukaemia and MDS had a high risk of severe, debilitating and fatal bleeding episodes in the ICU and lower platelet counts appeared to be a risk factor for bleeding. Preventing severe bleeding episodes appears to be crucial, and close daily monitoring of minor bleedings and increasing platelet dependency might aid this goal. Further research is warranted in order to avoid debilitating and fatal bleeding without increasing the risk of thrombosis. It seems worthwhile to test the benefits and harms of therapeutic interventions, e.g. higher platelet trigger values in high-risk patients and alternatives to platelet transfusions to prevent bleeding as well as the benefits/risk of thrombosis prophylaxis in thrombocytopenic ICU patients with acute leukaemia and MDS.

Abbreviations
ALL: acute lymphoblastic leukaemia; AML: acute myeloid leukaemia; CI: confidence interval; CT: computered tomography; FFP: fresh frozen plasma; GI: gastrointestinal; HSCT: haematopoietic stem cell transplantation; ICH: intracranial haemorrhage; ICU: intensive care unit; IQR: interquartile range; LMWH: low molecular weight heparin; MDS: myelodysplastic syndrome; OR: odds ratio; PLADO: platelet dose study; RBC: red blood cell; SAPS: Simplified Acute Physiology Score; SOFA: Sequential Organ Failure Assessment; TOPPS: trial of prophylactic platelets; WBC: white blood cell; WHO: World Health Organisation.

Authors' contributions
LR, LK, JS and AP designed the study; LR performed the statistical analyses and wrote the initial draft of the manuscript; AP and LH contributed substantially to interpretation of the data and writing the manuscript; all authors revised the manuscript for important intellectual content; all authors read and approved the final manuscript.

Author details
[1] Department of Intensive Care 4131, Copenhagen University Hospital, Rigshospitalet, Blegdamsvej 9, 2100 Copenhagen, Denmark. [2] Copenhagen Academy for Medical Education and Simulation, University of Copenhagen and The Capital Region of Denmark, Copenhagen, Denmark. [3] Department of Haematology, Copenhagen University Hospital, Rigshospitalet, Copenhagen, Denmark. [4] Section for Transfusion Medicine, Capital Region Blood Bank, Copenhagen University Hospital, Rigshospitalet, Copenhagen, Denmark. [5] Department of Anaesthesia, Centre of Head and Orthopaedics, Copenhagen University Hospital, Rigshospitalet, Copenhagen, Denmark.

Acknowledgements
The authors would like to thank Dr. Jan Bonde, Head of the Department of Intensive Care at Rigshospitalet for his support of this study. We would also like to thank Guy Williams for valuable help in creating the figures for this article.

Competing interests
We have read and understood AIC's policy on declaration of interests and declare that we have no competing interests.

Funding
None of the authors received any funding for the work related to this study.

References

1. Azoulay É, Thiéry G, Chevret S, et al. The prognosis of acute respiratory failure in critically ill cancer patients. Med Baltim. 2004;83(6):360–70.
2. Park HY, Suh GY, Jeon K, et al. Outcome and prognostic factors of patients with acute leukemia admitted to the intensive care unit for septic shock. Leuk Lymphoma. 2008;49(10):1929–34.
3. Lengliné E, Raffoux E, Lemiale V, et al. Intensive care unit management of patients with newly diagnosed acute myeloid leukemia with no organ failure. Leuk Lymphoma. 2012;53(7):1352–9.
4. Schellongowski P, Staudinger T, Kundi M, et al. Prognostic factors for intensive care unit admission, intensive care outcome, and post-intensive care survival in patients with de novo acute myeloid leukemia: a single center experience. Haematologica. 2011;96(2):231–7.
5. Azoulay E, Mokart D, Pène F, et al. Outcomes of critically ill patients with hematologic malignancies: prospective multicenter data from France and Belgium—a groupe de recherche respiratoire en réanimation onco-hématologique study. J Clin Oncol. 2013;31(22):2810–8.
6. Khassawneh BY, White P, Anaissie EJ, Barlogie B, Hiller FC. Outcome from mechanical ventilation after autologous peripheral blood stem cell transplantation. Chest. 2002;121:185–8.
7. Landolfi R, Di Gennaro L. Thrombosis in myeloproliferative and myelodysplastic syndromes. Hematology. 2012;17(Suppl 1):S174–6. https://doi.org/10.1179/102453312X13336169156898.
8. Crespo-Solís E. Thrombosis and acute leukemia. Hematology. 2012;17(Suppl 1):S169–73.
9. Slichter SJ, Kaufman RM, Assmann SF, et al. Dose of prophylactic platelet transfusions and prevention of hemorrhage. N Engl J Med. 2010;362(7):600–13.
10. Stanworth SJ, Estcourt LJ, Powter G, et al. A no-prophylaxis platelet-transfusion strategy for hematologic cancers. N Engl J Med. 2013;368(19):1771–80.
11. Webert KE, Cook RJ, Sigouin CS, Rebulla P, Heddle NM. The risk of bleeding in thrombocytopenic patients with acute myeloid leukemia. Haematologica. 2006;91(11):1530–7.
12. Haase N, Ostrowski SR, Wetterslev J, et al. Thromboelastography in patients with severe sepsis: a prospective cohort study. Intensive Care Med. 2014;41(1):77–85.
13. Drews RE. Critical issues in hematology: anemia, thrombocytopenia, coagulopathy, and blood product transfusions in critically ill patients. Clin Chest Med. 2003;24(4):607–22.
14. Perner A, Smith SH, Carlsen S, Holst LB. Red blood cell transfusion during septic shock in the ICU. Acta Anaesthesiol Scand. 2012;56(6):718–23.
15. McIntyre L, Tinmouth AT, Fergusson DA. Blood component transfusion in critically ill patients. Curr Opin Crit Care. 2013;19(4):326–33.
16. Wandt H, Schaefer-Eckart K, Wendelin K, et al. Therapeutic platelet transfusion versus routine prophylactic transfusion in patients with haematological malignancies: an open-label, multicentre, randomised study. Lancet. 2012;380(9850):1309–16.
17. Mirouse A, Resche-Rigon M, Lemiale V, et al. Red blood cell transfusion in the resuscitation of septic patients with hematological malignancies. Ann Intensive Care. 2017;7(1):62.
18. Miller AB, Hoogstraten B, Staquet M, Winkler A. Reporting results of cancer treatment. Am Cancer Soc. 1981;47(1):207–14.
19. Estcourt LJ, Heddle N, Kaufman R, et al. The challenges of measuring bleeding outcomes in clinical trials of platelet transfusions. Transfusion. 2013;53(7):1531–43.
20. Heddle NM, Cook RJ, Tinmouth A, et al. A randomized controlled trial comparing standard- and low dose strategies for transfusion of platelets (SToP) to patients with thrombocytopenia. Blood. 2009;113(7):1564–73.
21. Le Gall J, Lemeshow S, Saulnier F. A new Simplified Acute Physiology Score (SAPS II) based on a European/North American multicenter study. JAMA. 1993;270:2957–63.
22. Vincent J, Moreno R, Takala J, et al. The SOFA (Sepsis-related Organ Failure Assessment) score to describe organ dysfunction/failure. On behalf of the Working Group on Sepsis-Related Problems of the European Society of Intensive Care Medicine. Intensive Care Med. 1996;22(7):707–10.
23. Levy MM, Fink MP, Marshall JC, et al. 2001 SCCM/ESICM/ACCP/ATS/SIS international sepsis definitions conference. Crit Care Med. 2003;31(4):1250–6.
24. Lieberman F, Villgran V, Normolle D, Boyiadzis M. Intracranial hemorrhage in patients newly diagnosed with acute myeloid leukemia and hyperleukocytosis. Acta Haematol. 2017;138(2):116–8.
25. Taylor FJ, Toh C, Hoots W, Wada H, Levi M. Scientific and standardization committee communications towards definition, clinical and laboratory criteria, and a scoring system for disseminated intravascular coagulation* On behalf of the Scientific Subcommittee on Disseminated Intravascular Coagul. Thromb Haemost. 2001;86(5):1327–30.
26. Russell L, Madsen MB, Dahl M, Kampmann P, Perner A. Prediction of bleeding and thrombosis by standard biochemical coagulation variables in haematological intensive care patients. Acta Anaesthesiol Scand. 2017. https://doi.org/10.1111/aas.13036.
27. Pène F, Aubron C, Azoulay E, et al. Outcome of critically ill allogeneic hematopoietic stem-cell transplantation recipients: a reappraisal of indications for organ failure supports. J Clin Oncol. 2006;24(4):643–9.
28. Roze des Ordons AL, Chan K, Mirza I, Townsend DR, Bagshaw SM. Clinical characteristics and outcomes of patients with acute myelogenous leukemia admitted to intensive care: a case-control study. BMC Cancer. 2010;10:516.
29. Rabbat A, Chaoui D, Montani D, et al. Prognosis of patients with acute myeloid leukaemia admitted to intensive care. Br J Haematol. 2005;129(3):350–7.
30. Benoit DD, Depuydt PO, Vandewoude KH, et al. Outcome in severely ill patients with hematological malignancies who received intravenous chemotherapy in the intensive care unit. Intensive Care Med. 2006;32(1):93–9.
31. Benoit DD, Vandewoude KH, Decruyenaere JM, Hoste EA, Colardyn FA. Outcome and early prognostic indicators in patients with a hematologic malignancy admitted to the intensive care unit for a life-threatening complication. Crit Care Med. 2003;31:104–12.
32. Crowther MA, Cook DJ, Meade MO, et al. Thrombocytopenia in medical-surgical critically ill patients: prevalence, incidence, and risk factors. J Crit Care. 2005;20(4):348–53.
33. Dhainaut J-F, Shorr AF, Macias WL, et al. Dynamic evolution of coagulopathy in the first day of severe sepsis: relationship with mortality and organ failure. Crit Care Med. 2005;33(2):341–8.
34. Vandijck DM, Blot SI, De Waele JJ, Hoste EA, Vandewoude KH, Decruyenaere JM. Thrombocytopenia and outcome in critically ill patients with bloodstream infection. Heart Lung. 2010;39(1):21–6.
35. Akca S, Haji-Michael P, De Mendonça A, Suter P, Levi M, Vincent J. Time course of platelet counts in critically ill patients. Crit Care Med. 2002;30(4):753–6.
36. Shalansky SJ, Verma AK, Levine M, Spinelli JJ, Dodek PM. Risk markers for thrombocytopenia in critically ill patients: a prospective analysis. Pharmacotherapy. 2002;22(7):803–13.
37. Vanderschueren S, De Weerdt A, Malbrain M, et al. Thrombocytopenia and prognosis in intensive care. Crit Care Med. 2000;28(6):1871–6.
38. Thiolliere F, Serre-Sapin AF, Reignier J, et al. Epidemiology and outcome of thrombocytopenic patients in the intensive care unit: results of a prospective multicenter study. Intensive Care Med. 2013;39(8):1460–8.
39. Caruso P, Ferreira AC, Laurienzo CE, et al. Short- and long-term survival of patients with metastatic solid cancer admitted to the intensive care unit: prognostic factors. Eur J Cancer Care Engl. 2010;19(2):260–6.

40. Strauss R, Wehler M, Mehler K, Kreutzer D, Koebnick C, Hahn EG. Thrombocytopenia in patients in the medical intensive care unit: bleeding prevalence, transfusion requirements, and outcome. Crit Care Med. 2002;30(8):1765–71.

41. Ben Hamida C, Lauzet J-Y, Rézaiguia-Delclaux S, et al. Effect of severe thrombocytopenia on patient outcome after liver transplantation. Intensive Care Med. 2003;29(5):756–62.

42. Perner A, Haase N, Guttormsen AB, et al. Hydroxyethyl starch 130/0.42 versus Ringer's acetate in severe sepsis. N Engl J Med. 2012;367(2):124–34.

43. Haase N, Wetterslev J, Winkel P, Perner A. Bleeding and risk of death with hydroxyethyl starch in severe sepsis: post hoc analyses of a randomized clinical trial. Intensive Care Med. 2013;39(12):2126–34.

44. Del Principe MI, Del Principe D, Venditti A. Thrombosis in adult patients with acute leukemia. Curr Opin Oncol. 2017;29(6):448–54.

45. Gade I, Brækkan S, Næss IA, et al. Epidemiology of venous tromboembolism in hematological cancers: the Scandinavian Thrombosis and Cancer (STAC) Cohort. Thromb Res. 2017;158:157–60.

46. Choudhry A, DeLoughery TG. Bleeding and thrombosis in acute promyelocytic leukemia. Am J Hematol. 2012;87(6):596–603.

47. Rickles FR, Falanga A, Montesinos P, Sanz MA, Brenner B, Barbui T. Bleeding and thrombosis in acute leukemia: what does the future of therapy look like? Thromb Res. 2007;120(Suppl 2):99–106.

48. Colombo R, Gallipoli P, Castelli R. Thrombosis and hemostatic abnormalities in hematological malignancies. Clin Lymphoma Myeloma Leuk. 2014;14(6):441–50.

49. Falanga A, Rickles F. Pathogenesis and management of the bleeding diathesis in acute promyelocytic leukaemia. Best Pract Res Clin Haematol. 2003;16(3):463–82.

50. Rickles FR, Falanga A. Molecular basis for the relationship between thrombosis and cancer. Thromb Res. 2001;102:215–24.

51. Falanga A, Barbui T, Rickles FR. Hypercoagulability and tissue factor gene upregulation in hematologic malignancies. Semin Thromb Hemost. 2008;34(2):204–10.

52. Mooberry MJ, Key NS. Microparticle analysis in disorders of hemostasis and thrombosis. Cytom Part A. 2016;89(2):111–22.

53. Bruserud Ø, Foss B, Ulvestad E, Hervig T. Effects of acute myelogenous leukemia blasts on platelet release of soluble P-selectin and platelet-derived growth factor. Platelets. 1998;9(6):352–8.

54. Yan M, Jurasz P. The role of platelets in the tumor microenvironment: from solid tumors to leukemia. Biochim Biophys Acta. 2016;1863(3):392–400.

55. Cortelezzi A, Moia M, Falanga A, et al. Incidence of thrombotic complications in patients with haematological malignancies with central venous catheters: a prospective multicentre study. Br J Haematol. 2005;129(6):811–7.

56. Refaei M, Fernandes B, Brandwein J, Goodyear MD, Pokhrel A, Wu C. Incidence of catheter-related thrombosis in acute leukemia patients: a comparative, retrospective study of the safety of peripherally inserted versus centrally inserted central venous catheters. Ann Hematol. 2016;95(12):2057–64.

57. Del Principe MI, Buccisano F, Maurillo L, et al. Infections increase the risk of central venous catheter-related thrombosis in adult acute myeloid leukemia. Thromb Res. 2013;132(5):511–4.

58. Cook D, Crowther M, Meade M, et al. Deep venous thrombosis in medical-surgical critically ill patients: prevalence, incidence, and risk factors. Crit Care Med. 2005;33(7):1565–71.

59. Attia J, Ray JG, Cook DJ, Douketis J, Ginsberg JS, Geerts WH. Deep vein thrombosis and its prevention in critically ill adults. Arch Intern Med. 2001;161:1268–79.

60. Couban S, Goodyear M, Burnell M, et al. Randomized placebo-controlled study of low-dose warfarin for the prevention of central venous catheter-associated thrombosis in patients with cancer. J Clin Oncol. 2005;23(18):4063–9.

17

Increase in intra-abdominal pressure during airway suctioning-induced cough after a successful spontaneous breathing trial is associated with extubation outcome

Yasuhiro Norisue[1,2,4*] , Jun Kataoka[1], Yosuke Homma[1], Takaki Naito[2], Junpei Tsukuda[2], Kentaro Okamoto[2], Takeshi Kawaguchi[2], Lonny Ashworth[3], Shimada Yumiko[1], Yuiko Hoshina[1], Eiji Hiraoka[1] and Shigeki Fujitani[2]

Abstract

Background: A patient's ability to clear secretions and protect the airway with an effective cough is an important part of the pre-extubation evaluation. An increase in intra-abdominal pressure (IAP) is important in generating the flow rate necessary for a cough. This study investigated whether an increase from baseline in IAP during a coughing episode induced by routine pre-extubation airway suctioning is associated with extubation outcome after a successful spontaneous breathing trial (SBT).

Methods: Three hundred thirty-five (335) mechanically ventilated patients who passed an SBT were enrolled. Baseline IAP and peak IAP during successive suctioning-induced coughs were measured with a fluid column connected to a Foley catheter.

Results: Extubation was unsuccessful in 24 patients (7.2%). Unsuccessful extubation was 3.40 times as likely for patients with a delta IAP (ΔIAP) of $\leq$ 30 cm H_2O than for those with a ΔIAP > 30 cm H_2O, after adjusting for APACHE II score (95% CI, 1.39–8.26; $p = .007$).

Conclusion: ΔIAP during a coughing episode induced by routine pre-extubation airway suctioning is significantly associated with extubation outcome in patients with a successful SBT.

Keywords: Cough, Airway suctioning, Extubation, Intra-abdominal pressure, Mechanical ventilation

Background

Although cough strength for clearing secretions is important in successful extubation, it is not routinely objectively evaluated in daily practice after a successful spontaneous breathing trial (SBT). The inability to produce an adequate cough—because of muscle weakness or pain—increases the risks of atelectasis, oxygen desaturation, re-intubation, and, possibly, pneumonia [1–3].

Cough strength, as measured by voluntary and involuntary cough peak expiratory flow (CPEF), has been proposed as an independent predictor of successful extubation [4–10]. Previous studies reported that an involuntary CPEF of < 60 L/min was significantly associated with increased risk of extubation failure [5, 9, 10]. In addition to methods that focus on CPEF, clinicians desire a procedure that would allow evaluation of involuntary cough strength among patients who are unable or unwilling to produce maximal cough effort without special devices. Ideally, this procedure would not require disconnecting the patient from the ventilator circuit during routine pre-extubation airway suctioning, as this almost always induces cough.

*Correspondence: norisue.yasuhiro@gmail.com
[4] Department of Pulmonary and Critical Care Medicine, Tokyo Bay Urayasu Ichikawa Medical Center, 3-4-32 Todaijima, Urayasu, Chiba 2790001, Japan
Full list of author information is available at the end of the article

Physiologically, a cough begins with a deep inspiratory phase, followed by an expiratory phase of bursts of intercostal and abdominal muscle contractions [11]. This results in "the compressive phase" and an abrupt rise in intrapleural and intra-abdominal pressure (IAP) [12] with the relaxed diaphragm. IAP is then transmitted into intrapleural pressure [13], which abruptly increases airway pressure and cough. The increase in intra-abdominal pressure (ΔIAP) during an episode of continuous coughing is thus positively correlated with cough strength [13–16]. Use of a Foley catheter to measure bladder pressure during cough is straightforward and can be performed in most centers. We tested the hypothesis that low ΔIAP is associated with extubation failure after a successful SBT.

Methods

Study design

This is a single-center, prospective, cohort study. The study was approved by the Institutional Review Board at Tokyo Bay Urayasu Ichikawa Medical Center (TBUIMC). A waiver of informed consent was obtained because the study exposed patients to less than minimal risk.

Patients

The study was performed in the medical–surgical ICU during the period from April 2015 through November 2015. All mechanically ventilated patients 18 years or older who had been endotracheally intubated and had passed an SBT of longer than 30 min were eligible for inclusion. The SBT was conducted on pressure support ventilation with a pressure support of 5 cm H_2O, a positive end-expiratory pressure (PEEP) of ≤ 8 cm H_2O, and a fraction of inspiratory oxygen (FiO_2) of ≤ 0.50. Patients were excluded from the study if they had "comfort care" or "do not re-intubate" status or had been previously extubated during the same hospitalization. Patients were also excluded if they had documented or suspected upper airway obstruction, end-stage renal disease requiring hemodialysis, or no Foley catheter at the time of extubation. Successful completion of an SBT was determined using the standard Tokyo Bay Urayasu Ichikawa Medical Center (TBUIMC) Respiratory Care Weaning Protocols (no evidence of severe anxiety, dyspnea, or excessive accessory muscle use; a rapid shallow breathing index [RSBI] of ≤ 105 breaths/min/L; and adequate gas exchange, i.e., $SaO_2 \geq 90\%$ with $FiO_2 \leq 0.50$ and PEEP ≤ 8 cm H_2O).

Observations and measurements

A water-column technique was used to measure IAP [17], which was determined in the ICU by resident physicians using the following protocol, after all sedatives and analgesics were discontinued for at least 60 min: (1) the drainage tube of the patient's Foley bladder catheter was clamped; (2) sterile normal saline (20 ml) was instilled into the bladder via the aspiration port of the Foley catheter with a needleless connection system; (3) a fluid column consisting of two extension tubes (length 75 cm, inner diameter 3.1 mm; Terumo, Tokyo, Japan) was constructed, connected to the aspiration port of the Foley catheter, and then placed at the level of the mid-axillary line; (4) with the patient in supine position, fluid level in the absence of cough at end expiration was marked on the extension tube and recorded as the baseline bladder pressure; (5) airway suctioning was performed by advancing the closed-system suction catheter while the patient was connected to the ventilator, which is part of the standard pre-extubation procedure; and (6) the recorder observed changes in fluid level and marked the highest fluid level on the extension tube during successive coughs, which was recorded as the highest bladder pressure. The patient was extubated within 10 min after IAP measurement. Attending physicians and fellows responsible for clinical decisions, including extubation, were blinded to the results of the IAP and ΔIAP measurements.

Definitions of extubation success and failure

Successful extubation was defined as the absence of the need for re-intubation within 72 h after extubation. Extubation failure was defined as re-intubation within 72 h after extubation. Patients were followed until hospital discharge or death. The use of prophylactic or therapeutic noninvasive positive pressure ventilation without consequent re-intubation was not considered as extubation failure.

Sample size

Because at least 10 episodes of extubation failure were required in order to conduct multiple regression analysis adjusted for APACHE II score—the most important confounding factor for extubation outcomes—the estimated minimum sample size needed for the statistical analysis was 135 with a predicted extubation failure rate of 8%, as indicated by the past extubation failure rate in this ICU [18]. With a planned study duration of 9 months, the predicted number of patients to be recruited in the study was 400, assuming an average of approximately 45 extubations per month in our ICU.

Statistical analysis

The primary outcome of this study was extubation failure. Secondary outcomes included in-hospital mortality, ICU days, and length of hospital stay. A ΔIAP cutoff value for extubation failure was estimated with receiver operator characteristic (ROC) analysis. A multivariable-adjusted logistic regression model was used to calculate the odds ratio for extubation failure based on ΔIAP adjusted for APACHE II score. Mean baseline IAP, ΔIAP, and other variables were compared in relation to extubation success and failure. The Student *t* test was used to compare the means for variables. The Fisher exact test was used to compare grouped data such as sex, Confusion Assessment Method for the Intensive Care Unit (CAM-ICU), and mortality. For measures of association, 95% confidence intervals (CI) were computed, and statistical significance was defined as a two-tailed *p* value of less than .05. Using a multivariable-adjusted logistic regression model,

we estimated the odds ratio (OR) for re-intubation adjusted for APACHE II score. We also conducted a secondary analysis to investigate the relationship between ΔIAP and extubation outcomes in patients who were mechanically ventilated for longer than 72 h. All statistical analyses, except for sample size estimation, were performed with the IBM Statistical Package for the Social Sciences version 22.0 (IBM, Corp, Armonk, NY, USA).

Results

Patients

A total of 335 patients were included in the analyses (Fig. 1), 24 (7.2%) of whom were re-intubated within 72 h after extubation. Tables 1 and 2 show patient baseline characteristics and indications for intubation, respectively. Univariate analysis showed that CAM-ICU, APACHE II score, Simplified Acute Physiology Score II score, intubation days, length of ICU stay, length of hospital stay, 28-day mortality, and in-hospital mortality were significantly higher, and P/F ratio was significantly lower, in the extubation failure group than in the extubation success group. Figures 2 and 3 show the distributions of baseline IAP and ΔIAP for the patients. The median (interquartile range) baseline IAP was 8 (4–11) cm H_2O, and the median (interquartile range) ΔIAP was 38 (23–55) cm H_2O (range, 0–120 cm H_2O).

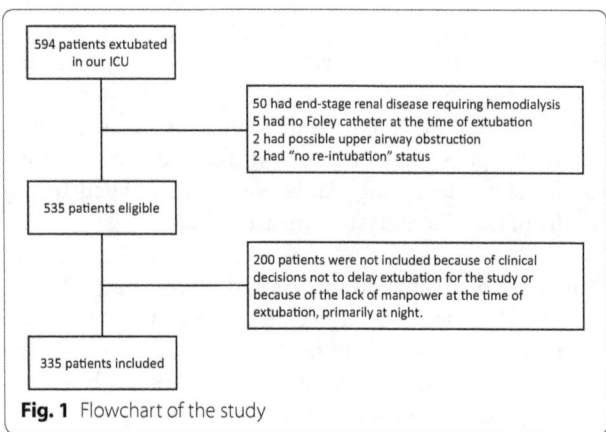

Fig. 1 Flowchart of the study

Table 1 Baseline characteristics of patients in each group

Characteristics	Extubation success	Extubation failure	p value
Number of patients, n	311	24	
Male sex, n (%)	193 (62.1)	17 (70.8)	0.512
Age, median (IQR)	71 (62–79)	72 (64–78)	0.581
BMI, median (IQR)	22.7 (20.3–25.2)	21.05 (17.3–24.8)	0.115
GCS, median (IQR)	11 (10–11)	11 (10–11)	0.667
CAM-ICU, positive (%)	40 (12.9)	8 (33.3)	0.012
APACHE II score, median (IQR)	20 (17–24)	24 (22–28)	<0.001
SAPS II score, median (IQR)	41 (32–51)	51 (46–59)	<0.001
In–out balance, median ml (IQR)	2959 (1000–5322)	2676 (793–4500)	0.701
Intubation days, median (IQR)	2 (1–3)	4 (2–6)	0.001
P/F ratio, median (IQR)	300 (250–367)	275 (218–326)	0.036
TV, median L (IQR)	0.44 (0.36–0.55)	0.47 (0.40–0.66)	0.139
MV, median L (IQR)	6.90 (5.60–8.19)	7.90 (5.76–9.75)	0.087
RSBI, median breaths/min/L (IQR)	37.2 (26.4–48.9)	38.2(16.9-51.3)	0.691
Length of ICU stay, median (IQR)	4 (2–6)	12 (6–16)	<0.001
Length of hospital stay, median (IQR)	20 (14–36)	48 (27–55)	<0.001
28-Day mortality, n (%)	3 (1.0)	3 (12.5)	0.006
In-hospital mortality, n (%)	10 (3.2)	5 (20.8)	0.002
Baseline IAP, mm H_2O, median (IQR)	7.9 (4.0–10.0)	8.0 (5.7–13.0)	0.19
ΔIAP, mm H_2O, median (IQR)	39.0 (24.0–57.0)	25.5 (19.8–38.3)	0.012

Table 2 Indications for intubation in each group

Indications for intubation	Extubation success (n)	Extubation failure (n)	p value
Emergent abdominal surgery	13	1	0.22
Emergent non-abdominal surgery	48	5	
Elective abdominal surgery	10	1	
Elective non-abdominal surgery	110	3	
Altered mental status	3	0	
Acute myocardial infarction	7	1	
Congestive heart failure	19	0	
Asthma	1	0	
Pneumonia	13	1	
Sepsis	22	3	
COPD	2	1	
Drug intoxication	5	0	
Hemorrhagic stroke	9	1	
Ischemic stroke	2	0	
Gastrointestinal bleeding	4	0	
Status epilepticus	6	1	
Others	37	6	

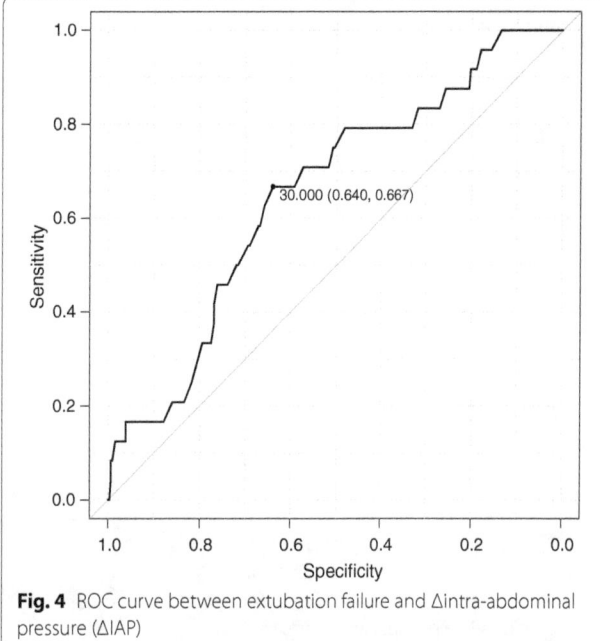

Fig. 4 ROC curve between extubation failure and Δintra-abdominal pressure (ΔIAP)

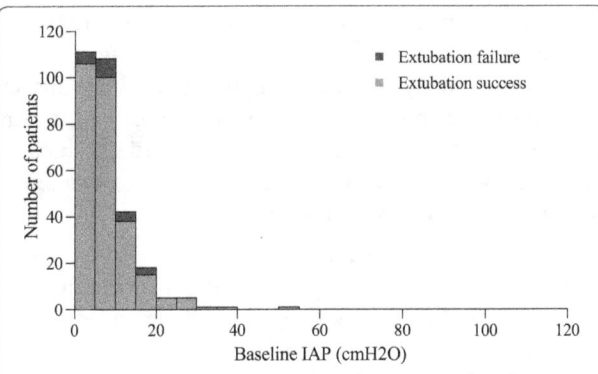

Fig. 2 Histogram showing the number of patients and baseline intra-abdominal pressure (IAP)

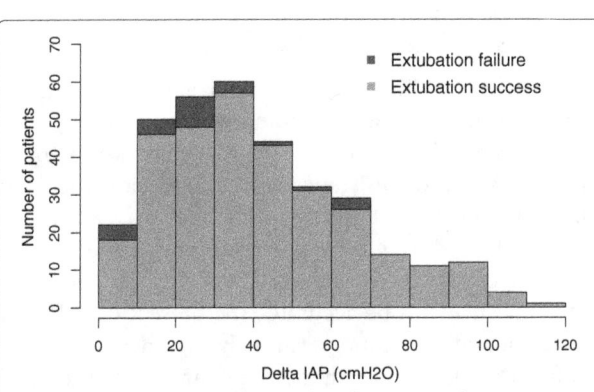

Fig. 3 Histogram showing the number of patients and Δintra-abdominal pressure (ΔIAP)

Table 3 Unadjusted and adjusted odds ratio of low ΔIAP for extubation failure

	OR	95% CI	p value
Unadjusted	3.56	1.47–8.55	0.005
Adjusted*	3.40	1.39–8.26	0.007

*Adjusted for APACHE II score

ΔIAP and outcome measures

ΔIAP was significantly higher in the extubation success group than in the extubation failure group ($p = 0.012$; median, 39.00 vs 25.50 cm H_2O, respectively). Figure 4 shows the ROC curve between ΔIAP and extubation failure. The area under the ROC curve was 0.654 (95% CI 0.544–0.764), and the cutoff value was 30 cm H_2O (sensitivity, 64%; specificity, 67%). ΔIAP was classified as ≤ 30 cm H_2O (low ΔIAP group) or > 30 cm H_2O (high ΔIAP group). Table 3 shows that low ΔIAP was significantly associated with extubation failure after adjusting for APACHE II score (adjusted OR, 3.40; 95% CI, 1.39–8.26, $p = .007$). The positive predictive value and negative predictive value of a ΔIAP value of ≤ 30 cm H_2O for extubation failure were 1.85 and 0.52, respectively.

ΔIAP and outcome measures in patients who were mechanically ventilated for longer than 72 h

A secondary analysis including only patients who were mechanically ventilated for longer than 72 h (124 patients with successful extubation and 17 patients with extubation failure) yielded an AUC of 0.708 (95% CI

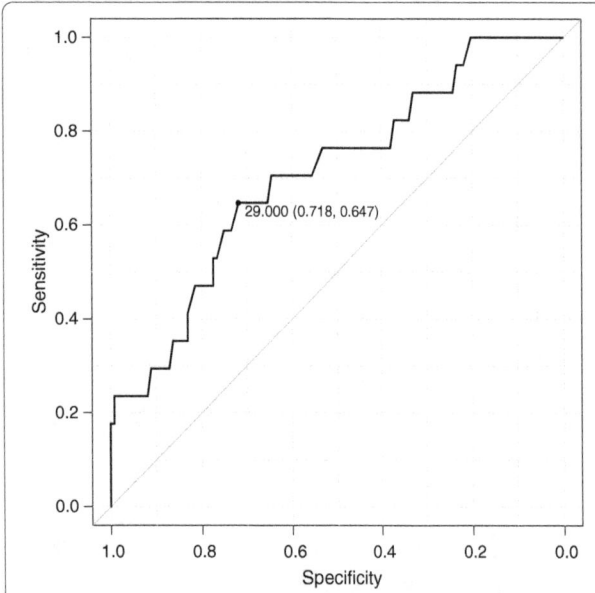

Fig. 5 ROC curve between extubation failure and Δintra-abdominal pressure (ΔIAP) in patients who were mechanically ventilated for more than 72 h

Table 4 Unadjusted and adjusted odds ratio of low ΔIAP for extubation failure in patients were mechanically ventilated for more than 72 h

	OR	95% CI	p value
Unadjusted	3.93	1.39–11.20	0.01
Adjusted*	3.79	1.32–10.75	0.01

*Adjusted for APACHE II score

0.571–0.845) with a cutoff value of 29 cm H_2O (Fig. 5). Multiple regression analysis (Table 4) showed that a low ΔIAP (≤ 29 cm H_2O) was significantly associated with extubation failure, after adjusting for APACHE II score (adjusted OR, 3.79; 95% CI, 1.32–10.75, $p = 0.01$). The positive predictive value and negative predictive value of a ΔIAP value of ≤ 29 cm H_2O for extubation failure were 2.21 and 0.56, respectively.

Discussion

This study showed that diminished ΔIAP during coughing induced by routine pre-extubation suctioning was significantly associated with extubation failure. Expiratory muscle strength is important in producing a successful cough [19]. However, CPEF is the only widely accepted method of evaluating pre-extubation expiratory muscle strength during cough production. Smina et al. [5] reported that a CPEF ≤ 60 L/min yielded an AUC of 0.7 (sensitivity 69%; specificity 74%) in predicting extubation

failure. Our ΔIAP data indicated similar predictive values, especially in patients mechanically ventilated for longer than 72 h. These findings suggest that ΔIAP is a potentially useful parameter for assessing expiratory muscle strength.

The cough reflex protects the airway by means of a continuous series of expiratory coughs with subsequent inspiratory efforts [20–22]. The continuous increase in IAP during such an episode provides sustained expiratory force [14]. The present results are consistent with these physiological characteristics of the cough reflex and support the hypothesis that an inability to increase IAP predicts extubation failure. Moreover, our secondary analysis of patients intubated for longer than 72 h yielded a better AUC in predicting extubation failure. The present results are attributable to the significant association between duration of mechanical ventilation and ICU-acquired weakness (ICUAW) [23]; thus, our method might be more relevant and useful for patients at high risk of ICUAW, including expiratory muscle weakness.

The proposed method of estimating cough strength has several practical strengths. Most mechanically ventilated patients already have a Foley catheter, and IAP measurement is feasible in most ICUs. Second, airway suctioning is part of the pre-extubation process; therefore, ΔIAP measurement can be included in routine pre-extubation evaluation. Finally, cough strength induced by airway suctioning does not depend on patient effort and is thus feasible for most mechanically ventilated patients, including those who are uncooperative because of dementia, delirium, or altered mental status.

Future studies should investigate how to apply ΔIAP to clinical decision making. For example, a patient who has passed an SBT but has a low ΔIAP may need appropriate preparation for possible re-intubation. Unlike the present patients with a low ΔIAP, none of those with a ΔIAP > 70 cm H_2O had extubation failure (Fig. 3). Thus, a ΔIAP > 70 cm H_2O may be potentially used to exclude the possibility of extubation failure in patients with a successful SBT and no airway obstruction.

This study has limitations that warrant mention. ΔIAP was measured with a fluid column rather than by connecting the Foley catheter to a digital pressure transducer. Because of resistance in the extension tube, the fluid level might not have reached the true maximum pressure level during a coughing episode. Moreover, the accuracy of visual IAP measurement has not been validated and may not be accurate. The present cutoff value might therefore be more accurately regarded as a cutoff value for the fluid column method than as the true ΔIAP cutoff value.

Conclusion

In conclusion, ΔIAP during a coughing episode induced by routine pre-extubation airway suctioning is significantly associated with extubation outcome in patients with a successful SBT.

Abbreviations

APACHE: Acute Physiology and Chronic Health Evaluation; CAM-ICU: Confusion Assessment Method for the Intensive Care Unit; CI: confidence interval; ESRD: end-stage renal disease; FiO2: fraction of inspired oxygen; GCS: Glasgow Coma Scale; IAP: intra-abdominal pressure; ICU: intensive care unit; OR: odds ratio; PEEP: positive end-expiratory pressure; PEF: peak expiratory flow; ROC: receiver operator characteristic; RSBI: rapid shallow breathing index; SBT: spontaneous breathing trial; SAPS: Simplified Acute Physiology Score; TBUIMC: Tokyo Bay Urayasu Ichikawa Medical Center.

Author contributions

YN is the guarantor of the content of the manuscript, including the data and analysis. YN had full access to all study data and takes responsibility for the integrity of the data and the accuracy of the data analysis. YN, TN, JT, KO, TK, EH, and SF substantially contributed to the study design, YH, YH, YS, LA, and JT contributed to data interpretation and drafting of the manuscript. YH, JK, and YH analyzed the data.

Author details

[1] Department of Emergency and Critical Care Medicine, Tokyo Bay Urayasu Ichikawa Medical Center, 3-4-32 Todaijima, Urayasu, Chiba 2790001, Japan. [2] Department of Emergency and Critical Care Medicine, St. Marianna University Hospital, 2-16-1 Sugao, Kawasaki, Kanagawa 2168511, Japan. [3] Department of Respiratory Care, Boise State University, 1910 W University Drive, Boise, ID 83725, USA. [4] Department of Pulmonary and Critical Care Medicine, Tokyo Bay Urayasu Ichikawa Medical Center, 3-4-32 Todaijima, Urayasu, Chiba 2790001, Japan.

Acknowledgements

We thank Professor Daniel Talmor for his valuable advice on this study and for reviewing the manuscript.

Competing interests

The authors declare that they have no competing interests.

References

1. Wang ZY, Bai Y. Cough-another important factor in extubation readiness in critically ill patients. Crit Care. 2012;16(6):461.
2. Jiang C, Esquinas A, Mina B. Evaluation of cough peak expiratory flow as a predictor of successful mechanical ventilation discontinuation: a narrative review of the literature. J Intensive Care. 2017;5:33.
3. Krinsley JS, Reddy PK, Iqbal A. What is the optimal rate of failed extubation? Crit Care. 2012;16(1):111.
4. Khamiees M, Raju P, DeGirolamo A, Amoateng-Adjepong Y, Manthous CA. Predictors of extubation outcome in patients who have successfully completed a spontaneous breathing trial. Chest. 2001;120(4):1262–70.
5. Smina M, Salam A, Khamiees M, Gada P, Amoateng-Adjepong Y, Manthous CA. Cough peak flows and extubation outcomes. Chest. 2003;124(1):262–8.
6. Duan J, Liu J, Xiao M, Yang X, Wu J, Zhou L. Voluntary is better than involuntary cough peak flow for predicting re-intubation after scheduled extubation in cooperative subjects. Respir Care. 2014;59(11):1643–51.
7. Bai L, Duan J. Use of cough peak flow measured by a ventilator to predict re-intubation when a spirometer is unavailable. Respir Care. 2017;62(5):566–71.
8. Beuret P, Roux C, Auclair A, Nourdine K, Kaaki M, Carton MJ. Interest of an objective evaluation of cough during weaning from mechanical ventilation. Intensive Care Med. 2009;35(6):1090–3.
9. Salam A, Tilluckdharry L, Amoateng-Adjepong Y, Manthous CA. Neurologic status, cough, secretions and extubation outcomes. Intensive Care Med. 2004;30(7):1334–9.
10. Su WL, Chen YH, Chen CW, Yang SH, Su CL, Perng WC, Wu CP, Chen JH. Involuntary cough strength and extubation outcomes for patients in an ICU. Chest. 2010;137(4):777–82.
11. Grelot L, Milano S. Diaphragmatic and abdominal muscle activity during coughing in the decerebrate cat. NeuroReport. 1991;2(4):165–8.
12. McCool FD. Global physiology and pathophysiology of cough: ACCP evidence-based clinical practice guidelines. Chest. 2006;129(1 Suppl):48S–53S.
13. Irwin RS, Rosen MJ, Braman SS. Cough. A comprehensive review. Arch Intern Med. 1977;137(9):1186–91.
14. Addington WR, Stephens RE, Phelipa MM, Widdicombe JG, Ockey RR. Intra-abdominal pressures during voluntary and reflex cough. Cough. 2008;4:2.
15. Luginbuehl H, Baeyens JP, Kuhn A, Christen R, Oberli B, Eichelberger P, Radlinger L. Pelvic floor muscle reflex activity during coughing—an exploratory and reliability study. Ann Phys Rehabil Med. 2016;59(5–6):302–7.
16. Stephens RE, Addington WR, Miller SP, Anderson JW. Videofluoroscopy of the diaphragm during voluntary and reflex cough in humans. Am J Phys Med Rehabil. 2003;82(5):384.
17. Malbrain ML, Cheatham ML, Kirkpatrick A, Sugrue M, Parr M, De Waele J, Balogh Z, Leppaniemi A, Olvera C, Ivatury R, et al. Results from the international conference of experts on intra-abdominal hypertension and abdominal compartment syndrome. I. Definitions. Intensive Care Med. 2006;32(11):1722–32.
18. Peduzzi P, Concato J, Kemper E, Holford TR, Feinstein AR. A simulation study of the number of events per variable in logistic regression analysis. J Clin Epidemiol. 1996;49(12):1373–9.
19. Epstein SK. Decision to extubate. Intensive Care Med. 2002;28(5):535–46.
20. Korpáš J. Tomori Zn: cough and other respiratory reflexes. Basel: S. Karger; 1979.
21. Tatar M, Hanacek J, Widdicombe J. The expiration reflex from the trachea and bronchi. Eur Respir J. 2008;31(2):385–90.
22. Widdicombe J, Fontana G. Cough: what's in a name? Eur Respir J. 2006;28(1):10–5.
23. Hermans G, Van den Berghe G. Clinical review: intensive care unit acquired weakness. Crit Care. 2015;19:274.

18

Practical approach to diastolic dysfunction in light of the new guidelines and clinical applications in the operating room and in the intensive care

F. Sanfilippo[1]* ⓘ, S. Scolletta[2], A. Morelli[3] and A. Vieillard-Baron[4]

Abstract

There is growing evidence both in the perioperative period and in the field of intensive care (ICU) on the association between left ventricular diastolic dysfunction (LVDD) and worse outcomes in patients. The recent American Society of Echocardiography and European Association of Cardiovascular Imaging joint recommendations have tried to simplify the diagnosis and the grading of LVDD. However, both an often unknown pre-morbid LV diastolic function and the presence of several confounders—i.e., use of vasopressors, positive pressure ventilation, volume loading—make the proposed parameters difficult to interpret, especially in the ICU. Among the proposed parameters for diagnosis and grading of LVDD, the two tissue Doppler imaging-derived variables e' and E/e' seem most reliable. However, these are not devoid of limitations. In the present review, we aim at rationalizing the applicability of the recent recommendations to the perioperative and ICU areas, discussing the clinical meaning and echocardiographic findings of different grades of LVDD, describing the impact of LVDD on patients' outcomes and providing some hints on the management of patients with LVDD.

Keywords: Diastolic function, Systolic function, Weaning failure, Sepsis, Critical care

Background

The study of left ventricular (LV) diastolic function and the impact of decreased LV compliance and impaired relaxation has received growing interest. This is certainly due to not only the high incidence of LV diastolic dysfunction (LVDD) in the general population and its sensible impact on patients outcomes [1], but also the growing use of echocardiography, which remains the sole clinical tool allowing the estimation of LV diastolic function. A cross-sectional survey of over 2000 randomly selected Minnesota residents aged 45 years or older found an incidence of LVDD almost five times higher than LV systolic dysfunction (28 vs. 6%, respectively), which was a strong

predictor of mortality (hazard ratio ranging from 8.3 for mild LVDD to 10.2 for at-least-moderate LVDD) [1]. Up to 50% of patients presenting to the hospital with pulmonary edema and hypertension have unchanged LV systolic function and normal mitral valve apparatus, when compared during and after the acute episode [2]. Similarly, the incidence of isolated LVDD may be higher than 50% in patients hospitalized for heart failure (HF) [3].

The importance of LVDD is strongly emerging in the perioperative setting [4] and in critically ill patients [5–8], and the present review highlights the knowledge in the field. Moreover, since pharmacological strategies for improving LV diastolic function are limited and are more likely to produce results only in the long term [9], we provide a focused summary of the literature followed by key approaches that may help clinicians in the optimization and management of the patient with LVDD.

*Correspondence: filipposanfi@yahoo.it
[1] Department of Anesthesia and Intensive Care, IRCCS-ISMETT (Istituto Mediterraneo per i Trapianti e Terapie ad alta specializzazione), Palermo, Italy

Practical approach to diastolic dysfunction in light of the new guidelines and clinical applications...

169

Main text

Recent guidelines and their applicability in the perioperative and intensive care settings

The most recent American Society of Echocardiography and European Association of Cardiovascular Imaging (ASE/EACVI) joint recommendations for the diagnosis and assessment of LVDD [10] made substantial changes compared with the previous recommendations [11]. One of the main aims of the new guidelines was to simplify the approach of clinicians to grading of LVDD, which in the previous version was deemed too complex because many parameters were included. Such recently revised guidelines have changed the methodology for determining LVDD, recommending an assessment mainly based on the following four variables: tricuspid regurgitation (TR) jet velocity, left atrial (LA) volume, e' wave and E/e' ratio. The e' and E/e' ratio are two parameters derived by tissue Doppler imaging (TDI) analysis, measuring longitudinal fiber lengthening during early diastole at level of mitral valve annulus using a modified pulsed wave Doppler setting (high amplitude, low velocity). The e' maximal velocity reflects LV relaxation rate, while E/e' correlates with the LV filling pressures and a ratio above 13–15 is associated with pulmonary arterial occlusion pressures > 18 mmHg [10]. The cutoffs for the four variables recommended by the guidelines are summarized in Table 1.

In patients with normal LV systolic function, abnormalities of more than half of measurable parameters (i.e., a patient may have no TR) define the presence of LVDD. On the other hand, the new guidelines support that patients with structural abnormalities, known ischemic heart disease or abnormal LV systolic function will have impaired myocardial relaxation, and thus, echocardiography examination may focus on the assessment of LV filling pressures and diastolic dysfunction grade.

Once diagnosis of LVDD is made, the following step is to proceed with grading of the dysfunction itself. The four parameters indicated in Table 1 and the E/A ratio are used to grade LVDD and can be found in the recently published recommendations [10], but LVDD grading is not the aim of the present review, which is not intended for cardiologists or experts in echocardiography. Of note, an interesting retrospective cohort study by Almeida and Colleagues conducted on 1000 individuals aged $\geq$ 45 years and with normal systolic function found poor concordance between the new and the previous versions of the guidelines (published in 2009) for the evaluation of LV diastolic function [10, 11]. In this study, the new guidelines resulted in a significantly lower incidence of LVDD (1.4 vs. 38.1% of 2009 recommendations) [12].

Unfortunately, assessing LVDD is not always easy and the guidelines' authors themselves state "...*the guidelines are not necessarily applicable to children or in the perioperative setting*." The fact that applicability of these guidelines to the perioperative setting represents a challenge is not surprising. Indeed, patients undergoing major surgery are mechanically ventilated and exposed to drugs with vasoactive effects, and they easily fluctuate from hyper- to hypovolemia due to perioperative fasting, fluid shift, hemorrhage, etc. Moreover, the use of transthoracic echocardiography (TTE) is limited in the operating room, and the applicability of e' and E/e' ratio with transesophageal echocardiography (TEE) should consider the importance of obtaining a good alignment of TDI signal.

On the other hand, it is somewhat surprising that the authors did not mention the limitations of such new guidelines in the critically ill patients. Same limitations as the ones described in the perioperative setting may be also present. Moreover, in this population of patients, the TR jet velocity may worsen under the negative influence of mechanical ventilation on right ventricular (RV) function and there are a large number of factors that may increase pulmonary pressure at pre-capillary level, making the reliability of TR jet velocity at least questionable. Among these factors, pulmonary vascular resistances may increase with elevated airway pressures, although it should be kept in mind that the transmission of pleural pressure itself is reduced when lung compliance is low (i.e., acute respiratory distress syndrome). Additionally, the effects of mechanical ventilation on LV diastolic function are not negligible, and one study in cardiac surgery patients showed that increasing levels of positive end-expiratory pressure (PEEP) reduced significantly both septal and lateral e' values, possibly representing an impaired LV relaxation due to worse RV function (and possibly RV dilatation) [13]. In other words, the observed LVDD may not be related to the disease itself, but driven by the conditions of mechanical ventilation. One could say that LVDD is associated with a worst prognosis when reflecting a specific injury of the myocardium, while probably this is not the case when LVDD is mainly induced by ventilation settings and clinical management.

With respect to the second parameter listed in Table 1, the LA volume is influenced by loading conditions and critically ill patients are certainly exposed to sudden changes of circulating volume for either absolute or relative hypovolemia (i.e., trauma and/or sepsis). More importantly, patients with sepsis or septic shock are characterized not only by vasoplegia with reduction in LV afterload, but they also show myocardial depression (septic cardiomyopathy) [14]. Furthermore, as clarified in the recent guidelines, LA enlargement is observed when LVDD is chronic and cannot probably be used in more acute situations, as frequently observed in the intensive care unit (ICU). How acutely the LA can dilate during

Table 1 Four main parameters used to define left ventricular diastolic dysfunction and their cutoffs

Parameter	Abnormal value	Mode of measurement	Limitation/confounders
TR jet velocity	> 2.8 m/s	Parasternal and apical 4-ch view with CFD to get highest velocity aligned with CWD. Adjust gain and contrast to display complete spectral envelope (no signal spikes or feathering) Analysis: peak modal velocity during systole at leading edge of spectral wave-form	Indirect estimate of LA pressure; adequate recording of full envelope not always possible; in some cases accuracy of calculation is dependent on reliable estima-tion of right atrial systolic pressure
LA volume	> 34 mL/m²	Apical 4-ch and 2-ch: acquire freeze frames (1–2 frames before MV opening). LA volume measured in dedicated views (length and transverse diameters maximized) Analysis: method of disks or area-length method; correct for body surface area. Do not include LA appendage or pulmonary veins in tracings	LA dilatation is seen in bradycardia, high-output states, heart transplants, atrial flutter/fibrillation, significant MV disease, despite normal LV diastolic function; LA dilatation occurs in well-trained athletes; suboptimal image quality (i.e., fore-shortening) precludes accurate tracings; it can be difficult to quantify in patients with aortic aneurysms or in patients with large inter-atrial septal aneurysms
e'	Septal < 7 cm/s Lateral < 10 cm/s	Apical 4-ch view: PWD sample volume (usually 5–10 mm axial size) at lateral or septal basal regions. Use ultrasound system presets for wall filter and lowest signal gain. Optimal spectral waveforms should be sharp (no signal spikes, feathering or ghosting) Analysis: peak modal velocity in early diastole at the leading edge of spectral waveform	Limited accuracy in patients with CAD and RWMAs, significant MAC, surgical rings or prosthetic MV, pericardial disease; need to sample at least two sites; different cutoffs depending on sampling site; age dependent (decreases with aging)
E/e' ratio	Average > 14 Septal > 15 Lateral > 13	E wave: apical 4-ch with CFD imaging for optimal alignment of PWD with blood flow. PWD sample volume (1–3 mm axial size) between mitral leaflet tips. Use low wall filter setting (100–200 MHz) and low signal gain. Optimal spectral waveforms should not display spikes or feathering Analysis: peak modal velocity in early diastole at the leading edge of spectral waveform e': see above Analysis: E velocity divided by e' velocity	Not accurate in normal subjects, patients with MAC, pericardial disease; "gray zone" of values in which LV filling pressures are indeterminate; accuracy reduced in CAD and RWMAs; different cutoff values depending on the site used for measurement

4-ch, four-chamber; 2-ch, two-chamber; CAD, coronary artery disease; CFD, color flow Doppler; CWD, continuous wave Doppler; LA, left atrium; LV, left ventricle; MAC, mitral annulus calcifications; MV, mitral valve; PWD, pulsed wave Doppler; RWMAs regional wall motion abnormalities; TR, tricuspid regurgitation

the early stages of critical illness is a matter of future research. A recent study evaluated early changes in LA volume after acute myocardial infarction. At 4-month follow-up the authors found that 35% of patients had LA remodeling, defined as LA volume index ≥ 10 ml/m^2. However, at 1-month follow-up there was a mean change of 6 ml/m^2, with no significant differences between patients with or without LA remodeling [15]. Therefore, it seems that changes in LA volume can happen in a relatively short-term but not so acutely as it matters in the case of critically ill patients. Interestingly, another study demonstrated that magnitude and pattern of LA appendage emptying/filling velocities are dependent on loading conditions and that velocities are influenced mainly by changes in LV rather than in LA appendage function [16]. In light of the above, estimation of LA volume as for the prediction of acute changes of LV diastolic function in critically ill patients seems a physiologically imprecise parameter. Moreover, it is important to note that the LA volume is not precisely quantifiable with TEE, which adds further limitations for patients necessitating an echocardiographic assessment but having poor acoustic windows for a transthoracic examination, for whatever reason (i.e., due to mechanical ventilation). Another significant issue in the ICU regards the inability of echocardiographic evaluation to diagnose whether the LVDD is a new acute finding, mainly related to the critical illness (e.g. sepsis for instance) and then possibly reversible, or if LVDD pre-existed to the ICU admission, considering the amount of admission of older and older patients carrying a significant burden of comorbidities. The only way to differentiate between both is to repeat echocardiographic evaluation longitudinally until the discharge and maybe after full recovery, but this approach would be very time- and resource-consuming. However, observing a LA dilatation could help physicians determine whether diastolic dysfunction existed prior to admission in the ICU.

For the above reasons it becomes challenging the assessment of sepsis-related changes in LV diastolic function according to fluctuations in LA volume and/or TR jet velocities, while the two TDI parameters (e' and E/e', see Table 1) probably remain the only reliable approach, due to their relative independency from the loading state [17]. Importantly, a recent meta-analysis by Sanfilippo et al. [5] showed that such parameters are associated with survival in septic patients.

Clinical and echocardiographic findings of different grades of LVDD

Hereby, we provide a simplified interpretation to the progression from normal LV diastolic function to different degrees of LVDD. In this context, it should be kept in mind that LV diastolic properties and LV filling pressure are closely related. In particular, Fig. 1 shows the relationship between left-sided pressures (LA and LV, Fig. 1a) and the corresponding echocardiographic findings for each stage in terms of transmitral blood flow (Fig. 1b) and of TDI mitral annular displacement (Fig. 1c). In the outpatient setting, once diagnosis of LVDD is made (i.e., patients with reduced LV systolic function and/or structural cardiomyopathy and/or fulfilling 3–4 parameters shown in Table 1), the grading of dysfunction is assessed according to the E/A ratio (and eventually E wave velocity). Figure 2 shows an algorithm for grading of LVDD in the outpatients according to the ASE/EACVI 2016 guidelines.

From physiological perspectives, in patients with normal LV diastolic function, the LV fills smoothly in the presence of low LA pressures and thus with a relatively small LA-to-LV gradient (in the order of few mmHg). The corresponding echocardiographic appearance in the transmitral blood flow is a dominant early (E) wave over the atrial (A or late) wave, and the corresponding TDI e' and a' waves demonstrate a similar ratio (first column from the left in Fig. 1).

With regard to the interpretation of transmitral blood flow, at initial stages of LVDD the LV becomes stiffer with impaired LV relaxation and the LA-to-LV gradient becomes smaller. Therefore, the early filling wave gradually decreases and the atrial wave becomes dominant ($E < A$ wave): This is the classical features of LVDD grade I (second column from the left in Fig. 1).

The subsequent progression of LVDD with further relaxation impairment causes physiological mechanisms of adaptation (i.e., fluid retention and changed loading conditions) with a consequent increase in LA pressure in order to restore a "pseudo-normal" LA-to-LV gradient (LVDD grade II). Thus, during this stage of LVDD there is a "pseudo-normalization" of transmitral flow pattern ($E > A$ wave) due to the reactive increase in LA pressures in response to worsening LVDD (third column from the left in Fig. 1).

Finally, when the LV chamber becomes poorly compliant and increasingly stiff (LVDD grade III), only a certain amount of blood can flow from the LA to the LV at each diastole. Importantly, such reduced amount of blood flowing into the LV during the early phase of diastole (E wave) quickly boosts the LV end-diastolic pressure at very high level so that the subsequent atrial contraction is unable to generate a decent filling (usually in the order of very few ml of blood). Consequently, the E wave is very dominant and the E/A ratio is usually > 2 (last column from the left in Fig. 1). The LVDD grade III has been further divided into reversible and irreversible, but performing such distinction is challenging, it requires patient's collaboration (i.e.,

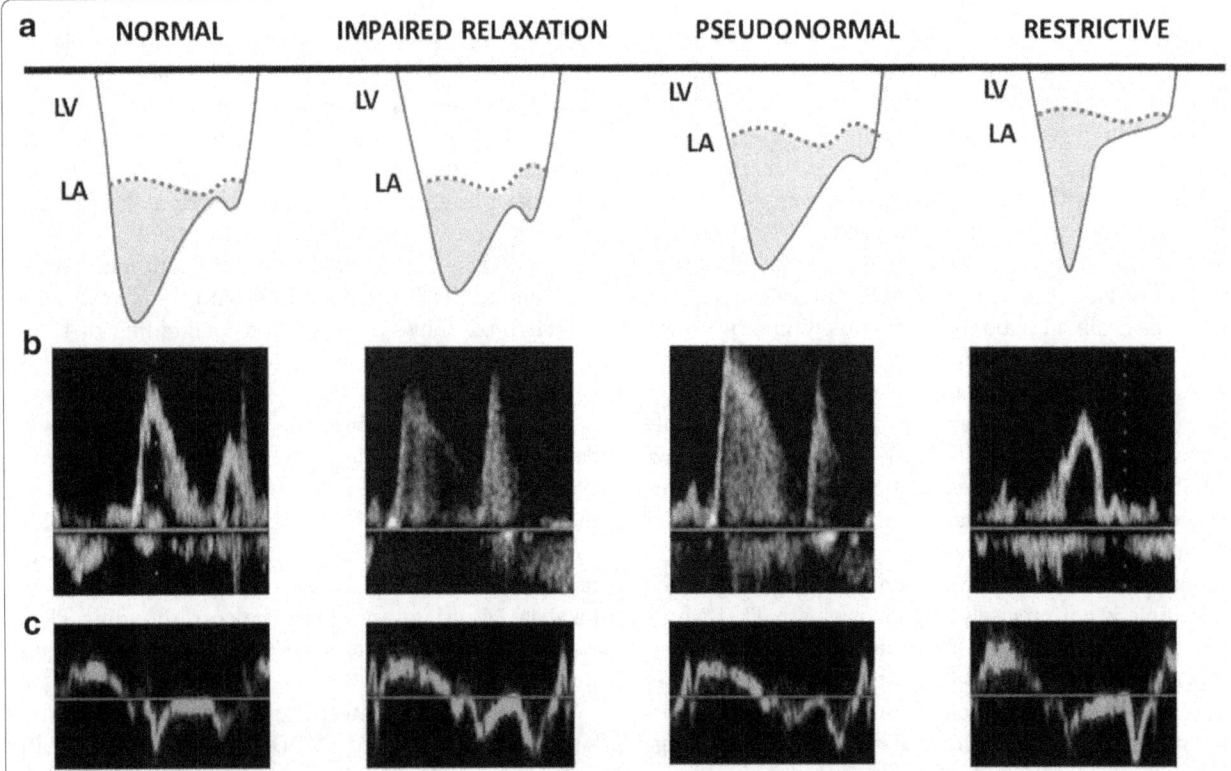

Fig. 1 Progression from normal diastolic function to worsening degrees of left ventricular diastolic dysfunction (LVDD). The top row **a** illustrates the respective changes in left atrial (LA) and left ventricular (LV) pressures with the progression of LVDD. The middle and bottom rows show examples of the patterns of transmitral blood flow (**b**) and of tissue Doppler imaging of the mitral annulus (**c**). These patterns are shown for each stage of LVDD, with corresponding changes of the E and e' (early), and A and a' (atrial) waves. From left to right, 2a: normal diastolic function ($E > A$; $e' > a'$); 2b: LVDD grade I ($E < A$; $e' < a'$); 2c: LVDD grade II ($E > A$; $e' < a'$); 2d: LVDD grade III ($E \gg A$; $e' \ll a'$)

performing Valsalva manoeuver), and more importantly it is probably more useful in the cardiology outpatient setting rather than in the operating room or in the ICU patients.

On the other hand, as shown in Fig. 1c, changes in TDI waves e' and a' are more unidirectional with the development of LVDD. The a' is an excellent marker of global atrial contraction and has similar values at septal and lateral levels [18]. It correlates very well with LA ejection fraction, LA ejection force and LA kinetic energy [19], being independent from the flow of blood filling the LV. For this reason the a' does not become smaller, but rather increases with progression of LV diastolic dysfunction and with more vigorous LA contraction in adaptation to the increased pressures. Only with advanced LA dilatation reaching a threshold of fiber length, LA shortening and contractility begin to decline, similar to what happens for the LV (Frank–Starling curve) [20–23]. On the other hand, the decline in A wave is likely to happen earlier in the progression of LVDD, because it is related to the reduction in transmitral blood flow in the presence of very high LV filling pressure.

Therefore, there is a progressive decrease in e' and a consequent increase in a' so that the e'/a' ratio moves gradually from > 1 to < 1 values; however, while $e'/a' > 1$ usually denotes a normal LV diastolic function and $e'/a' \ll 1$ is of restrictive pattern, it is more difficult to use the e'/a' ratio for the distinction between LVDD grades I and II.

In general, this paragraph provides a summary that may help readers in understanding the relationships between the LA-to-LV gradient and the changes in transmitral blood flow and mitral annular TDI displacement. It is mandatory to keep in mind that the interpretation of such parameters should take into account factors like patient's history (i.e., chronic atrial fibrillation—AF—may cause LA enlargement) and physiological factors (i.e., age influences cutoff for E wave). Moreover, the assessment becomes even more challenging in the ICU where the echocardiographic parameters can be affected by several confounders. For instance, the heart rate (especially tachycardia) and the use of vasopressors and/or inotropes influence the LV

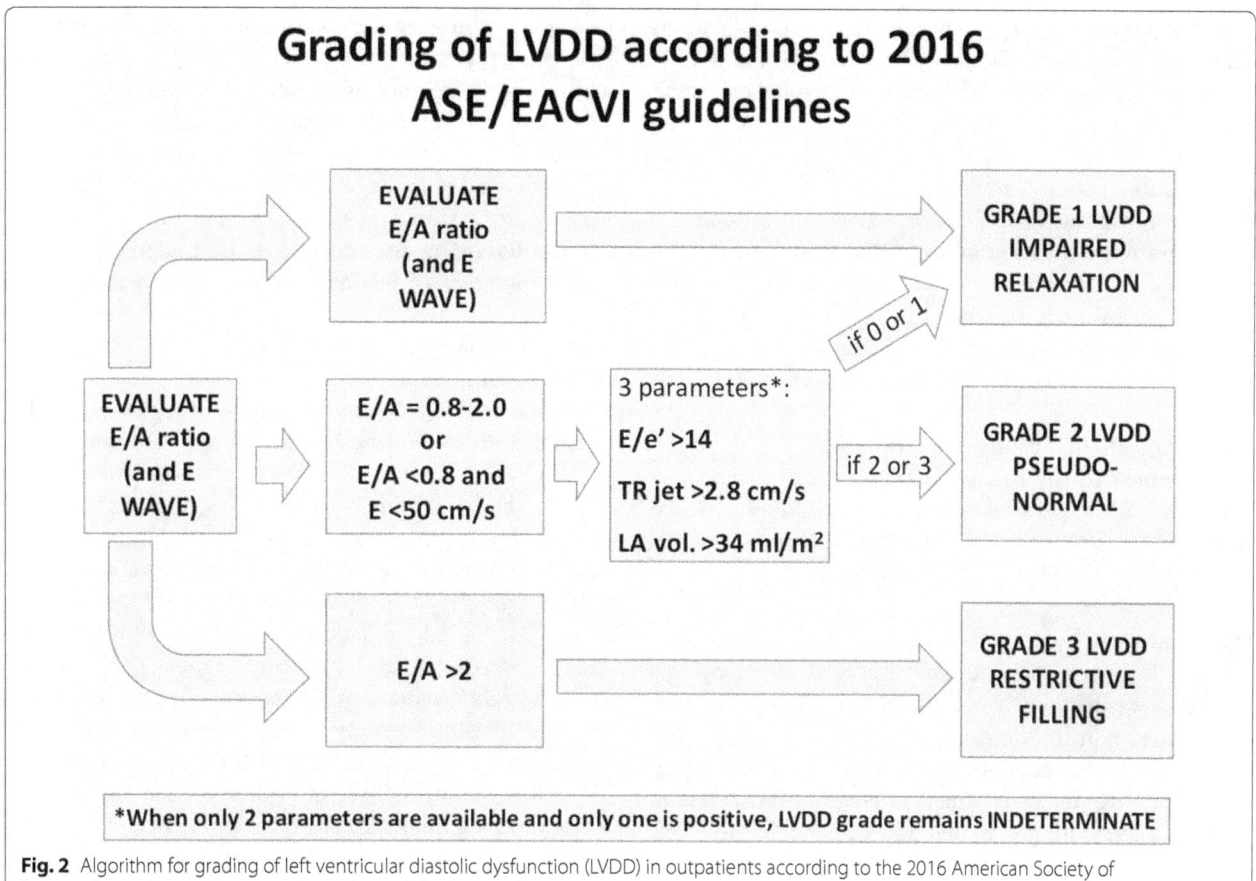

Fig. 2 Algorithm for grading of left ventricular diastolic dysfunction (LVDD) in outpatients according to the 2016 American Society of Echocardiography and European Association of Cardiovascular Imaging (ASE/EACVI) guidelines

diastolic properties; the *E/A* ratio may vary according to non-hemodynamic factors such as mechanical ventilation; and it is also of limited value in patients with significant mitral and/or aortic valve disease, or before fluid resuscitation has been carried out in critically ill patients.

Impact of LVDD in the perioperative setting

Nowadays, surgery is performed without a true "age cut-off" with older and older patients undergoing surgical procedures. Such patients have a large burden of comorbidities, including LVDD. However, the vast majority of literature of LVDD in the perioperative setting includes patients undergoing cardiac surgery or vascular surgery, since these patients generally present a larger spectrum of comorbidities, especially from cardiovascular perspectives. Moreover, such patients are frequently monitored perioperatively with TEE and thus real-time estimation and monitoring of LVDD could be feasible, although it should be kept in mind that TDI measures have not yet been fully validated with TEE.

In patients undergoing cardiac surgery, LVDD correlates with difficult weaning from cardiopulmonary bypass

and higher inotropic needs [24, 25]. Moreover, there is some evidence of correlation between advanced LVDD and postoperative AF after cardiac surgery [26, 27].

In patients undergoing major vascular surgery, preoperative isolated LVDD is more frequent than isolated LV systolic dysfunction (43 vs. 8%, respectively) and, importantly, LVDD is an independent predictor of postoperative HF and prolonged hospital stay, and it is associated with postoperative adverse cardiovascular events and long-term cardiovascular mortality [28, 29].

While the impact of preoperative LVDD in these high-risk surgical specialties is not unexpected, more uncertainty reigns on the importance of LVDD in patient's outcome in other surgical specialties. In this regard, one of the issues is the ethical concerns and potential value in performing intraoperative TEE in patients with isolated LVDD undergoing non-high-risk surgery. Cabrera-Schulmeyer and Arriaza conducted an interesting study in patients with cardiac comorbidities and undergoing non-cardiac/non-vascular (abdominal, urological and orthopedic) surgery. The authors stratified patients according to preoperative normal (< 8), borderline (8–15) and high (> 15) *E/e'* ratio. Patients with borderline and high *E/e'* had a higher incidence of perioperative complications (higher incidence of pulmonary edema at 24 h and 48 h, arrhythmias) and longer ICU stay and hospital stay than patients with normal E/e'. Moreover, patients with high E/e' had significantly higher mortality as compared to normal ratio (8 vs. 0%, respectively) [4].

While preoperative LVDD correlates with outcome, a postoperative evaluation of patient's diastolic function should consider ruling out first the influence of stressors that may worsen diastolic function (i.e., pain-related tachycardia reduces diastolic time, hypo- and hypervolemia may influence LV filling pressures, etc.).

Impact of LVDD in the intensive care

With respect to the role of LVDD in (non-cardiac surgery) critically ill patients, the greater amount of research is related to the role of LVDD in the outcome of sepsis and in the weaning from mechanical ventilation.

LVDD and sepsis

Septic shock is characterized by intense vasoplegia requiring vasoactive therapy to restore blood pressure [30]; however, it has become more evident over the past years that septic patients are affected by pronounced myocardial dysfunction, which is possibly the result of increased circulating cytokine and catecholamine levels [14, 31]. We emphasize that, in case of overt septic shock and in the absence of signs of other causes of shock, fluid resuscitation should not be delayed in order to get information on LV diastolic function from an advanced critical care echocardiography examination or by requesting cardiology consultation. It is also likely that in patients with pronounced hypovolemia (and vasoplegia), the parameters used for the evaluation of LV diastolic function will undergo dramatic changes according to fluid resuscitation and/or the start of vasopressor infusion. It is pivotal understanding that assessment of LV diastolic function cannot be dissociated from evaluation of LV filling pressure, which in certain group of patients undergoes sudden clinical variations.

The so-defined septic cardiomyopathy may involve either the LV, the RV, or both, affecting systolic and/or diastolic function. With all the limitations coming from the use of LV ejection fraction (LVEF) for the evaluation of systolic function, a meta-analysis found no association between LV or RV systolic dysfunction and mortality in patients with severe sepsis or septic shock [32]. On the other hand, a subsequent meta-analysis demonstrated a strong association between LVDD and mortality in the same population of critically ill patients and confirmed also the absence of association between LV systolic dysfunction and mortality [6, 7]. Moreover, the same group of authors recently showed that worse TDI parameters

(lower e' and higher E/e' ratio) are associated with mortality in septic patients [5]. Interestingly, another meta-analysis investigated the value of speckle tracking echocardiography in the prognostic evaluation of septic cardiomyopathy, showing that worse values of LV strain are associated with negative outcome in septic patients [33]. More research is warranted for speckle tracking echocardiography to understand if it could represent a better marker of intrinsic LV function in critically ill patients.

The association between LVDD and outcome in patients with severe sepsis and septic shock may be explained looking at the pathophysiology of sepsis. In patients with LVDD, the LV filling benefits from maintenance of adequate preload, sinus rhythm and avoidance of tachycardia, while sepsis causes sequential disturbances at such levels since patients become relatively hypovolemic, tachycardic and frequently develop arrhythmias, with AF described in up to 23% of patients with septic shock [34, 35]. Septic patients are relatively hypovolemic due to vasoplegia and increased capillary permeability and higher venous capacitance. In fact, the recommended first-line therapy for the treatment of sepsis is to restore preload. In patients with LVDD and increased LV filling pressures there is probably a narrow window for optimizing fluid status. In these patients, even under condition of theoretical "fluid-responsiveness," a little amount of fluid may precipitate pulmonary edema or cause a hemodynamic collapse. Therefore, without any delay in the initial fluid resuscitation of septic patients, the subsequent preload optimization may benefit by the knowledge of his/her LVDD conditions, too, which should be integrated with other variables. For instance, patients with acute respiratory distress syndrome and/ or acute or pulmonale may not benefit from fluid due to both hydrostatic worsening of non-cardiogenic pulmonary edema and further RV dilatation. Patients with severe RV dysfunction may suffer from extra amount of fluids because the RV dilatation together with paradoxical septal motion hampers LV filling creating a "LVDD-like" condition by pushing the septal region and reducing LV compliance. However, using an experimental model of lung injury and high airway pressures, Katira et al. [36] reported very low augmentation of LV filling pressure as a consequence of RV failure, possibly as a consequence of decreased venous return and/or increased pulmonary vascular permeability.

Similarly, patients with at-least-moderate mitral regurgitation may worsen their pulmonary function if an extra amount of fluid is administered [37]. Not only preload but afterload too affects negatively the evaluation of LV diastolic function. In this regard, LV diastolic function worsens as a consequence of increased afterload due to hypertension [38] or related pharmacological [39] and non-pharmacological (increased intra-abdominal pressure [40]) factors. However, the main issues in this matter are represented by the difficulty of directly and reliably quantifying the LV afterload with echocardiography.

Another factor that further worsens LV filling is tachycardia, mainly disproportionally reducing the LV diastolic time. Although healthy individuals compensate for by accelerating the LV relaxation process (frequency-dependent acceleration of relaxation [41]), this process is impaired during sepsis [42]. The LV filling is further worsened by the development of AF and the consequent loss of efficacious atrial contraction. In this respect, although speculative, it is possible that the use of beta-blockade may produce more benefits in septic patients with LVDD for their ability to reduce heart rate and for their anti-arrhythmic properties [43, 44]. Another hypothesis which has to be evaluated in the future is the fact that septic patients with LVDD may have a worst tolerance to fluid expansion.

Concerning the incidence of LVDD in sepsis, it is worth noting that a recent study by Clancy et al. [45] found that the application of new guidelines for the evaluation of LV diastolic function identified a significantly higher incidence of LVDD as compared to the previous 2009 guidelines. This finding is interesting since a study in the general population found opposite results (much lower incidence of LVDD with new guidelines as compared to the 2009 version), as previously discussed [12].

LVDD and weaning from mechanical ventilation
During mechanical ventilation, LV preload and afterload are decreased, and the transition from positive to negative pressure (spontaneous breathing) creates unfavorable LV loading conditions and may also trigger myocardial ischemia [46]. There is growing evidence that the largest amount of weaning failures are of cardiac origin.

A recent study investigated the value of a combined integrated thoracic sonographic evaluation (respiratory, cardiac and diaphragmatic) in predicting early post-extubation respiratory distress. The detection of lung interstitial water was the most relevant parameter detected during thoracic ultrasound, while among factors studied by echocardiography, the estimation of LV filling pressure was predictive of post-extubation distress. On the contrary, indexes of systolic function and diaphragmatic excursion had poor impact over the prediction of respiratory failure [47].

One study showed an association between weaning failure and both lower LVEF and higher E/e' [48], but another one failed to show an association between LVEF and weaning failure [49]. The presence of LVDD seems more strongly associated with weaning failure as shown

by several studies. Konomi et al. [50] found an independent association between LVDD and weaning failure (odds ratio 11.2), while Papanikolaou et al. [51] found lateral E/e' as the only factor independently associated with weaning failure possibly reflecting the association between a higher degree of LVDD and weaning failure. Moschietto et al. [49] found higher E/e' and lower e' in the failing group and interestingly that e' velocity increased in patients successfully weaned, while it remained unchanged in those failing.

The largest study on this topic recently showed that the vast majority of patients failing a spontaneous breathing trial (SBT) and weaning from mechanical ventilation develop weaning-induced pulmonary edema (WiPO) and that structural cardiopathy, chronic obstructive pulmonary disease and obesity are the main risk factors for WiPO [52]. In a subgroup of patients with cardiac output monitoring, the authors were able to show that WiPO is associated with *preload-independence* and that a subsequent SBT is more likely to succeed after diuretic therapy and a more negative fluid balance (achieving *preload-dependence*). This study found similar LVEF and fluid balance between patients with WiPO and non-WiPO, but the first group had significantly higher E/e' ratio, possibly reflecting a worse diastolic function [8]. In support of this hypothesis, WiPO failure patients monitored with cardiac output showed an increase in both global end-diastolic volume and extra-vascular lung water as compared to non-WiPO failures where these remained unchanged. Such findings highlight the risk of the transition from positive to negative pressure ventilation, where an increase in LV preload cannot be accommodated in patients with high LV filling pressures.

How to manage the patient with LVDD
The management of patients with LVDD can be challenging, and unfortunately, there is no magic bullet that rapidly improves LV diastolic function, pharmacologically or non-pharmacologically. A graphical summary of suggestions to manage the critically ill patients with LVDD is provided in Fig. 3. Moreover, no study exists to demonstrate that improving LVDD in the critically ill patients could beneficially impact the prognosis. Only few drugs have shown some improvements of LVDD. Among them beta-blockers are an example. Indeed, it is known their ability to ameliorate LVDD in HF with preserved LVEF [9], and beta-blockade also improves LV filling pressures and coronary flow reserve in patients with uncomplicated arterial hypertension [53]. It is worth noting the results of the first large randomized study on beta-blockers in patients with septic shock, with beneficial effects of esmolol infusion as shown by a significant improvement in cardiac performance, lower inotropic requirements

and higher survival as compared to placebo. Both negative chronotropic and anti-arrhythmic effects of esmolol may have had positive influence on LV diastolic function, although the authors did not present echocardiographic data and this hypothesis remains speculative.The same group of authors recently showed an improved LV filling pattern and ventriculo-arterial coupling after esmolol infusion in septic patients [54]; moreover, immune, metabolic and coagulative effects of beta-blockers treatment may result advantageous in patients with sepsis [44]. Another therapeutically plausible option for patients with heart failure could be represented by the use of angiotensin-converting enzyme inhibitors, which may reduce LV remodeling and improve diastolic function [55–58]. However, the effects of this class of drugs are evident in the long run only and their efficacy is not demonstrated for LVDD in the acute setting. A potentially interesting drug that may ameliorate the hemodynamic profile of septic patients may be represented by dexmedetomidine (α-2 agonist), a sedative drug that has shown a possible reduction in catecholamines release associated with increased blood pressure response to exogenous vasopressors in experimental models of septic shock [59–62]. A clinical study has completed its enrollment (ClinicalTrials.gov Identifier: NCT02638545), but more research is warranted before drawing any conclusion. Another drug that has shown improvements of LV diastolic function is levosimendan [63], and its properties are unique if compared to catecholamines (which usually worsen LV diastolic function [64]) and phosphodiesterase inhibitors (LV diastolic function remaining grossly unchanged) [65]. However, levosimendan has specific pharmacokinetic and pharmacodynamic properties that make it not ideal when the effect is needed rapidly.

In general, although LVDD can be potentially reversed or reduced in its magnitude with appropriate treatment in the long run, this seems rather difficult in the acute critically ill patients; since the pharmacological approach to the optimization of diastolic function does not offer rapid solutions at present, clinicians should probably focus on the maintenance of the best loading conditions for the patient with established LVDD. From a clinical perspective, patients with LVDD grade I are usually more easy to manage, but the dominance of the atrial filling ($E < A$, see Fig. 1) makes them very sensible to the loss of atrial filling (i.e., AF) in case of baseline reduced LVEF. Therefore, particular attention should be devoted to the avoidance of AF [66].

In case of patients with LVDD grade II, clinicians should carefully evaluate the volume status. Indeed, such patients are prone to develop pulmonary edema under condition of hypervolemia; on the other hand, in case of hypovolemia the LA pressure decreases and patients

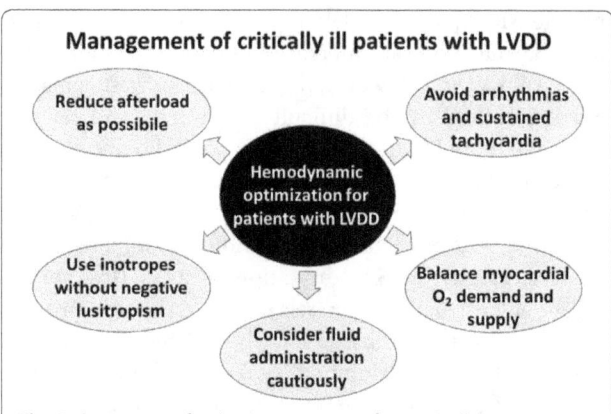

Fig. 3 Suggestions for the management of critically ill patients with left ventricular diastolic dysfunction (LVDD)

lose their compensatory mechanism to maintain a "normal" LA-to-LV gradient, and this situation can be further aggravated by AF (loss of atrial contribution).

Patients with LVDD grade III are generally very frail patients and, for instance, severe abnormalities in LV filling pattern can explain the case of patients with HF with preserved LVEF, where patients are symptomatic despite no gross alteration in LVEF. In the outpatients, these individuals benefit from cardiology consultation and optimization, and they may also be considered for cardiac resynchronization therapy in case of prolonged QRS [67]. However, this option may not be easy in the acute phase of critical illness [68]. It is the authors' opinion that, if an urgent intervention is needed, such patients should be possibly managed by anesthesiologists with experience in the cardiac setting and optimized using echocardiography across the perioperative period.

Finally, because diastolic function is affected early during myocardial ischemia (earlier than systolic function) [69], attention should be paid to the factors associated with myocardial hypoperfusion. Ensuring an appropriate oxygen delivery to the LV by maintaining adequate diastolic blood pressure (with careful approach especially in patients with reduced arterial elastance and with risk factors for—or known for—coronary artery disease), possibly reducing the heart rate and thus the myocardial oxygen demand, and balancing the right level of LV afterload should all be part of the clinician's considerations when approaching the patient with LVDD.

Conclusion

There is growing evidence on the contribution of diastolic function to patients' outcome both in the perioperative setting and in the ICU. The assessment and grading of diastolic dysfunction remains challenging in these patients, and the guidelines used in the outpatient setting are not fully applicable. While pharmacological optimization remains difficult, especially with time constraints

Practical approach to diastolic dysfunction in light of the new guidelines and clinical applications...

177

(urgency/emergency cases), a proactive management aiming at maintaining adequate loading conditions and an appropriate balance between myocardial oxygen demand and delivery could be the best strategies in managing patients with left ventricular diastolic dysfunction.

Abbreviations

LV: left ventricle; LVDD: left ventricular diastolic dysfunction; HF: heart failure; ASE: American Society of Echocardiography; EACVI: European Association of Cardiovascular Imaging; TR: tricuspid regurgitation; LA: left atrium; TDI: tissue Doppler imaging; TTE: transthoracic echocardiography; TEE: transesophageal echocardiography; RV: right ventricle; PEEP: positive end-expiratory pressure; AF: atrial fibrillation; LVEF: left ventricular ejection fraction; SBT: spontaneous breathing trial; WiPO: weaning-induced pulmonary edema.

Authors' contributions

All the authors discussed the idea of writing a review on this topic. FS wrote the first draft of the review. SS designed the figures. FS amended the draft according to the feedback from SS, AM and AVB. All authors read and approved the final manuscript.

Author details

[1] Department of Anesthesia and Intensive Care, IRCCS-ISMETT (Istituto Mediterraneo per i Trapianti e Terapie ad alta specializzazione), Palermo, Italy. [2] Unit of Intensive Care Medicine, Department of Medical Biotechnologies, University of Siena, Siena, Italy. [3] Department of Anaesthesiology and Intensive Care, University of Rome, "La Sapienza", Rome, Italy. [4] Hospital Ambroise Paré, Assistance Publique-Hôpitaux de Paris, Boulogne, France.

Acknowledgements

None.

Competing interests

The authors declare that they have no competing interests.

References

1. Redfield MM, Jacobsen SJ, Burnett JC Jr, Mahoney DW, Bailey KR, Rodeheffer RJ. Burden of systolic and diastolic ventricular dysfunction in the community: appreciating the scope of the heart failure epidemic. JAMA. 2003;289:194–202.
2. Gandhi SK, Powers JC, Nomeir AM, Fowle K, Kitzman DW, Rankin KM, Little WC. The pathogenesis of acute pulmonary edema associated with hypertension. N Engl J Med. 2001;344:17–22.
3. Yancy CW, Lopatin M, Stevenson LW, De Marco T, Fonarow GC, Committee ASA. Investigators: clinical presentation, management, and in-hospital outcomes of patients admitted with acute decompensated heart failure with preserved systolic function: a report from the Acute Decompensated Heart Failure National Registry (ADHERE) Database. J Am Coll Cardiol. 2006;47:76–84.
4. Cabrera Schulmeyer MC, Arriaza N. Good prognostic value of the intraoperative tissue Doppler-derived index E/e' after non-cardiac surgery. Minerva Anestesiol. 2012;78:1013–8.
5. Sanfilippo F, Corredor C, Arcadipane A, Landesberg G, Vieillard-Baron A, Cecconi M, Fletcher N. Tissue Doppler assessment of diastolic function and relationship with mortality in critically ill septic patients: a systematic review and meta-analysis. BJA: Br J Anaesth. 2017;119:583–94.
6. Sanfilippo F, Corredor C, Fletcher N, Landesberg G, Benedetto U, Foex P, Cecconi M. Erratum to: Diastolic dysfunction and mortality in septic patients: a systematic review and meta-analysis. Intensive Care Med. 2015;41:1178–9.
7. Sanfilippo F, Corredor C, Fletcher N, Landesberg G, Benedetto U, Foex P, Cecconi M. Diastolic dysfunction and mortality in septic patients: a sys-

tematic review and meta-analysis. Intensive Care Med. 2015;41:1004–13.
8. Sanfilippo F, Santonocito C, Burgio G, Arcadipane A. The importance of diastolic dysfunction in the development of weaning-induced pulmonary oedema. Crit Care. 2017;21:29.
9. Bergstrom A, Andersson B, Edner M, Nylander E, Persson H, Dahlstrom U. Effect of carvedilol on diastolic function in patients with diastolic heart failure and preserved systolic function. Results of the Swedish Doppler-echocardiographic study (SWEDIC). Eur J Heart Fail. 2004;6:453–61.
10. Nagueh SF, Smiseth OA, Appleton CP, Byrd BF III, Dokainish H, Edvardsen T, Flachskampf FA, Gillebert TC, Klein AL, Lancellotti P, Marino P, Oh JK, Alexandru Popescu B, Waggoner AD. Recommendations for the evaluation of left ventricular diastolic function by echocardiography: an update from the American Society of Echocardiography and the European Association of Cardiovascular imaging. Eur Heart J Cardiovasc Imaging. 2016;29:277–314.
11. Nagueh SF, Appleton CP, Gillebert TC, Marino PN, Oh JK, Smiseth OA, Waggoner AD, Flachskampf FA, Pellikka PA, Evangelisa A. Recommendations for the evaluation of left ventricular diastolic function by echocardiography. Eur J Echocardiogr. 2009;10:165–93.
12. Almeida JG, Fontes-Carvalho R, Sampaio F, Ribeiro J, Bettencourt P, Flachskampf FA, Leite-Moreira A, Azevedo A. Impact of the 2016 ASE/EACVI recommendations on the prevalence of diastolic dysfunction in the general population. Eur Heart J Cardiovasc Imaging. 2017;19:380–6.
13. Juhl-Olsen P, Hermansen JF, Frederiksen CA, Rasmussen LA, Jakobsen CJ, Sloth E. Positive end-expiratory pressure influences echocardiographic measures of diastolic function: a randomized, crossover study in cardiac surgery patients. Anesthesiology. 2013;119:1078–86.
14. Vieillard-Baron A, Cecconi M. Understanding cardiac failure in sepsis. Intensive Care Med. 2014;40:1560–3.
15. Bakkestrom R, Andersen MJ, Ersboll M, Bro-Jeppesen J, Gustafsson F, Kober L, Hassager C, Moller JE. Early changes in left atrial volume after acute myocardial infarction. Relation to invasive hemodynamics at rest and during exercise. Int J Cardiol. 2016;223:717–22.
16. Hoit BD, Shao Y, Gabel M. Influence of acutely altered loading conditions on left atrial appendage flow velocities. J Am Coll Cardiol. 1994;24:1117–23.
17. Ho CY, Solomon SD. A clinician's guide to tissue Doppler imaging. Circulation. 2006;113:e396–8.
18. Lindstrom L, Wranne B. Pulsed tissue Doppler evaluation of mitral annulus motion: a new window to assessment of diastolic function. Clin Physiol. 1999;19:1–10.
19. Khankirawatana B, Khankirawatana S, Peterson B, Mahrous H, Porter TR. Peak atrial systolic mitral annular velocity by Doppler tissue reliably predicts left atrial systolic function. J Am Soc Echocardiogr. 2004;17:353–60.
20. Blondheim DS, Osipov A, Meisel SR, Frimerman A, Shochat M, Shotan A. Relation of left atrial size to function as determined by transesophageal echocardiography. Am J Cardiol. 2005;96:457–63.
21. Okamoto M, Tsubokura T, Morishita K, Nakagawa H, Yamagata T, Kawagoe T, Hondo T, Tsuchioka Y, Matsuura H, Kajiyama G. Effects of volume loading on left atrial systolic time intervals. J Clin Ultrasound. 1991;19:405–11.
22. Prioli A, Marino P, Lanzoni L, Zardini P. Increasing degrees of left ventricular filling impairment modulate left atrial function in humans. Am J Cardiol. 1998;82:756–61.
23. Triposkiadis F, Tentolouris K, Androulakis A, Trikas A, Toutouzas K, Kyriakidis M, Gialafos J, Toutouzas P. Left atrial mechanical function in the healthy elderly: new insights from a combined assessment of changes in atrial volume and transmittal flow velocity. J Am Soc Echocardiogr. 1995;8:801–9.
24. Bernard F, Denault A, Babin D, Goyer C, Couture P, Couturier A, Buithieu J. Diastolic dysfunction is predictive of difficult weaning from cardiopulmonary bypass. Anesth Analg. 2001;92:291–8.
25. Licker M, Cikirikcioglu M, Inan C, Cartier V, Kalangos A, Theologou T, Cassina T, Diaper J. Preoperative diastolic function predicts the onset of left ventricular dysfunction following aortic valve replacement in high-risk patients with aortic stenosis. Crit Care. 2010;14:R101.
26. Chua SK, Shyu KG, Lu MJ, Hung HF, Cheng JJ, Lee SH, Lin CH, Chao HH, Lo HM. Association between renal function, diastolic dysfunction, and postoperative atrial fibrillation following cardiac surgery. Circ J. 2013;77:2303–10.

27. Lacalzada J, Jimenez JJ, Iribarren JL, de la Rosa A, Martin-Cabeza M, Izquierdo MM, Mari-Lopez B, Garcia-Gonzalez MJ, Jorge-Perez P, Barragan A, Laynez I. Early transthoracic echocardiography after cardiac surgery predicts postoperative atrial fibrillation. Echocardiography. 2016;33:1300–8.

28. Flu WJ, van Kuijk JP, Hoeks SE, Kuiper R, Schouten O, Goei D, Elhendy A, Verhagen HJ, Thomson IR, Bax JJ, Fleisher LA, Poldermans D. Prognostic implications of asymptomatic left ventricular dysfunction in patients undergoing vascular surgery. Anesthesiology. 2010;112:1316–24.

29. Matyal R, Hess PE, Subramaniam B, Mitchell J, Panzica PJ, Pomposelli F, Mahmood F. Perioperative diastolic dysfunction during vascular surgery and its association with postoperative outcome. J Vasc Surg. 2009;50:70–6.

30. Antonelli M, Bonten M, Chastre J, Citerio G, Conti G, Curtis JR, De Backer D, Hedenstierna G, Joannidis M, Macrae D, Mancebo J, Maggiore SM, Mebazaa A, Preiser JC, Rocco P, Timsit JF, Wernerman J, Zhang H. Year in review in Intensive Care Medicine 2011. II. Cardiovascular, infections, pneumonia and sepsis, critical care organization and outcome, education, ultrasonography, metabolism and coagulation. Intensive Care Med. 2012;38:345–58.

31. Beesley SJ, Weber G, Sarge T, Nikravan S, Grissom CK, Lanspa MJ, Shahul S, Brown SM. Septic cardiomyopathy. Crit Care Med. 2018;46:625–34.

32. Huang SJ, Nalos M, McLean AS. Is early ventricular dysfunction or dilatation associated with lower mortality rate in adult severe sepsis and septic shock? A meta-analysis. Crit Care. 2013;17:R96.

33. Sanfilippo F, Corredor C, Fletcher N, Tritapepe L, Lorini FL, Arcadipane A, Vieillard-Baron A, Cecconi M. Left ventricular systolic function evaluated by strain echocardiography and relationship with mortality in patients with severe sepsis or septic shock: a systematic review and meta-analysis. Crit Care. 2018;22:183.

34. Kuipers S, Klein Klouwenberg PM, Cremer OL. Incidence, risk factors and outcomes of new-onset atrial fibrillation in patients with sepsis: a systematic review. Crit Care. 2014;18:688.

35. Makrygiannis SS, Margariti A, Rizikou D, Lampakis M, Vangelis S, Ampartzidou OS, Katsifa K, Tselioti P, Foussas SG, Prekates AA. Incidence and predictors of new-onset atrial fibrillation in noncardiac intensive care unit patients. J Crit Care. 2014;29(697):e1–5. https://doi.org/10.1016/j.jcrc.2014.03.029 **Epub 2014 Apr 4**.

36. Katira BH, Giesinger RE, Engelberts D, Zabini D, Kornecki A, Otulakowski G, Yoshida T, Kuebler WM, McNamara PJ, Connelly KA, Kavanagh BP. Adverse heart–lung interactions in ventilator-induced lung injury. Am J Respir Crit Care Med. 2017;196:1411–21.

37. Sanfilippo F, Scolletta S. Fluids in cardiac surgery: sailing calm on a stormy sea? Common sense is the guidance. Minerva Anestesiol. 2017;83:537–9.

38. Krzesinski P, Uzieblo-Zyczkowska B, Gielerak G, Stanczyk A, Kurpaska M, Piotrowicz K. Global longitudinal two-dimensional systolic strain is associated with hemodynamic alterations in arterial hypertension. J Am Soc Hypertens. 2015;9:680–9.

39. Ros M, Azevedo ER, Newton GE, Parker JD. Effects of nitroprusside on cardiac norepinephrine spillover and isovolumic left ventricular relaxation in the normal and failing human left ventricle. Can J Cardiol. 2002;18:1211–6.

40. Alfonsi P, Vieillard-Baron A, Coggia M, Guignard B, Goeau-Brissonniere O, Jardin F, Chauvin M. Cardiac function during intraperitoneal CO2 insufflation for aortic surgery: a transesophageal echocardiographic study. Anesth Analg. 2006;102:1304–10.

41. Janssen PM, Periasamy M. Determinants of frequency-dependent contraction and relaxation of mammalian myocardium. J Mol Cell Cardiol. 2007;43:523–31.

42. Joulin O, Marechaux S, Hassoun S, Montaigne D, Lancel S, Neviere R. Cardiac force-frequency relationship and frequency-dependent acceleration of relaxation are impaired in LPS-treated rats. Crit Care. 2009;13:R14.

43. Morelli A, Ertmer C, Westphal M, Rehberg S, Kampmeier T, Ligges S, Orecchioni A, D'Egidio A, D'Ippoliti F, Raffone C, Venditti M, Guarracino F, Girardis M, Tritapepe L, Pietropaoli P, Mebazaa A, Singer M. Effect of heart rate control with esmolol on hemodynamic and clinical outcomes in patients with septic shock: a randomized clinical trial. JAMA. 2013;310:1683–91. https://doi.org/10.1001/jama.2013.278477.

44. Sanfilippo F, Santonocito C, Morelli A, Foex P. Beta-blocker use in severe sepsis and septic shock: a systematic review. Curr Med Res Opin. 2015;31:1817–25.

45. Clancy DJ, Scully T, Slama M, Huang S, McLean AS, Orde SR. Application of updated guidelines on diastolic dysfunction in patients with severe sepsis and septic shock. Ann Intensive Care. 2017;7:121.

46. Dres M, Teboul JL, Anguel N, Guerin L, Richard C, Monnet X. Passive leg raising performed before a spontaneous breathing trial predicts weaning-induced cardiac dysfunction. Intensive Care Med. 2015;41:487–94.

47. Silva S, Ait Aissa D, Cocquet P, Hoarau L, Ruiz J, Ferre F, Rousset D, Mora M, Mari A, Fourcade O, Riu B, Jaber S, Bataille B. Combined thoracic ultrasound assessment during a successful weaning trial predicts postextubation distress. Anesthesiology. 2017;127:666–74.

48. Caille V, Amiel JB, Charron C, Belliard G, Vieillard-Baron A, Vignon P. Echocardiography: a help in the weaning process. Crit Care. 2010;14:R120.

49. Moschietto S, Doyen D, Grech L, Dellamonica J, Hyvernat H, Bernardin G. Transthoracic echocardiography with Doppler tissue imaging predicts weaning failure from mechanical ventilation: evolution of the left ventricle relaxation rate during a spontaneous breathing trial is the key factor in weaning outcome. Crit Care. 2012;16:R81.

50. Konomi I, Tasoulis A, Kaltsi I, Karatzanos E, Vasileiadis I, Temperikidis P, Nanas S, Routsi CI. Left ventricular diastolic dysfunction—an independent risk factor for weaning failure from mechanical ventilation. Anaesth Intensive Care. 2016;44:466–73.

51. Papanikolaou J, Makris D, Saranteas T, Karakitsos D, Zintzaras E, Karabinis A, Kostopanagiotou G, Zakynthinos E. New insights into weaning from mechanical ventilation: left ventricular diastolic dysfunction is a key player. Intensive Care Med. 2011;37:1976–85.

52. Liu J, Shen F, Teboul JL, Anguel N, Beurton A, Bezaz N, Richard C, Monnet X. Cardiac dysfunction induced by weaning from mechanical ventilation: incidence, risk factors, and effects of fluid removal. Crit Care. 2016;20:369.

53. Galderisi M, D'Errico A, Sidiropulos M, Innelli P, de Divitiis O, de Simone G. Nebivolol induces parallel improvement of left ventricular filling pressure and coronary flow reserve in uncomplicated arterial hypertension. J Hypertens. 2009;27:2108–15.

54. Morelli A, Singer M, Ranieri VM, D'Egidio A, Mascia L, Orecchioni A, Piscioneri F, Guarracino F, Greco E, Peruzzi M, Biondi-Zoccai G, Frati G, Romano SM. Heart rate reduction with esmolol is associated with improved arterial elastance in patients with septic shock: a prospective observational study. Intensive Care Med. 2016;42:1528–34.

55. Chang NC, Shih CM, Bi WF, Lai ZY, Lin MS, Wang TC. Fosinopril improves left ventricular diastolic function in young mildly hypertensive patients without hypertrophy. Cardiovasc Drugs Ther. 2002;16:141–7.

56. Siegmund T, Schumm-Draeger PM, Antoni D, Bibra HV. Beneficial effects of ramipril on myocardial diastolic function in patients with type 2 diabetes mellitus, normal LV systolic function and without coronary artery disease: a prospective study using tissue Doppler. Diab Vasc Dis Res. 2007;4:358–64.

57. Yalcin F, Aksoy FG, Muderrisoglu H, Sabah I, Garcia MJ, Thomas JD. Treatment of hypertension with perindopril reduces plasma atrial natriuretic peptide levels, left ventricular mass, and improves echocardiographic parameters of diastolic function. Clin Cardiol. 2000;23:437–41.

58. Zhang Q, Chen Y, Liu Q, Shan Q. Effects of renin-angiotensin-aldosterone system inhibitors on mortality, hospitalization, and diastolic function in patients with HFpEF. A meta-analysis of 13 randomized controlled trials. Herz. 2016;41:76–86.

59. Geloen A, Chapelier K, Cividjian A, Dantony E, Rabilloud M, May CN, Quintin L. Clonidine and dexmedetomidine increase the pressor response to norepinephrine in experimental sepsis: a pilot study. Crit Care Med. 2013;41:e431–8.

60. Hernandez G, Tapia P, Alegria L, Soto D, Luengo C, Gomez J, Jarufe N, Achurra P, Rebolledo R, Bruhn A, Castro R, Kattan E, Ospina-Tascon G, Bakker J. Effects of dexmedetomidine and esmolol on systemic hemodynamics and exogenous lactate clearance in early experimental septic shock. Crit Care. 2016;20:234.

61. Lankadeva YR, Booth LC, Kosaka J, Evans RG, Quintin L, Bellomo R, May CN. Clonidine restores pressor responsiveness to phenylephrine and angiotensin II in ovine sepsis. Crit Care Med. 2015;43:e221–9.

62. Miranda ML, Balarini MM, Bouskela E. Dexmedetomidine attenuates the microcirculatory derangements evoked by experimental sepsis. Anesthesiology. 2015;122:619–30.

63. Malik V, Subramanian A, Hote M, Kiran U. Effect of levosimendan on diastolic function in patients undergoing coronary artery bypass grafting: a comparative study. J Cardiovasc Pharmacol. 2015;66:141–7.

64. Tarvasmaki T, Lassus J, Varpula M, Sionis A, Sund R, Kober L, Spinar J, Parissis J, Banaszewski M, Silva Cardoso J, Carubelli V, Di Somma S, Mebazaa A, Harjola VP. Current real-life use of vasopressors and inotropes in cardiogenic shock—adrenaline use is associated with excess organ injury and mortality. Crit Care. 2016;20:208.

65. Couture P, Denault AY, Pellerin M, Tardif JC. Milrinone enhances systolic, but not diastolic function during coronary artery bypass grafting surgery. Can J Anaesth. 2007;54:509–22.

66. Vieillard-Baron A, Boyd J. Non-antiarrhythmic interventions in new onset and paroxysmal sepsis-related atrial fibrillation. Intensive Care Med. 2018;44:94–7.

67. Cleland JG, Daubert JC, Erdmann E, Freemantle N, Gras D, Kappenberger L, Tavazzi L. The effect of cardiac resynchronization on morbidity and mortality in heart failure. N Engl J Med. 2005;352:1539–49.

68. Rinaldi C, Auricchio A, Prinzen F. Left ventricular endocardial pacing for the critically ill. Intensive Care Med. 2018;44:915–7.

69. Schwarzl M, Huber S, Maechler H, Steendijk P, Seiler S, Truschnig-Wilders M, Nestelberger T, Pieske BM, Post H. Left ventricular diastolic dysfunction during acute myocardial infarction: effect of mild hypothermia. Resuscitation. 2012;83:1503–10.

19

Video laryngoscopy versus direct laryngoscopy for first-attempt tracheal intubation in the general ward

Moon Seong Baek[1], MyongJa Han[2], Jin Won Huh[1], Chae-Man Lim[1], Younsuck Koh[1] and Sang-Bum Hong[1*]

Abstract

Background: Recent trials showed that video laryngoscopy (VL) did not yield higher first-attempt tracheal intubation success rate than direct laryngoscopy (DL) and was associated with higher rates of complications. Tracheal intubation can be more challenging in the general ward than in the intensive care unit. This study aimed to investigate which laryngoscopy mode is associated with higher first-attempt intubation success in a general ward.

Methods: This is a retrospective study of tracheal intubations conducted at a tertiary academic hospital. This analysis included all intubations performed by the medical emergency team in the general ward during a 48-month period.

Results: For the 958 included patients, the initial laryngoscopy mode was video laryngoscopy in 493 (52%) and direct laryngoscopy in 465 patients (48%). The overall first-attempt success rate was 69% (664 patients). The first-attempt success rate was higher with VL (79%; 391/493) than with DL (59%; 273/465, $p < 0.001$). The first-attempt intubation success rate was higher among experienced operators (83%; 266/319) than among inexperienced operators (62%; 398/639, $p < 0.001$). In multivariate logistic regression analyses, VL, pre-intubation heart rate, pre-intubation $SpO_2 > 80\%$, a non-predicted difficult airway, experienced operator, and Cormack–Lehane grade were associated with first-attempt intubation success in the general ward. Over all intubation-related complications were not different between two groups (27% for VL vs. 25% for DL). However, incidence of a post-intubation $SpO_2 < 80\%$ was higher with VL than with DL (4% vs. 1%, $p = 0.005$), and in-hospital mortality was also higher (53.8% vs. 43%, $p = 0.001$).

Conclusion: In a general ward setting, the first-attempt intubation success rate was higher with video laryngoscopy than with direct laryngoscopy. However, video laryngoscopy did not reduce intubation-related complications. Furthers trials on best way to perform intubation in the emergency settings are required.

Keywords: Laryngoscopy, Intubation, Critical illness

Background

Tracheal intubation can be a hazardous procedure outside of the operating room, as it tends to be performed by inexperienced junior trainees and involves physiologically unstable patients. Accordingly, tracheal intubation outside of the operating room is associated with a higher rate of complications than the corresponding procedure inside the operating room [1–3]. Furthermore,

*Correspondence: sbhong@amc.seoul.kr
[1] Department of Pulmonary and Critical Care Medicine, Asan Medical Centre, University of Ulsan College of Medicine, 88 Olympic-ro 43-gil, Songpa-gu, Seoul 05505, Republic of Korea

a successful first-attempt intubation is important in the emergency setting [4] because related complications are associated with multiple intubation attempts [5, 6].

A video laryngoscope, defined as a laryngoscopic device to which a camera has been attached to the tip of the blade, could assist airway management by improving visualisation of the glottis in critically ill patients [7–10]. According to a few studies, video laryngoscopy yields a greater rate of first-attempt intubation success than direct laryngoscopy [7, 11]. However, a recent randomised clinical trial in an intensive care unit (ICU) setting found that video laryngoscopy did not yield higher first-attempt tracheal intubation success rate than direct laryngoscopy and was associated with higher rates of complications [12]. Therefore, the superior device for first-attempt intubation success in critically ill patients remains controversial. Furthermore, limited data are available regarding tracheal intubation in general ward settings [5, 13].

The objective of this study was to investigate which laryngoscopy mode is associated with higher first-attempt intubation success in a general ward. We hypothesised that tracheal intubation with the video laryngoscope would be associated with increased successful intubation on first attempt compared with the direct laryngoscopy.

Methods

Study design and eligible patients

This retrospective study of tracheal intubations was conducted at Asan Medical Centre, a tertiary referral hospital in Korea. Tracheal intubation data between January 2012 and December 2015 were collected. The primary outcome was first-attempt success and secondary outcome was intubation-related complications. All patients aged $\geq$ 19 years who had been intubated in the ward by medical emergency team (MET) were eligible. Exclusion criteria were as follow: (1) tracheal intubations performed during cardiac arrest because the success of first-attempt intubation might have been affected by cardiopulmonary resuscitation, (2) patients who initially used supraglottic airway devices because the study aimed to compare the direct laryngoscopy and video laryngoscopy, (3) patients whose records were unavailable, 4) duplicated cases.

The institutional review board of the Asan Medical Centre approved this study (approval no. 2016-0599) and granted a waiver of patient consent because of the retrospective nature of the study.

Study setting

The MET provides airway management to general ward patients who require immediate or cardiopulmonary resuscitation. A MET comprises attending critical care physicians, critical care medicine fellows, internal medicine residents, and critical care qualified nurses and is available 24 h per day, 7 days per week. If the MET is activated via a screening or calling system, the team members proceed to the intubation location with a portable airway bag. This bag contains a video laryngoscope, capnograph, i-gel (Intersurgical Ltd, Wokingham, Berkshire, UK), laryngeal tube (VBM Medizintechnik, Sulz, Germany), gum elastic bougie, tracheal tube exchanger (Cook airway exchange catheter), and percutaneous cricothyroidotomy kit (Melker Emergency Cricothyrotomy Kit, Cook Critical Care, Bloomington, Indiana). The laryngeal tube is one of the supraglottic airway devices that consists of an airway tube with a small cuff attached at the tip

and a larger balloon cuff at the middle part of the tube. The i-gel is also a supraglottic airway device that features a non-inflatable cuff and the possibility to introduce a gastric catheter. Direct laryngoscopes were contained in the emergency trolley each general ward. Before starting rotations in ICU, medical residents received airway management programme, consisted with direct laryngoscopy and video laryngoscopy and i-gel, laryngeal tube. Airway management training programme for critical care medicine fellows is provided by attending physician once a month. The curriculum is designed with basic skills with direct laryngoscopy and video laryngoscopy and more difficult scenarios requiring execution with alternative techniques, including i-gel, laryngeal tube, gum elastic bougie, bronchoscopy, and cricothyroidotomy.

In this study, the intubation procedure was conducted in accordance with general guidelines for the airway management of critically ill patients [14, 15]. Although fentanyl (1–3 μg kg^{-1}) and etomidate (0.3 mg kg^{-1}) were the preferred pre-treatment and induction agents, the operators selected the sedatives and dosages after considering each patient's condition. A sedative was administered 2 min after pre-treatment agent injection, and tracheal intubation was performed 20–30 s later. The operators chose either a curved Macintosh laryngoscope with metal reusable blade or a GlideScope video laryngoscope (Verathon, Bothell, WA, USA) as the initial device. Tracheal intubation was supervised by an experienced operator when performed by an inexperienced operator. If the second intubation attempt was unsuccessful, the experienced operator performed the third attempt. However, for the patient safety, supervisors tended to intubate directly if the patient was expected to have difficult airway or hemodynamically unstable. It is presumed that relatively less severe patients were intubated by inexperienced operators and with direct laryngoscopy for the training purpose. Correct tracheal tube placement was assessed using careful auscultation, end-tidal carbon dioxide measurement, and chest radiography. The end-tidal carbon dioxide level was measured using an EMMA Emergency Capnograph (Masimo Corp., Irvine, CA, USA). After each tracheal intubation, intubation-related information was recorded on a data collection sheet by MET nurses, and all tracheal intubations were reviewed in regular weekly meetings.

Data collection and definition

The following information was recorded on the intubation data collection sheet: patient demographics, operator specialty, time and location of tracheal intubation, reason for intubation, number of intubation attempts, device(s) used, medications (pre-treatment agents, sedatives, and paralytics), complications during tracheal intubation, characteristics of the predicted difficult airway, Cormack–Lehane grade, and vital signs pre- and post-tracheal intubation.

We defined intubation duration as the time interval between infusion of the pre-treatment agent (or sedative if the patient did not receive a pre-treatment agent) and confirmation of tracheal tube placement by capnography. The board-certified physician or surgeon in the ICU (attending physician and fellow) was considered an experienced operator, while a medical or surgical resident-in-training was considered an inexperienced operator. A tracheal intubation attempt was defined as insertion of the laryngoscopy blade into the oral cavity, regardless of whether tracheal tube insertion was attempted. A first-attempt success was defined as the placement of a tracheal tube on the first attempt and difficult intubation was defined as more than two attempts of intubation [16].

Several factors were investigated before intubation to predict difficult airways. These factors included blood/vomitus/secretion in the airway, cervical immobilisation, neck trauma/mass or vocal cord palsy, the 3-3-2 rule, short neck, obesity, limited mouth opening, small mouth, and large tongue. The 3-3-2 rule was defined as an inter-incisor distance of < 3 fingers, a hyoid-mental distance of < 3 fingers, and a hyoid-thyroid cartilage distance of < 2 fingers.

An event occurring within 30 min after tracheal intubation was considered intubation-related complications. These events included hypotension (systolic arterial pressure < 90 mmHg despite adequate volume loading or inotrope use), severe desaturation (oxygen saturation < 80%), oesophageal intubation, dental injury (tooth extraction), oral bleeding, aspiration of gastric contents, and cardiac arrest/arrhythmia [17].

Statistical analysis

Continuous variables are presented as median (interquartile range) or mean (standard deviation). Categorical variables are presented as number (percentage). Differences among categorised groups were compared using either the Chi-square test or Fisher's exact test, and data for continuous variables were compared using the independent Student's t test or Mann–Whitney U test. Univariate and multivariate logistic regressions using backward elimination method were performed to identify the factors associated with first-attempt intubation success and intubation-related complications. Calibration of the models was evaluated with the Hosmer–Lemeshow goodness-of-fit test. All statistical comparisons were two-sided, and a p value of < 0.05 was considered statistically significant. Data were analysed using the Statistical Package for the Social Sciences (SPSS), version 22.0

(IBM Corporation, Armonk, NY, USA). To reduce the effect of treatment-selection bias and potential confounding factors in an observational study, we performed an adjustment for differences in baseline characteristics of patients using a propensity-score matching (Additional file 1: Table S1). Compounding factors were age, sex, medical department, pre-intubation blood pressure, pre-intubation heart rate, pre-intubation oxygen saturation, predicted difficult airway, level of operator experience, pre-treatment agent, sedatives, and paralytic agents. Using these methods we could reduce or eliminate confounding by those measured covariates. A power analysis was performed with reference to similar studies conducted in an intensive care unit setting [7, 9, 18]. We determined the power of the study by assuming a first-pass success rate of 65% (direct laryngoscopy) and 80% (video laryngoscopy).

Results

During the study period, 1312 tracheal intubations were performed in general ward. A total of 354 patients were excluded which received tracheal intubation during cardiac arrest, 4 younger than 19 years, 4 which initially received tracheal intubation using a supraglottic airway device, 4 which records were unavailable. Because thirty-nine patients were intubated twice, and one patient was intubated three times, 41 cases also excluded. Among the 958 intubations, the initial laryngoscopy mode was video laryngoscopy in 493 (52%) and direct laryngoscopy in 465 (48%) (Fig. 1). As the alternative techniques, an i-gel and a laryngeal tube was used. Gum elastic bougie was used in four cases for 102 failures at first pass in the video laryngoscopy group and was not used for 192 failures in the direct laryngoscopy group. Tracheostomy was conducted in three patients. One tracheostomy was conducted after a failure of cricothyroidotomy. The other two tracheostomies were performed after failures of tracheal intubation because oxygen saturation was maintained at > 90%. One patient died after a failure of emergency cricothyroidotomy in a 'cannot intubate, cannot oxygenate' situation.

Hypoxic respiratory failure (59%) was the most common reason for intubation in the general ward. A predicted difficult airway was present in 202 intubations (20%), and this incidence was higher in the video laryngoscopy group (27%) than the direct laryngoscopy group (13%, $p < 0.001$; Table 1). The first intubation attempt was conducted by inexperienced operators in 67% of patients and by experienced operators in 33% of patients (Table 2). Video laryngoscopy was chosen by 62% (198/319) of experienced operators and by 46% (295/639, $p < 0.001$) of inexperienced operators. Overall, 20.7% of patients received NMB (Table 2).

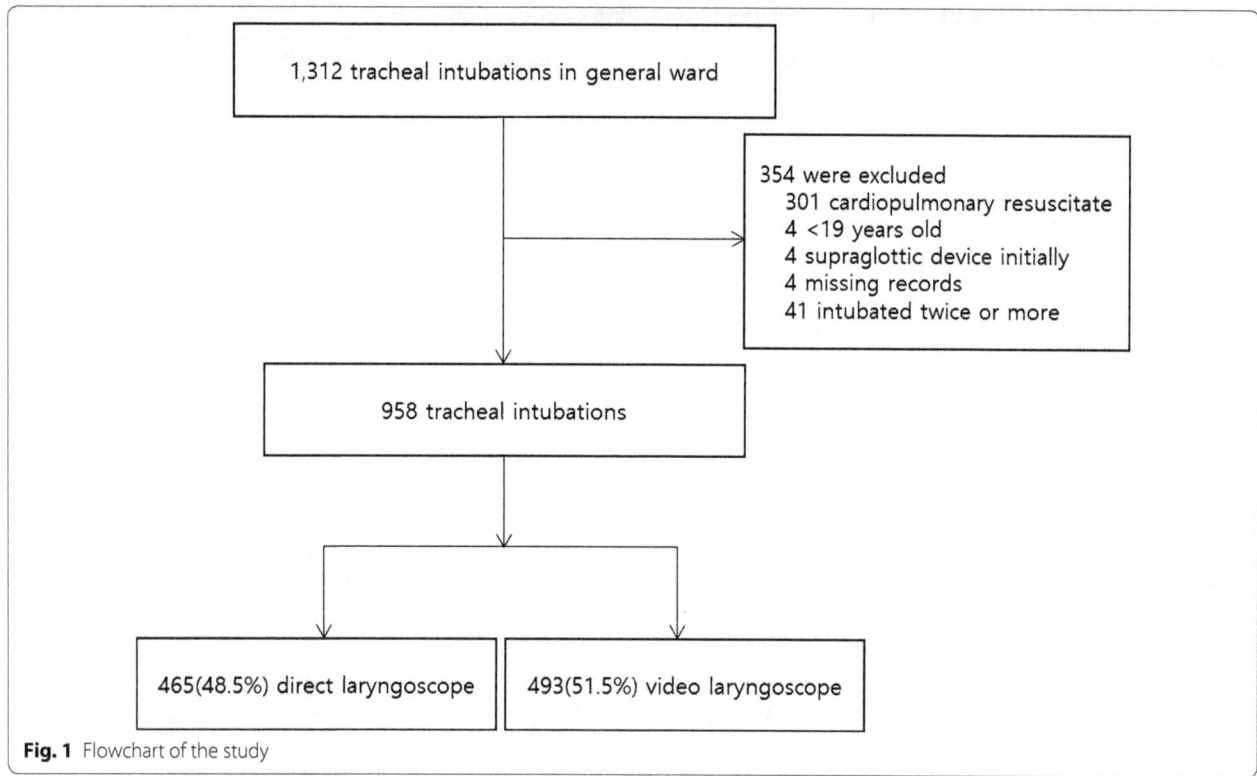

Fig. 1 Flowchart of the study

The overall first-attempt intubation success rate was 69%, with rates of 79% and 59% in the video laryngoscopy and direct laryngoscopy groups, respectively (Fig. 2). Among 192 unsuccessful tracheal intubation with direct laryngoscopy, second intubation attempt was performed by 90 (47%) video laryngoscopy. On the contrary, 102 unsuccessful tracheal intubation with video laryngoscopy changed to 7 (7%) direct laryngoscopy. Among inexperienced operators, the first-attempt intubation success rate was higher with video laryngoscopy (75%) than with direct laryngoscopy (52%, $p < 0.001$; Table 7). The incidence of difficult intubation was 294 (31%). The incidence of difficult intubation was higher in the direct laryngoscopy group (41%) than in the video laryngoscopy group (21%, $p < 0.001$; Table 3).

A Cormack–Lehane grade of 3 or 4 (poor glottis visualisation) was more frequent in the direct laryngoscopy group (6% vs. 4%, $p = 0.024$). The number of intubation attempts was fewer with video laryngoscopy than with direct laryngoscopy, with an absolute difference of 0.32 (95% CI: 0.21–0.42, $p < 0.001$). The intubation duration was also shorter with video laryngoscopy than with direct laryngoscopy, with an absolute difference of 0.74 min (95% CI: 0.31–1.20, $p = 0.001$). No significant differences were observed in intubation-related complications according to the device used (27% in the video laryngoscopy group vs. 25% in the direct laryngoscopy

group, $p = 0.573$; Table 4). The incidence of a pre-intubation $SpO_2 < 80\%$ was higher in the video laryngoscopy group (11% vs. direct laryngoscopy group, 7%; $p = 0.029$); similarly, the incidence of a post-intubation $SpO_2 < 80\%$ was also higher with video laryngoscopy (4% vs. 1%, $p = 0.005$; Table 4).

In multivariate logistic regression analyses, video laryngoscopy (odds ratio, 95% CI 3.058, 2.192–4.267, $p < 0.001$), pre-intubation heart rate (1.006, 1.000–1.011, $p = 0.044$), pre-intubation $SpO_2 < 80\%$ (0.521, 0.316–0.861, $p = 0.011$), a predicted difficult airway (0.344, 0.230–0.514, $p < 0.001$), experienced operator (3.319, 2.284–4.823, $p < 0.001$), and Cormack–Lehane grade (0.459, 0.352–0.599, $p < 0.001$) were associated with first-attempt intubation success in the general ward (Table 5). The use of sedatives (OR, 95% CI: 2.377, 1.224–4.616, $p = 0.011$), paralytic agents (OR, 95% CI: 0.449, 0.293–0.687, $p < 0.001$), and the number of intubation attempts (OR, 95% CI: 1.535, 1.291–1.825, $p < 0.001$) were associated with intubation-related complications (Table 6). In the propensity-score matching, video laryngoscopy group has increased odds of first-attempt intubation success (OR, 95% CI: 2.450, 1.696, 3.539, $p < 0.001$; Additional file 2: Table S2). After propensity-score matching, the first-attempt success rate was 60% (181/300) in direct laryngoscopy group, and 80% (239/300) in video laryngoscopy group. The procedure-related complication rate

Table 1 Baseline clinical characteristics of the patients according to intubation device

Variable	Total $n = 958$	Direct laryngoscopy $n = 465$	Video laryngoscopy $n = 493$	p
Age (years)	63 [53, 73]	66 [56, 74]	61 [51, 71]	< 0.001
Male, n (%)	621 (64.8)	318 (68.4)	303 (61.5)	0.025
Medical department*, n (%)	713 (74.4)	293 (63.0)	420 (85.2)	< 0.001
Reason for intubation, n (%)				
Airway protection	138 (14.4)	67 (14.4)	71 (14.4)	0.998
Hypercapnic respiratory failure	91 (9.5)	49 (10.5)	42 (8.5)	0.287
Hypoxic respiratory failure	567 (59.2)	273 (58.7)	294 (59.6)	0.771
Shock	44 (4.6)	22 (4.7)	22 (4.5)	0.843
Metabolic acidosis	84 (8.8)	33 (7.1)	51 (10.3)	0.076
Others	34 (3.5)	21 (4.5)	13 (2.6)	0.116
Pre-intubation				
Systolic blood pressure (mmHg)	125 ± 33	127 ± 34	122 ± 33	0.022
Diastolic blood pressure (mmHg)	72 ± 23	73 ± 22	71 ± 23	0.227
Heart rate (beats per minute)	120 ± 28	120 ± 28	121 ± 28	0.385
Oxygen saturation (%)	94 [88, 98]	94 [89, 98]	93 [88, 98]	0.003
Severe desaturation (SpO$_2$ < 80%), n (%)	76 (8.6)	28 (6.5)	48 (10.6)	0.029
Pre-oxygenation devices, n (%)				< 0.001
Nasal cannula	154 (17.5)	79 (18.6)	75 (16.5)	
Venture mask	103 (11.7)	62 (14.6)	41 (9.0)	
Simple mask	14 (1.6)	7 (1.6)	7 (1.5)	
Reservoir mask	424 (48.2)	206 (48.5)	218 (47.9)	
High-flow nasal cannula	163 (18.5)	55 (12.9)	108 (23.7)	
BiPAP	22 (2.5)	16 (3.8)	6 (1.3)	
Predicted difficult airway, n (%)	194 (20.3)	59 (12.7)	135 (27.4)	< 0.001
Blood, vomitus, or secretion in airway	18 (1.9)	6 (1.3)	12 (2.4)	0.193
Cervical immobilisation	21 (2.2)	6 (1.3)	15 (3.0)	0.064
Neck trauma/mass or vocal cord palsy	47 (4.9)	15 (3.2)	32 (6.5)	0.019
Evaluate the 3-3-2 rule	37 (3.9)	7 (1.5)	30 (6.1)	< 0.001
Short neck	74 (7.7)	25 (5.4)	49 (9.9)	0.008
Obesity	32 (3.3)	9 (1.9)	23 (4.7)	0.019
Limited mouth opening/small mouth	59 (6.2)	15 (3.2)	44 (8.9)	< 0.001
Large tongue	16 (1.7)	8 (1.7)	8 (1.6)	0.906

Values are expressed as median (interquartile range), mean (standard deviation), or n (%)

SpO$_2$ Oxygen saturation

* Departments were divided into two groups: medical and surgical departments

showed 27% in direct laryngoscopy group, and 26% in video laryngoscopy group. Table 7 demonstrated that subgroup analysis of the outcomes. In the inexperienced operators, video laryngoscopy group had higher first-attempt success rate than direct laryngoscopy group. On the other hand, there was no significant difference on the intubation-related complications in the experienced operators. In the patients without predicted difficult airway, video laryngoscopy group had greater first-intubation success rate than direct laryngoscopy group.

In the power analysis referent to previous studies, we achieved a statistical power of 99–100% for our study populations (493 in the video laryngoscopy group and 465 in the direct laryngoscopy group). Therefore, our study has an adequate sample size and appropriate power. Hosmer–Lemeshow goodness-of-fit testing revealed that multivariate models were well fitted ($\chi^2 = 6.419$, $p = 0.600$ for first-attempt intubation success; $\chi^2 = 1.666$, $p = 0.948$ for intubation-related complications, respectively).

Discussion

To our knowledge, this is the first study of the efficacy of video laryngoscopy when performed by non-anaesthesiologists in a general ward setting. The results of this study

Table 2 Characteristics of the physicians and types of hypnotic medication and neuromuscular blocker

Variable	Total $n=958$	Direct laryngoscopy $n=465$	Video laryngoscopy $n=493$	p
Level of operator experience*, n (%)				< 0.001
Inexperienced	639 (66.7)	344 (74.0)	295 (59.8)	
Experienced	319 (33.3)	121 (26.0)	198 (40.2)	
Pre-treatment agent, n (%)				
Fentanyl	722 (75.4)	335 (72.0)	387 (78.5)	0.021
Sedatives, n (%)	877 (91.5)	427 (91.8)	450 (91.3)	0.760
Etomidate	814 (85.0)	384 (82.6)	430 (87.2)	0.045
Ketamine	24 (2.5)	12 (2.6)	12 (2.4)	0.885
Midazolam	58 (6.1)	49 (10.5)	9 (1.8)	< 0.001
Other†	10 (1.0)	4 (0.9)	6 (1.2)	0.754
Paralytic agents, n (%)	198 (20.7)	125 (26.9)	73 (14.8)	< 0.001
Succinylcholine	150 (15.7)	106 (22.8)	44 (8.9)	< 0.001
Rocuronium	9 (0.9)	5 (1.1)	4 (0.8)	0.746
Other‡	41 (4.3)	15 (3.2)	26 (5.3)	0.118

Values are expressed as n (%)

IM internal medicine

* Operators were divided into two groups by the level of experience at the first intubation attempt. An experienced operator was defined as a board-certified physician or surgeon working in a critical care unit; an inexperienced operator was defined as a medical or surgical resident-in-training

† Included propofol and Ativan

‡ Included atracurium and cisatracurium

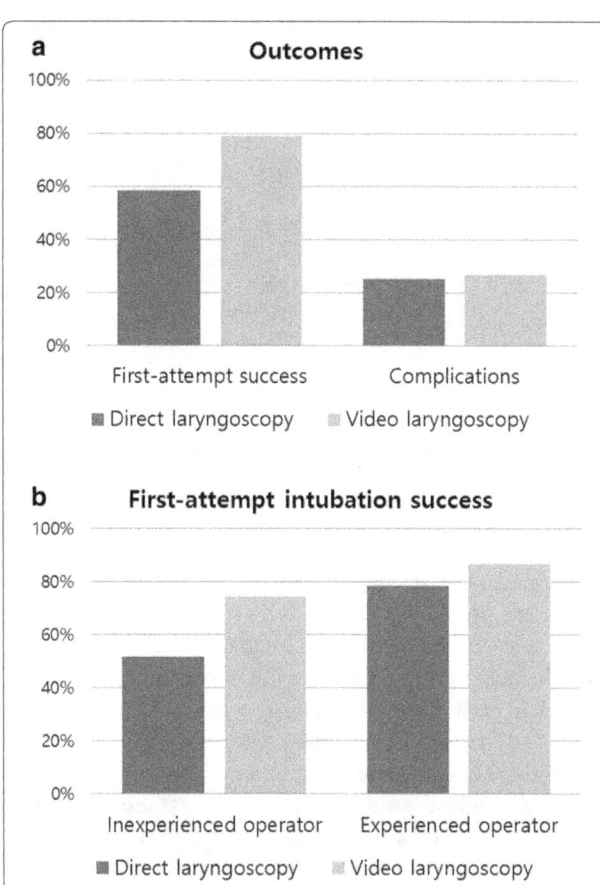

Fig. 2 Main results of the study. **a** Outcomes, **b** first-attempt intubation success

showed a higher first-attempt intubation success rate with video laryngoscopy than with direct laryngoscopy. However, there was no significant association of video laryngoscopy with lower intubation-related complications. Additionally, the number of intubation attempts was significantly lower in the video laryngoscopy group. Video laryngoscopy was also associated with improved visualisation of the glottis when compared with direct laryngoscopy.

In the general ward, tracheal intubation tends to be performed by less experienced operators and without capnography. Several studies have demonstrated that residents conducted 76–83% of first intubation attempts in critically ill patients [12, 19]. Bowles et al. reported that capnography was used in only 20% of general ward intubations [13]. In our hospital, all general ward tracheal intubations performed by inexperienced operators were supervised, involved capnography, and featured assistance by highly trained MET nurses. Accordingly, our study observed an overall first-attempt success rate of 69%, which is comparable to the rates of 56–75% reported for the ICU and emergency department (ED) [7, 9, 12, 20]. Furthermore, intubation-related complications were observed in 26% of the patients, and this was lower than the rates of 28–39% in the ICU and ED [1–3, 20–22].

Previous studies have reported an association of video laryngoscopy with an improved first-attempt success rate

Table 3 Outcomes according to intubation device

Variable	Total $n=958$	Direct laryngoscopy $n=465$	Video laryngoscopy $n=493$	p
First-attempt success, n (%)	664 (69.3)	273 (58.7)	391 (79.3)	<0.001
Difficult intubation*, n (%)	294 (30.7)	192 (41.3)	102 (20.7)	<0.001
Cormack–Lehane grade†, n (%)				0.024
1	721 (76.8)	328 (72.6)	393 (80.7)	
2	170 (18.1)	95 (21.0)	75 (15.4)	
3	38 (4.0)	22 (4.9)	16 (3.3)	
4	10 (1.1)	7 (1.5)	3 (0.6)	
No. of intubation attempts	1 [1, 2]	1 [1, 2]	1 [1, 1]	<0.001
Intubation duration‡ (min)	4 [3, 6]	4 [3, 7]	4 [3, 5]	<0.001

Values are expressed as median (interquartile range) or n (%)

* Defined as more than two attempts of intubation

† Reflects glottis visualisation, with a score range of 1 (good) to 4 (no glottis visualisation)

‡ Defined as the time between the infusion of induction medication and confirmation of endotracheal tube placement by capnography or chest radiography

Table 4 Complications according to intubation device

Variable	Total $n=958$	Direct laryngoscopy $n=465$	Video laryngoscopy $n=493$	p
Complications, n (%)	251 (26.2)	118 (25.4)	133 (27.0)	0.573
Hypotension*	181 (18.9)	94 (20.2)	87 (17.6)	0.310
Severe desaturation†	24 (2.6)	5 (1.1)	19 (4.1)	0.005
Oesophageal intubation	1 (0.1)	1 (0.2)	0 (0.0)	0.485
Dental trauma	4 (0.4)	1 (0.2)	3 (0.6)	0.625
Oral bleeding	42 (4.4)	18 (3.9)	24 (4.9)	0.451
Aspiration	3 (0.3)	2 (0.4)	1 (0.2)	0.614
Others‡	12 (1.3)	3 (0.6)	9 (1.8)	0.101
Length of hospital stay (days)	32 [17, 58]	32 [18, 58]	31 [16, 59]	0.640
In-hospital mortality (%)	465 (48.5)	200 (43.0)	265 (53.8)	0.001

* Defined as a systolic blood pressure < 90 mmHg

† Defined as an oxygen saturation < 80%

‡ Included cardiopulmonary resuscitation or bradycardia

for difficult intubation cases; [10] in the ICU [7, 8, 18, 23, 24], ED [25, 26], and pre-hospital settings; [27] and in cases of in-hospital cardiac arrest [28]. However, recent randomised clinical trials (RCTs) [12, 20, 29] in ICU settings found that video laryngoscopy did not yield higher first-attempt tracheal intubation success rate than direct laryngoscopy. The MACMAN trial [12] emphasised that improved glottis visualisation with video laryngoscopy did not translate into an improved first-attempt success rate. The authors suggested that tracheal catheterisation under indirect vision was more difficult. However, our analysis suggests that first-attempt intubation success depends on complex interactions of the mode of laryngoscopy, level of operator experience, and prediction of difficult airways. In the MACMAN trial [12], 83%

of tracheal intubations were performed by non-expert operators. Although another RCT by Janz et al. [20]. included tracheal intubations conducted by pulmonary and critical care medicine fellows, the fellows had each performed fewer than 5 tracheal intubations with video laryngoscopy during the study period and had a previous experience of only 10 tracheal intubations using video laryngoscopy. Also, in a single-centre pilot RCT by Griesdale et al. [29], video laryngoscopy did not yield an improved first-attempt success rate. However, that study included only 40 tracheal intubations conducted by novices (e.g. medical students or non-anaesthesiology residents), with an overall first-attempt success rate of 38%. Although there is an argument to use of video laryngoscopy could shorten the learning curve, a recent study

Table 5 Factors associated with first-attempt intubation success

Variable	Univariate analysis OR (95% CI)	p	Multivariate analysis OR (95% CI)	p
Age	0.992 (0.982, 1.002)	0.102		
Female	1.031 (0.773, 1.375)	0.835		
Video laryngoscopy	2.696 (2.026, 3.587)	<0.001	3.058 (2.192, 4.267)	<0.001
Medical department	1.346 (0.990, 1.831)	0.058		
Systolic blood pressure (mmHg)	0.998 (0.994, 1.002)	0.380		
Diastolic blood pressure (mmHg)	1.000 (0.994, 1.006)	0.931		
Heart rate (beats per minute)	1.006 (1.001, 1.011)	0.021	1.006 (1.000, 1.011)	0.044
Oxygen saturation (%)	1.012 (0.999, 1.025)	0.076		
Severe desaturation (SpO$_2$ < 80%), n (%)	0.559 (0.347, 0.901)	0.017	0.521 (0.316, 0.861)	0.011
Predicted difficult airway	0.388 (0.280, 0.536)	<0.001	0.344 (0.230, 0.514)	<0.001
Experienced operator	3.039 (2.173, 4.250)	<0.001	3.319 (2.284, 4.823)	<0.001
Pre-treatment agent	1.127 (0.822, 1.545)	0.457		
Sedatives	0.722 (0.427, 1.220)	0.223		
Paralytic agents	0.857 (0.614, 1.197)	0.365		
Cormack–Lehane grade	0.384 (0.301, 0.489)	<0.001	0.459 (0.352, 0.599)	<0.001

OR odds ratio, *CI* confidence interval

Table 6 Factors associated with intubation-related complications

Variables	Univariate analysis OR (95% CI)	p	Multivariate analysis OR (95% CI)	p
Age	1.006 (0.996, 1.017)	0.250		
Female	0.993 (0.734, 1.343)	0.964		
Video laryngoscopy	1.086 (0.814, 1.450)	0.573	1.173 (0.865, 1.591)	0.306
Medical department	1.393 (0.986, 1.968)	0.060		
Systolic blood pressure (mmHg)	0.998 (0.994, 1.002)	0.366		
Diastolic blood pressure (mmHg)	0.995 (0.989, 1.002)	0.165		
Heart rate (beats per minute)	0.999 (0.994, 1.004)	0.747		
Oxygen saturation (%)	0.990 (0.977, 1.003)	0.134		
Severe desaturation (SpO$_2$ < 80%), n (%)	1.408 (0.851, 2.329)	0.183		
Predicted difficult airway	1.302 (0.920, 1.842)	0.136		
Experienced operator	0.939 (0.691, 1.277)	0.688		
Pre-treatment agent	1.346 (0.950, 1.908)	0.094		
Sedatives	2.398 (1.248, 4.606)	0.009	2.377 (1.224, 4.616)	0.011
Paralytic agents	0.476 (0.316, 0.717)	<0.001	0.449 (0.293, 0.687)	<0.001
Cormack–Lehane grade	1.168 (0.923, 1.477)	0.195		
No. of intubation attempts	1.460 (1.237, 1.723)	<0.001	1.535 (1.291, 1.825)	<0.001
Intubation duration	1.067 (1.025, 1.111)	0.002		

OR odds ratio, *CI* confidence interval

of the GlideScope device demonstrated that 76 attempts would be required to master intubation whereas traditional cut-off for direct laryngoscopy is set at 50 attempts [30]. In other words, these RCTs were limited by the lack of sufficient time for the operators to acquire a reliable level of experience with video laryngoscopy.

There is a concern of video laryngoscopy is associated with severe complications. The MACMAN trial demonstrated that video laryngoscopy was associated with severe life-threatening complications and higher incidence of severe desaturation [12]. The results of our study did not show that video laryngoscopy reduced intubation-related complications, and video laryngoscopy was

Table 7 Subgroup analysis

Variable	Total n=958	First-attempt success	p	Intubation-related complications	p
Inexperienced operator, n (%)	639 (66.7)	398 (62.3)	< 0.001	170 (26.6)	0.785
Direct laryngoscopy	344 (53.8)	178 (51.7)		90 (26.2)	
Video laryngoscopy	295 (46.2)	220 (74.6)		80 (27.1)	
Experienced operator, n (%)	319 (33.3)	266 (83.4)	0.068	81 (25.4)	0.470
Direct laryngoscopy	121 (37.9)	95 (78.5)		28 (23.1)	
Video laryngoscopy	198 (62.1)	171 (86.4)		53 (26.8)	
Without predicted difficult airway, n (%)	764 (79.7)	563 (73.7)	< 0.001	192 (25.1)	0.871
Direct laryngoscopy	406 (53.1)	256 (63.1)		103 (25.4)	
Video laryngoscopy	358 (46.9)	307 (85.8)		89 (24.9)	
Video laryngoscopy group	493 (51.5)	391 (79.3)	0.223	133 (27.0)	0.056
Paralytics	73 (14.8)	54 (74.0)		13 (17.8)	
No paralytics	420 (85.2)	337 (80.2)		120 (28.6)	

associated with more severe desaturation than direct laryngoscopy. However in our study, the incidence rates of a pre-intubation $SpO_2 < 80\%$ and predicted difficult airway were higher in the video laryngoscopy group. This may affect the rate of intubation-related complications (Additional file 3: Table S3).

In this study, hospital mortality was higher in the video laryngoscopy group than in the direct laryngoscopy group. However, meta-analysis of the 12 RCTs showed that in-hospital mortality was not significantly different between video laryngoscopy and direct laryngoscopy [31]. We think many factors such as disease severity, organ dysfunction, underlying disease and comorbidities also contribute to mortality.

There were similar complications associated with the video laryngoscope such as the insertion of a styletted endotracheal tube through the right palatopharyngeal arch [32, 33]. In addition, even small amounts of oropharyngeal blood or vomitus can easily contaminated the lens of the video laryngoscope [34]. The GlideScope with a hyper-angulated blade is not the best device to learn intubation skills and required stylet mandatory. We cannot guarantee whether other types of video laryngoscopes would yield similar results.

This study had several limitations. First, this was a retrospective analysis, and the operators chose the laryngoscopy mode according to their preference. Thus, the device used for the first intubation attempt was not randomly assigned. Accordingly, the level of operator experience may have influence the device success rates. However, we performed an adjustment for differences in baseline characteristics of patients using a propensity-score matching to reduce the effect of confounding factors. As we described in Additional file 2: Tables S2 and Additional file 4: Table S4, the results of the

propensity-score matching showed that the use of video laryngoscopy is associated with increased odds of successful intubation on first attempt compared with the direct laryngoscopy. Second, we did not demonstrate the Mallampati score and the percentage of glottis opening (POGO) score. Unfortunately, these variables were not routinely recorded in our intubation data collection sheet. Third, the experienced operators in our study may differ from those in other studies [7, 12, 20]. In previous studies, the authors defined an expert operator as a critical care medicine attending physician or anaesthesiologist. However, it is unlikely that every tracheal intubation in real-world general ward settings is performed under the supervision of such experts. In our hospital, an anaesthesiologist is not always available for tracheal intubation outside of the operating room. A rescue airway team, which includes an anaesthesiologist, is activated only in 'cannot intubate, cannot oxygenate' situations. In addition, the results of our analysis showed that the first-attempt success rate of experienced operators was sufficiently high to allow them to supervise inexperienced operators. Therefore, stratification of the level of operator experience according to board certification seems appropriate. Fourth, only 21% of patients received paralytics, which is associated with improved first-attempt success, improved Cormack–Lehane grade, and decreased procedure-related complications in critically ill patients [35]. Low rate of neuromuscular blockade use could have decreased the first-attempt success rate, and the video laryngoscopy group seems to be an awake intubation group which require expertise. However, in this study the first-intubation success rate was lower in direct laryngoscopy group, which usage of neuromuscular blockers was higher. In addition, after propensity-score matching, the first-attempt success rate was greater in video laryngoscopy group than direct laryngoscopy group. Therefore, further study is needed for this issue.

A strength of our study is the enrolment of a relatively large number of general ward patients who underwent tracheal intubation; accordingly, the results of our study will provide information to support the selection of intubation devices in a general ward setting.

Conclusion

In this study, we observed a higher first-attempt intubation success rate with video laryngoscopy than with direct laryngoscopy in a general ward setting. However, video laryngoscopy did not reduce intubation-related complications. Furthers trials on best way to perform intubation in the emergency settings are required.

Abbreviations
ICU: intensive care unit; MET: medical emergency team; ED: emergency department; RCT: randomised clinical trial.

Authors' contributions
MSB and SBH conceived the study design and performed data collection, statistical analysis, and draft writing. MJH, JWH, CML, and YSK performed data collection and a critical revision of the manuscript. All authors read and approved the final manuscript.

Author details
[1] Department of Pulmonary and Critical Care Medicine, Asan Medical Centre, University of Ulsan College of Medicine, 88 Olympic-ro 43-gil, Songpa-gu, Seoul 05505, Republic of Korea. [2] Medical Emergency Team, Asan Medical Centre, University of Ulsan College of Medicine, Seoul, Republic of Korea.

Acknowledgements
We gratefully acknowledge all the following dedicated Asan Medical Centre (AMC) Medical Alert Team (MAT) nurses who working to improve patients' safety and care: Jin Mi Lee, MyongJa Han, Ju Ry Lee, Yu Jung Shin, Jeong Suk Son, Sun Hui Choi, Youn Kyung Jung, Eun-Joo Choi, Da Hye Kim.

Competing interests
The authors declare that they have no competing interests.

Funding
This research was supported by a grant of the Korea Health Technology R&D Project through the Korea Health Industry Development Institute (KHIDI), which was funded by the Ministry of Health & Welfare, Republic of Korea (Grant No. HI15C1106). The funders had no role in the study design, data collection and analysis, preparation of the manuscript, or decision to publish.

References

1. Simpson GD, Ross MJ, McKeown DW, Ray DC. Tracheal intubation in the critically ill: a multi-centre national study of practice and complications. Br J Anaesth. 2012;108:792–9.
2. Jaber S, Amraoui J, Lefrant JY, Arich C, Cohendy R, Landreau L, et al. Clinical practice and risk factors for immediate complications of endotracheal intubation in the intensive care unit: a prospective, multiple-center study. Crit Care Med. 2006;34:2355–61.
3. Griesdale DE, Bosma TL, Kurth T, Isac G, Chittock DR. Complications of endotracheal intubation in the critically ill. Intensive Care Med. 2008;34:1835–42.
4. Sakles JC, Chiu S, Mosier J, Walker C, Stolz U. The importance of first pass success when performing orotracheal intubation in the emergency department. Acad Emerg Med. 2013;20:71–8.
5. Mort TC. Emergency tracheal intubation: complications associated with repeated laryngoscopic attempts. Anesth Analg. 2004;99:607–13 (table of contents).
6. Hasegawa K, Shigemitsu K, Hagiwara Y, Chiba T, Watase H, Brown CA 3rd, et al. Association between repeated intubation attempts and adverse events in emergency departments: an analysis of a multicenter prospective observational study. Ann Emerg Med. 2012;60(749–754):e742.
7. Silverberg MJ, Li N, Acquah SO, Kory PD. Comparison of video laryngoscopy versus direct laryngoscopy during urgent endotracheal intubation: a randomized controlled trial. Crit Care Med. 2015;43:636–41.
8. De Jong A, Molinari N, Conseil M, Coisel Y, Pouzeratte Y, Belafia F, et al. Video laryngoscopy versus direct laryngoscopy for orotracheal intubation in the intensive care unit: a systematic review and meta-analysis. Intensive Care Med. 2014;40:629–39.
9. Mosier JM, Whitmore SP, Bloom JW, Snyder LS, Graham LA, Carr GE, et al. Video laryngoscopy improves intubation success and reduces esophageal intubations compared to direct laryngoscopy in the medical intensive care unit. Crit Care. 2013;17:R237.
10. Griesdale DE, Liu D, McKinney J, Choi PT. Glidescope(R) video-laryngoscopy versus direct laryngoscopy for endotracheal intubation: a systematic review and meta-analysis. Can J Anaesth. 2012;59:41–52.
11. Arulkumaran N, Lowe J, Ions R, Ruano MM, Bennett V, Dunser MW. Videolaryngoscopy versus direct laryngoscopy for emergency orotracheal intubation outside the operating room: a systematic review and meta-analysis. Br J Anaesth. 2018;120:712–24.
12. Lascarrou JB, Boisrame-Helms J, Bailly A, Le Thuaut A, Kamel T, Mercier E, et al. Video laryngoscopy vs direct laryngoscopy on successful first-pass orotracheal intubation among ICU patients: a randomized clinical trial. JAMA. 2017;317:483–93.
13. Bowles TM, Freshwater-Turner DA, Janssen DJ, Peden CJ. Out-of-theatre tracheal intubation: prospective multicentre study of clinical practice and adverse events. Br J Anaesth. 2011;107:687–92.
14. Sinclair RCF, Luxton MC. Rapid sequence induction. Contin Educ Anaesth Crit Care Pain. 2005;5:45–8.
15. Frerk C, Mitchell VS, McNarry AF, Mendonca C, Bhagrath R, Patel A, et al. Difficult Airway Society 2015 guidelines for management of unanticipated difficult intubation in adults. Br J Anaesth. 2015;115:827–48.
16. Apfelbaum JL, Hagberg CA, Caplan RA, Blitt CD, Connis RT, Nickinovich DG, et al. Practice guidelines for management of the difficult airway: an updated report by the American Society of Anesthesiologists Task Force on Management of the Difficult Airway. Anesthesiology. 2013;118:251–70.
17. Jaber S, Jung B, Corne P, Sebbane M, Muller L, Chanques G, et al. An intervention to decrease complications related to endotracheal intubation in the intensive care unit: a prospective, multiple-center study. Intensive Care Med. 2010;36:248–55.
18. Hypes CD, Stolz U, Sakles JC, Joshi RR, Natt B, Malo J, et al. Video laryngoscopy improves odds of first-attempt success at intubation in the intensive care unit. A propensity-matched analysis. Ann Am Thorac Soc. 2016;13:382–90.
19. Choi HJ, Kim YM, Oh YM, Kang HG, Yim HW, Jeong SH. GlideScope video laryngoscopy versus direct laryngoscopy in the emergency department: a propensity score-matched analysis. BMJ Open. 2015;5:e007884.

20. Janz DR, Semler MW, Lentz RJ, Matthews DT, Assad TR, Norman BC, et al. Randomized trial of video laryngoscopy for endotracheal intubation of critically ill adults. Crit Care Med. 2016;44:1980–7.

21. Cook TM, Woodall N, Harper J, Benger J. Major complications of airway management in the UK: results of the Fourth National Audit Project of the Royal College of Anaesthetists and the Difficult Airway Society. Part 2: intensive care and emergency departments. Br J Anaesth. 2011;106:632–42.

22. Walz JM, Zayaruzny M, Heard SO. Airway management in critical illness. Chest. 2007;131:608–20.

23. Lakticova V, Koenig SJ, Narasimhan M, Mayo PH. Video laryngoscopy is associated with increased first pass success and decreased rate of esophageal intubations during urgent endotracheal intubation in a medical intensive care unit when compared to direct laryngoscopy. J Intensive Care Med. 2015;30:44–8.

24. Kory P, Guevarra K, Mathew JP, Hegde A, Mayo PH. The impact of video laryngoscopy use during urgent endotracheal intubation in the critically ill. Anesth Analg. 2013;117:144–9.

25. Mosier JM, Stolz U, Chiu S, Sakles JC. Difficult airway management in the emergency department: GlideScope videolaryngoscopy compared to direct laryngoscopy. J Emerg Med. 2012;42:629–34.

26. Sakles JC, Mosier JM, Chiu S, Keim SM. Tracheal intubation in the emergency department: a comparison of GlideScope(R) video laryngoscopy to direct laryngoscopy in 822 intubations. J Emerg Med. 2012;42:400–5.

27. Jarvis JL, McClure SF, Johns D. EMS intubation improves with king vision video laryngoscopy. Prehosp Emerg Care. 2015;19:482–9.

28. Lee DH, Han M, An JY, Jung JY, Koh Y, Lim CM, et al. Video laryngoscopy versus direct laryngoscopy for tracheal intubation during in-hospital cardiopulmonary resuscitation. Resuscitation. 2015;89:195–9.

29. Griesdale DE, Chau A, Isac G, Ayas N, Foster D, Irwin C, et al. Video-laryngoscopy versus direct laryngoscopy in critically ill patients: a pilot randomized trial. Can J Anaesth. 2012;59:1032–9.

30. Cortellazzi P, Caldiroli D, Byrne A, Sommariva A, Orena EF, Tramacere I. Defining and developing expertise in tracheal intubation using a GlideScope((R)) for anaesthetists with expertise in Macintosh direct laryngoscopy: an in vivo longitudinal study. Anaesthesia. 2015;70:290–5.

31. Jiang J, Ma D, Li B, Yue Y, Xue F. Video laryngoscopy does not improve the intubation outcomes in emergency and critical patients: a systematic review and meta-analysis of randomized controlled trials. Crit Care. 2017;21:288.

32. Choo MK, Yeo VS, See JJ. Another complication associated with videola-ryngoscopy. Can J Anaesth. 2007;54:322–4.

33. Cooper RM. Complications associated with the use of the GlideScope videolaryngoscope. Can J Anaesth. 2007;54:54–7.

34. Rothfield KP, Russo SG. Videolaryngoscopy: should it replace direct laryn-goscopy? a pro-con debate. J Clin Anesth. 2012;24:593–7.

35. Wilcox SR, Bittner EA, Elmer J, Seigel TA, Nguyen NT, Dhillon A, et al. Neuromuscular blocking agent administration for emergent tracheal intubation is associated with decreased prevalence of procedure-related complications. Crit Care Med. 2012;40:1808–13.

20

Severe atypical pneumonia in critically ill patients

S. Valade[1,2*], L. Biard[2,3], V. Lemiale[1,2], L. Argaud[4], F. Pène[5], L. Papazian[6], F. Bruneel[7], A. Seguin[8], A. Kouatchet[9], J. Oziel[10], S. Rouleau[11], N. Bele[12], K. Razazi[13], O. Lesieur[14], F. Boissier[15], B. Megarbane[16], N. Bigé[17], N. Brulé[18], A. S. Moreau[19], A. Lautrette[20], O. Peyrony[21], P. Perez[22], J. Mayaux[23] and E. Azoulay[1,2]

Abstract

Background: *Chlamydophila pneumoniae* (CP) and *Mycoplasma pneumoniae* (MP) patients could require intensive care unit (ICU) admission for acute respiratory failure.

Methods: Adults admitted between 2000 and 2015 to 20 French ICUs with proven atypical pneumonia were retrospectively described. Patients with MP were compared to *Streptococcus pneumoniae* (SP) pneumonia patients admitted to ICUs.

Results: A total of 104 patients were included, 71 men and 33 women, with a median age of 56 [44–67] years. MP was the causative agent for 76 (73%) patients and CP for 28 (27%) patients. Co-infection was documented for 18 patients (viruses for 8 [47%] patients). Median number of involved quadrants on chest X-ray was 2 [1–4], with alveolar opacities ($n = 61$, 75%), interstitial opacities ($n = 32$, 40%). Extra-pulmonary manifestations were present in 34 (33%) patients. Mechanical ventilation was required for 75 (72%) patients and vasopressors for 41 (39%) patients. ICU length of stay was 16.5 [9.5–30.5] days, and 11 (11%) patients died in the ICU. Compared with SP patients, MP patients had more extensive interstitial pneumonia, fewer pleural effusion, and a lower mortality rate [6 (8%) vs. 17 (22%), $p = 0.013$]. According MCA analysis, some characteristics at admission could discriminate MP and SP. MP was more often associated with hemolytic anemia, abdominal manifestations, and extensive chest radiograph abnormalities. SP-P was associated with shock, confusion, focal crackles, and focal consolidation.

Conclusion: In this descriptive study of atypical bacterial pneumonia requiring ICU admission, mortality was 11%. The comparison with SP pneumonia identified clinical, laboratory, and radiographic features that may suggest MP or CP pneumonia.

Keywords: Pneumonia, Outcome, ICU, *Mycoplasma pneumoniae*, *Chlamydophila pneumoniae*

Background

Severe pneumonia remains the major reasons for admission to the intensive care unit (ICU), mainly related to *Streptococcus pneumoniae* (SP). Atypical pneumonia (AP) related, for instance, to *Chlamydophila pneumoniae* (CP) and *Mycoplasma pneumoniae* (MP) accounts for 1–30% of documented pneumonia in patients admitted to ICU [1–11]. Although AP is rarely severe, some patients with community-acquired AP require ICU admission. Several retrospective studies reported ICU admission for 2–16.3% of patients with AP [1–3, 8, 11–15]. In one study, even 38.8% of patients with AP, older than 65 years, were admitted to ICU [12]. Among ICU-admitted patients with AP, 0.3–11% required mechanical ventilation [4, 5], with acute respiratory distress syndrome (ARDS) for few patients [15, 16]. In previous studies, mortality rates were low, around 3% [5, 13, 14, 17], although a recent retrospective study found 29.4% mortality [12] in a population with high rates of co-infection and cardiac complications.

*Correspondence: sandrine.valade@aphp.fr
[1] AP-HP, Medical ICU, Hôpital Saint-Louis, 1 Avenue Claude Vellefaux, 75010 Paris, France
Full list of author information is available at the end of the article

In previous non-ICU studies, compared to bacterial pneumonia, AP was associated with younger age and fewer comorbidities, a lower risk of severe respiratory failure, and better outcome [4, 6, 13, 14, 18]. For patients admitted to ICU, studies remained rare.

The main objective of the study was to describe AP in patients admitted to ICU. Our secondary objective was to compare the diagnostic strategy and outcomes between *Mycoplasma pneumoniae*-related pneumonia (MP) and *Streptococcus pneumoniae*-related pneumonia (SP) admitted to ICU.

Methods

Patients with atypical pneumonia (AP)

This is a retrospective chart review of adults admitted to 20 ICUs in France with a diagnosis of AP over the 16-year period from 2000 to 2015 (Additional file 1: Figure S1). Inclusion criteria were pneumonia defined with sepsis and a new pulmonary infiltrate on the chest radiograph and either a positive specific polymerase chain reaction (PCR) test for MP or CP on respiratory specimens (noninvasive samples or bronchoalveolar lavage) or blood serologic tests suggesting acute MP or CP infection (elevated specific IgM or fourfold increase in IgG level between two time points or elevated anti-MP IgG combined with presence of cold agglutinins) [19].

This study was approved by a local ethic committee (Société de Réanimation de Langue Française, CE SRLF 18-01).

Data collection

Clinical and laboratory data at ICU admission were collected, as well as organ failure during ICU stay. The SAPS II score [20] was used to assess severity at ICU admission. We also collected extra-pulmonary symptoms; arthritis was defined as new inflammation with one or more joints, myocarditis with cardiac dysfunction and troponin elevation and cutaneous involvement with the onset of skin rash. Bacterial and/or viral co-infections at diagnosis were recorded.

Patients with *Streptococcus pneumoniae* pneumonia (SP-P)

Patients with MP-AP were compared to a group of consecutive patients with proven SP-P admitted to one of the study ICUs (Saint Louis Hospital, Paris) during the same period. SP-P was diagnosed based on sepsis with a new pulmonary infiltrate and identification of SP in at least one microbiological specimen (blood culture, respiratory specimen, or urinary antigen with no alternative diagnosis).

Statistical analysis

Categorical variables were described as n (%) and quantitative variables as median [25th–75th percentiles]. We first described the features in the patients with AP at ICU admission. Then, we conducted univariate analyses with a nonparametric test to compare the groups with MP-AP and SP-P. Finally, multiple correspondence analysis (MCA) was performed to identify the dimensions associated with the parameters at ICU admission (HIV, symptom duration, shock, confusion, diarrhea, physical chest findings, chest radiograph abnormalities, bilirubin level, and hemolytic anemia) and the causative organism, using the FactoMineR library in the R software platform. MCA is an extension of simple correspondence analysis designed to analyze relations among categorical variables. The aim is to redefine the principal dimensions or axes of the space in a way that captures the highest possible percentage of the inertia (which can be likened to the explained variance).

All tests were two-tailed. p values < 0.05 were considered significant. All statistical analyses were carried out using the R 2.13.1 statistical platform (http://www.R-project.org).

Results

Clinical findings in the patients with atypical pneumonia (AP)

We included 104 patients, 71 men and 33 women, with a median age of 56 [44–67] years (Additional file 2: Table S2). Acute respiratory failure was the main reason for ICU admission ($n=96$; 92%); other reasons were cardiovascular failure ($n=2$), neurological disorders ($n=3$), and miscellaneous reasons ($n=3$).

AP was more common in the fall and winter (Fig. 1). Furthermore, AP became more common over time, suggesting improved diagnosis after the introduction of PCR testing.

Table 1 and Additional file 3: Table S1 report the main features of the patients with AP. The most common comorbidity was chronic respiratory disease, which was present in 32 (31%) patients including 9 patients with chronic obstructive lung disease, 4 patients with asthma, and 4 patients with interstitial lung disease; of these 32 patients, 7 patients were on long-term oxygen therapy before ICU admission. Immunosuppression was noted in 21 patients including 10 (48%) with hematological malignancies (lymphoma, $n=6$), 7 with solid cancer, and 2 with HIV infection. Delay from respiratory symptoms onset to ICU admission was 5 [3–8] days. A fever defined with a body temperature above 38.5 °C was present in 77 patients (74%). At ICU admission, all patients were tachypneic (respiratory rate, 32 [26–37]/min) and

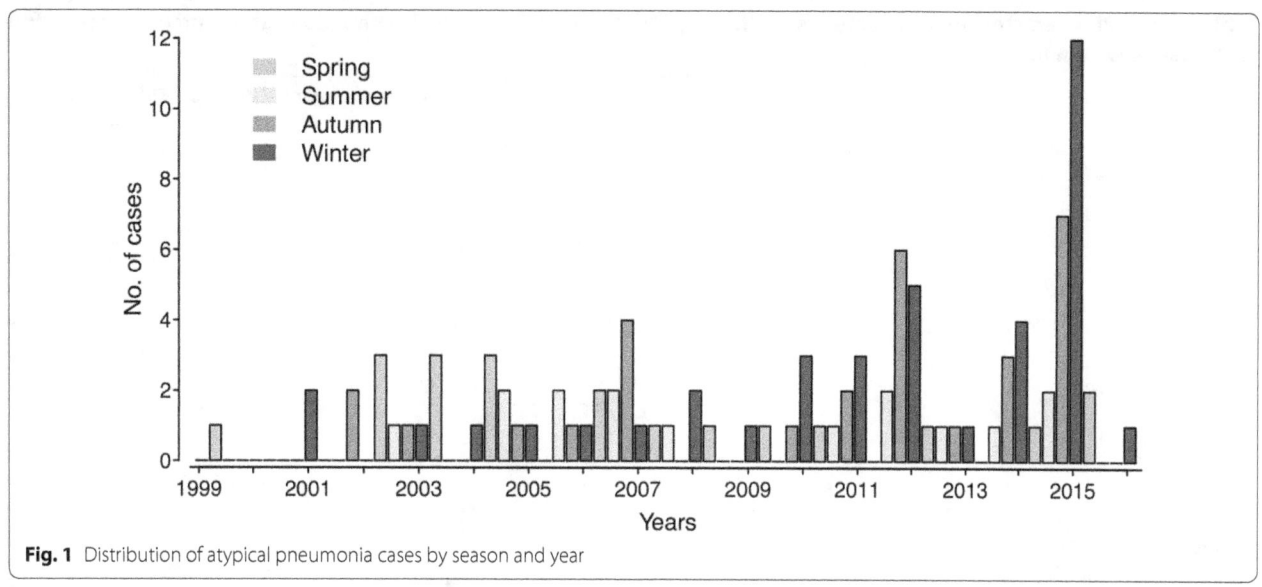

Fig. 1 Distribution of atypical pneumonia cases by season and year

48 (46%) had severe respiratory symptoms. Physical chest examination included crackles ($n=54$; 52%), rhonchi ($n=15$; 14%), wheezing ($n=12$; 11%), and signs of consolidation ($n=7$; 7%). No squeaks were reported. Extrapulmonary symptoms concerned 34 (33%) patients and included arthritis ($n=2$), myocarditis ($n=4$), and skin rash ($n=6$). Almost one-third of the patients ($n=32$; 31%) had neurological symptoms at ICU admission, mostly with an altered level of consciousness related to severity of sepsis or to hypoxemia. Confusion was the main symptom for 3 (3%) patients, and meningoencephalitis was diagnosed in 1 patient. Cold agglutinins assessed in case of hemolytic anemia were positive in 9 (9%) MP patients, cytolysis occurred in 11 (10%) patients, and rhabdomyolysis was present in 3 (3%) patients. At ICU admission, 10 (10%) patients had shock, the SOFA score was 5 [2–7], and the SAPS II was 33 [25–44].

Other findings in patients with atypical pneumonia (AP)

The most common findings by chest radiography were alveolar opacities ($n=61$, 59%), and interstitial opacities ($n=32$, 31%) in 2 [1–4] quadrants. Pleural effusion was rare ($n=6$, 6%).

The causative organism was MP in 76 (73%) patients and CP in 28 (27%) patients and was identified by serological testing (positive IgM or elevated IgG) in 71 patients, positive PCR on respiratory samples in 33 patients (18 on bronchoalveolar lavage, 10 on naso-pharyngeal aspirate, 2 on tracheal aspirate and 4 on nasal swab) and by both diagnostic methods in 5 patients. None of the collected variables differed between patients diagnosed with PCR, serology or both (Additional file 4: Table S3). Co-infection was found in 18 (20%) patients and was related to

viruses ($n=9$; influenza, rhinovirus, respiratory syncytial virus, coronavirus) or bacteria ($n=6$; *Haemophilus influenzae, Proteus mirabilis, Staphylococcus aureus, Serratia marcescens*) or *Pneumocystis jirovecii* ($n=3$). None of MP patients had co-infection with CP or SP.

ICU management of atypical pneumonia (AP)

Mechanical ventilation was required for 75 (72%) patients and lasted 13 [8–19] days. Of the 34 (45%) patients meeting criteria for ARDS, 4 required extracorporeal membrane oxygenation. Vasoactive agents were required for 41 (39%) patients, and renal replacement therapy was started for 10 (10%) patients.

The first-line antibiotics were active on MP and CP in 62 (60%) patients. Time from ICU admission to antibiotic initiation was 1 [0–4] day. Combination therapy was used in 61 (59%) patients and consisted to a third-generation cephalosporin (C3G) and a macrolide in 24 (39%) patients, a C3G and a quinolone in 13 (21%) patients, another betalactam and a macrolide in 16 (26%) patients, another betalactam and a quinolone in 6 (9%) patients, or another antibiotic and a macrolide in 2 (3%) patients. Antibiotics was adapted according to microbiology results with a macrolide ($n=72$), a quinolone ($n=24$) or a cycline ($n=3$).

Outcomes of atypical pneumonia (AP)

Eleven (11%) patients died in the ICU. ICU stay length was 16.5 [9.5–30.5] days. Persistent hypoxemia was present at ICU discharge in 60 (58%) patients. By univariate analysis, factors associated with mortality were age ≥ 65 years ($p=0.033$), signs of respiratory distress ($p=0.017$), and interstitial opacities on the chest

Table 1 Clinical characteristics of patients with atypical pneumonia at ICU admission and outcome according to the causative agent

N (%) or median [IQR]	Total (N = 104)	Mycoplasma pneumoniae (N = 76)	Chlamydophila pneumoniae (N = 28)
Demographics			
Age	56 [44–67]	54 [41–69]	64 [52–75]
Female gender	33 (32%)	26 (34%)	7 (25%)
Comorbidities			
Chronic respiratory disease	32 (31%)	22 (29%)	10 (36%)
Current smoker	30 (29%)	20 (38%)	10 (36%)
Immunosuppression	21 (20%)	17 (22%)	4 (14%)
HIV infection	2 (2%)	2 (3%)	0
Hematological malignancy	10 (10%)	9 (12%)	1 (3.5%)
Cancer	7 (7%)	4 (5%)	3 (11%)
Hypertension	32 (31%)	24 (32%)	8 (28%)
Reason for ICU admission			
Acute respiratory distress	96 (92%)	70 (92%)	26 (93%)
Cardiovascular failure	2 (2%)	2 (3%)	0
Neurological disorders	3 3%)	2 (3%)	1 (3.6%)
Other	3 (3%)	2 (3%)	1 (3.6%)
Clinical respiratory findings			
Respiratory rate	32 [26–37]	33 [27–38]	30 [26–33]
Signs of respiratory failure	48 (46%)	33 (49%)	15 (54%)
Rhonchi	15 (14%)	9 (15%)	6 (21%)
Crackles	54 (52%)	36 (47%)	18 (64%)
Signs of consolidation	7 (7%)	5 (9%)	2 (7%)
Decreased vesicular breath sounds	14 (13%)	10 (17%)	4 (14%)
Clinical presentation			
Time since symptom onset (days)	5 [3–8]	6 [4–9]	4 [2–7]
Fever	77 (74%)	58 (83%)	19 (68%)
Shock	10 (10%)	6 (8%)	4 (14%)
Neurological symptoms	32 (31%)	19 (25%)	13 (46%)
Gastrointestinal symptoms	1 (1%)	1 (1%)	0
Extra-pulmonary signs			
≥ 1 extra-pulmonary symptom	34 (33%)	27 (36%)	7 (25%)
Arthritis	2 (2%)	1 (1%)	1 (3.5%)
Myocarditis	4 (4%)	4 (5%)	0
Treatments in the ICU			
Mechanical ventilation	75 (72%)	50 (66%)	25 (89%)
Duration of ventilation	13 [8–19]	12.5 [8–22.5]	13.5 [8.5–19]
Vasopressors	41 (39%)	26 (34%)	15 (54%)
Renal replacement therapy	10 (9.5%)	7 (9%)	3 (11%)
Outcomes			
Death in the ICU	11 (10%)	6 (8%)	5 (18%)
Length of ICU stay (days)			
Discharged alive	15 [8–26]	15 [8–27]	19 [12–24]
ICU death	39 [25–49]	37 [26–47]	39 [25–90]

HIV human immunodeficiency virus, *ICU* intensive care unit

radiograph ($p = 0.017$). For MP patients, 26 (34%) did not receive adequate antibiotic at ICU admission. Among them 2 patients died.

Comparison to *Streptococcus pneumoniae* pneumonia (SP-P)

Tables 2 and 3 reports univariate analysis comparing patients with MP-AP and SP-P. Factors significantly associated with SP-P were HIV infection [12 (16%) vs. 2 (3%), $p = 0.009$], neurological symptoms [20 (26%) vs. 1 (1%), $p < 0.0001$], and gastrointestinal symptoms [15 (20%) vs. 1 (1%), $p = 0.0003$]. Factors significantly associated with MP were hemolytic anemia or cold agglutinins [0 (0%) vs. 9 (12%), $p = 0.003$]. Also, 6 patients with SP-P had co-infection (influenza A, $n = 3$; *Haemophilus influenzae*, $n = 2$; *Streptococcus constellatus*, $n = 1$).

SP-P was associated with a shorter length of respiratory symptoms before ICU admission (3 days [2–7] vs. 6 days [4–9], $p = 0.0008$). At ICU admission SAPS II score was higher for SP-P (42 [30–55] vs. 32 [22–41], $p = 0.005$), shock was more frequent (32% vs. 8%; $p = 0.0004$), creatinine level was higher (101 [69.5–168.8] μmol/L vs. 77 [57.5–108] μmol/L, $p = 0.008$), and lactate level was high (2.3 [1.8–3.4] mmol/l vs. 1 [0.07–2.7] mmol/l; $p = 0.003$).

Signs of consolidation and decreased breath sounds were more common in SP-P than in MP-AP (30% vs. 9% and 38% vs. 17%, respectively). MP-AP involved 4 quadrants on chest X-ray (26% vs. 8%, $p = 0.013$) but less frequently pleural space (5% vs. 11%, $p = 0.007$). The bilirubin level was higher in the patients with SP-P (15 [9.2–24.5] μmol/L vs. 8.4 [5.8–13] μmol/L, $p = 0.0006$). MP-AP was associated with the use of mechanical ventilation (66% vs. 50%, $p = 0.049$). ICU length of stay (LOS) seemed prolonged in case of MP-AP regardless of the ICU outcome (median LOS 37 vs. 5 days and 15 vs. 5 days, respectively, in patients who died in the ICU and in patients who were discharged alive). However, 28-day mortality was lower in the MP-AP group (5% vs. 20%, $p = 0.005$).

Figure 2 shows the MCA results for the clinical and radiological characteristics at admission. Several characteristics discriminated between MP and CP. MP was more often associated with hemolytic anemia, abdominal manifestations and extensive chest radiograph abnormalities. SP-P was associated with shock, confusion, focal crackles, and focal consolidation.

Discussion

This multicenter study is the largest one analyzing 104 AP patients admitted to ICU. Extra-pulmonary symptoms were seen for one-third of patients, corresponding to data on previous study for patients not admitted to ICU [21]. However, AP in non-ICU patients was described as mild [6], whereas a substantial proportion of our patients had severe acute pneumonia, with shock at ICU admission for 10% of patients and mechanical ventilation required for 72% of patients including 45% of patients with ARDS.

In previous studies, patients with MP-AP were younger and had fewer comorbidities, lower respiratory disease severity and better outcomes [4, 6, 13, 14, 18]. In our study, with ICU patients, age was similar for patients with MP-AP and SP-P.

Previous studies also compared clinical and radiological features according to the causative organism of pneumonia [8, 15, 18]. In a Japanese cohort, among patients with pneumonia and audible crackles, these were more often heard only in late inspiration in patients with AP and throughout inspiration in patients with other bacteria [22]. In our study, patients with MP-AP had no specific clinical findings, except signs of consolidation which were associated with SP-P. On radiological findings, compared to SP-P, MP-AP was more often responsible for ground-glass opacification, centrilobular nodules, bronchial wall thickening, and diffuse radiological abnormalities [1, 15, 18]. In our study, extensive interstitial pneumonia was more common in MP-AP than in SP-P.

The Japanese Respiratory Society published guidelines for identifying MP-AP [17] and established a scoring system based on six parameters: age < 60 years, minor or no comorbidities, stubborn cough, abnormal chest auscultation, the absence of sputum and of an etiological agent identifiable by rapid diagnostic testing, and peripheral white blood cell count < 10,000/μL. A score ≥ 4 indicates a high probability of MP-AP (sensitivity, 88.7%; and specificity, 77.5%). Another scoring system performed well in separating patients with pneumonia into three groups: pyogenic bacteria; MP, CP, or virus; and unknown agent [23]. Nevertheless, neither scoring system had been assessed in ICU patients. In our study, MCA provided insights into differences between MP-AP and SP-P. Hemolytic anemia, diffuse chest radiograph abnormalities, and interstitial opacities were associated with MP-AP. On the contrary, HIV infection, shock, neurological symptoms, gastrointestinal symptoms, signs of consolidation, shorter symptom duration, higher bilirubin level, and radiological alveolar opacities were strongly linked to SP-P.

Compared to patients with SP-P, those with MP-AP more often required mechanical ventilation and spent more time in the ICU yet had a lower risk of death. This lower mortality may be ascribable to the smaller number of MP-AP patients with extra-pulmonary organ failure (shock, neurological manifestations, acute renal failure) and to the lower SAPS II severity score in the MP-AP group (32 [22–41] vs. 42 [30–55], $p = 0.005$).

Table 2 Univariate analysis comparing clinical characteristics and outcomes of patients with *Mycoplasma pneumoniae* versus *Streptococcus pneumoniae* pneumonia

N (%) or median (IQR)	Total (N = 152)	Mycoplasma pneumoniae (N = 76)	Streptococcus pneumoniae (N = 76)	p value
Demographics				
Age	55 [43–69]	54 [41–69]	57 [44–73]	0.058
Female gender	51 (34%)	26 (34%)	25 (33%)	1
Comorbidities				
Chronic respiratory disease	36 (24%)	22 (29%)	14 (18%)	0.18
Current smoker	49 (41%)	20 (38%)	29 (43%)	
Immunosuppression	44 (29%)	17 (22%)	27 (36%)	0.11
HIV infection	14 (9%)	2 (3%)	12 (16%)	*0.009*
Hematological malignancy	18 (12%)	9 (12%)	9 (12%)	1
Cancer	12 (8%)	4 (5%)	8 (11%)	0.37
Hypertension	50 (33%)	24 (32%)	26 (34%)	0.86
Reason for ICU admission				
Acute respiratory distress	140 (92%)	70 (92%)	70 (92%)	0.59
Shock	6 (4%)	2 (3%)	4 (5%)	
Neurological symptoms	4 (3%)	2 (3%)	2 (3%)	
Other	2 (1%)	2 (3%)	0	
Clinical respiratory findings				
Respiratory rate	31 [26–38]	33 [27–38]	30 [26–36]	0.43
Signs of respiratory distress	67 (47%)	33 (49%)	34 (45%)	0.74
Rhonchi	21 (16%)	9 (15%)	12 (16%)	1
Crackles	79 (59%)	36 (61%)	44 (59%)	1
Signs of consolidation	27 (21%)	5 (9%)	22 (30%)	*0.008*
Decreased vesicular breath sounds	38 (28%)	10 (17%)	28 (38%)	*0.007*
Clinical presentation				
Time since symptom onset (days)	4 [2–7]	6 [4–9]	3 [2–7]	*0.0008*
Fever	112 (77%)	58 (83%)	54 (71%)	0.12
Shock	30 (20%)	6 (8%)	24 (32%)	*0.0004*
Neurological symptoms	21 (14%)	1 (1%)	20 (26%)	*< 0.0001*
Gastrointestinal symptoms	16 (11%)	1 (1%)	15 (20%)	*0.0003*
Extra-pulmonary signs				
≥ 1 extra-pulmonary sign	66 (43%)	27 (36%)	39 (51%)	0.071
Arthritis	1 (1%)	1 (1%)	0	1
Myocarditis	4 (3%)	4 (5%)	0	0.12
Treatments in the ICU				
Mechanical ventilation	88 (58%)	50 (66%)	38 (50%)	*0.049*
Duration of ventilation (days)				
Discharged alive	11 [7–19]	13 [8–23]	9 [6–16]	
ICU death	11 [3–18]	18 [17–34]	5 [2–15]	
Vasopressors	60 (39%)	26 (34%)	34 (45%)	0.26
Renal replacement therapy	17 (11%)	7 (9%)	10 (13%)	0.49
SAPS II	36 [24–47]	32 [22–41]	42 [30–55]	*0.0005*
Outcomes				
ICU stay length (days)				
Discharged alive	9 [5–19]	15 [8–27]	5 [3–10]	
ICU death	13 [4–27]	37 [26–47]	5 [3–14]	
28-day mortality	23 (15%)	6 (8%)	17 (22%)	*0.013*

HIV human immunodeficiency virus, *ICU* intensive care unit, *SAPS II* Simplified Acute Physiology Score version II

Table 3 Univariate analysis comparing laboratory findings in patients with *Mycoplasma pneumoniae* versus *Streptococcus pneumoniae* pneumonia

N (%) or median (IQR)	Total (N = 152)	Mycoplasma pneumoniae patients (N = 76)	Streptococcus pneumoniae patients (N = 76)	p value
Laboratory features				
Lactate (mmol/l)	2.2 [1.6–3.3]	1 [0.7–2.7]	2.3 [1.8–3.4]	0.003
P/F ratio	163 [92–267]	120 [88–236]	178 [114–280]	0.051
Serum sodium (mmol/L)	136 [133–139]	137 [135–140]	136 [132–139]	*0.028*
Creatinine (µmol/L)	87 [65–139.5]	77 [57.5–108]	101 [69.5–168.8]	*0.008*
CPK (IU/l)	122 [40–309]	138 [89–608]	108 [36–202]	0.093
ASAT (IU/l)	38 [23–80]	44 [24–81]	38 [22–77]	0.45
Bilirubin (µmol/l)	12.8 [8–21.7]	8.4 [5.8–13]	15 [9.2–24.5]	*0.0006*
Leukocytes	11,400 [7200–16,300]	11,140 [8100–17,000]	11,200 [5112–16,142]	0.63
Hemoglobin (g/dL)	11.6 [10–12.9]	11.3 [9.6–13.1]	11.6 [10.2–12.8]	0.89
Platelets (Giga/L)	217 [138–287]	262.5 [179.5–311.25]	204 [138–252]	*0.009*
Cytolysis	21 (14%)	8 (11%)	13 (17%)	0.35
Hemolytic anemia/cold agglutinins	9 (6%)	9 (12%)	0	*0.003*
Rhabdomyolysis	5 (3%)	2 (3%)	3 (4%)	1
Radiological features				
Number of quadrants involved				*0.013*
≤ 2	103 (68%)	37 (49%)	66 (87%)	
> 2	25 (16%)	16 (21%)	9 (12%)	
Alveolar opacities	111 (85%)	42 (75%)	19 (68%)	*0.013*
Interstitial opacities	26 (20%)	20 (36%)	12 (43%)	*0.0001*
Pleural effusion	20 (15%)	3 (5%)	3 (11%)	*0.007*

P/F ratio ratio of partial pressure of oxygen in arterial blood over fraction of inspired oxygen, *CPK* creatine phosphokinase, *ASAT* aspartate aminotransferase

Interestingly, intracellular pathogens are underdiagnosed like viruses, but under-covered despite the availability of therapeutic agents. These findings are in line with these from Menendez et al. [24] who reported a lack of antibiotic compliance in patients with CAP. Our descriptive data may be useful to help clinicians to discriminate SP-related pneumonia and MP-related pneumonia, even if a double antibiotherapy active against atypical pathogens is recommended in severe patients.

This study had several limitations. First, the study design was retrospective and patients were included within a 16-year period. ICU management may have changed over this period. ICU admissions criteria could be different according to the center and the year of admission. Atypical pneumonia remains rare, and the main objective of the study was to describe AP in the most severe patients. However, the study assessed mostly the clinical and radiological characteristics at admission which would be unlikely to change between the centers.

Secondarily, SP-P patients were included from only one single center, whereas AP patients were included from several centers. The main objective of the study was to describe patients at ICU admission. Although admission rules would be different between the centers,

the clinical presentation would not be affected. Thirdly, only patients with proven AP based on positive microbiologic samples were included. Half of the patients with MP-AP had their diagnosis based on serological testing. More recently only PCR was used to diagnose *Mycoplasma pneumoniae* infection. Positivity of IgM anti-MP is considered as the gold standard, and PCR sensitivity is equal [25]. Although some of the patients had serological tests with fourfold increase in IgG level between two time points, we believe that we included only proven MP-AP patients. Although different diagnostic tests were used within the study period and among the centers, those tests were enough sensitive and specific to include real MP-AP pneumonia.

Fourth, we did not include patients with *Legionella pneumophila* pneumonia, a more frequent atypical pneumonia. Although *Legionella pneumophila* pneumonia was associated with higher risk of ICU admission comparing to MP-AP and CP-AP, our goal was to focus on AP that is usually non-severe and only occasionally leads to ICU admission. Moreover, several studies analyzed *Legionella pneumophila* pneumonia. Similarly, we did not include more rare etiology of pneumonia as Q fever.

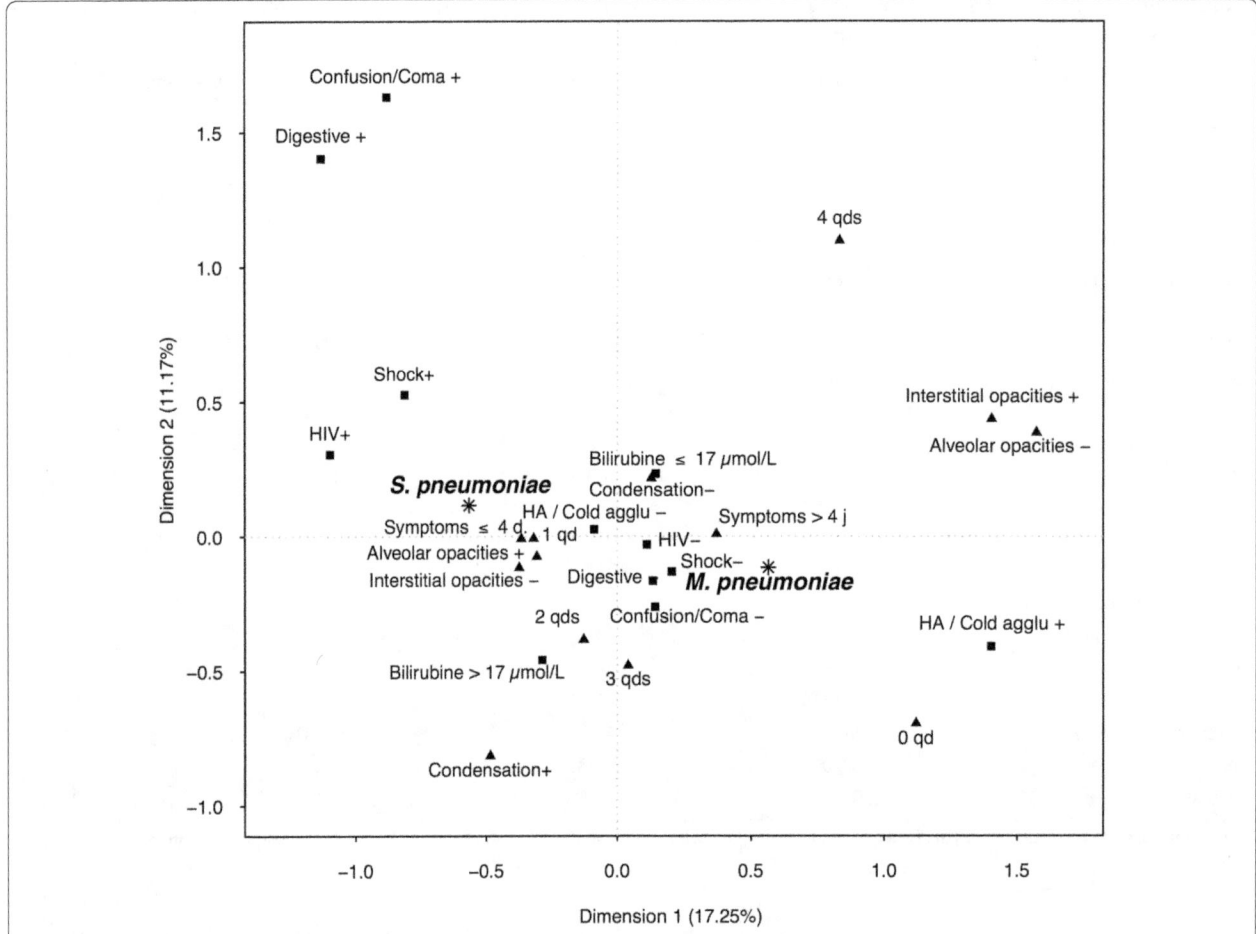

Fig. 2 Multiple correspondence analysis: the factors are mapped along two dimensions. Triangles indicate pulmonary signs and squares extra-pulmonary signs. *HA* hemolytic anemia, *Cold agglu+* presence of cold agglutinins, *QD* quadrants

Conclusion

Although considered as less severe pneumonia, atypical pneumonia requiring ICU admission remained associated with 11% mortality. At ICU admission, several clinical and radiological features could differ between MP-AP and SP-P, which may help physicians. Prospective studies are needed to validate clinical model to AP in ICU patients.

Abbreviations

AP: atypical pneumonia; ARDS: adult respiratory distress syndrome; CP: *Chlamydophila pneumoniae*; ICU: intensive care unit; MCA: multiple correspondence analysis; MP: *Mycoplasma pneumoniae*; MP-AP: atypical pneumonia due to *Mycoplasma pneumoniae*; PCR: polymerase chain reaction; SAPS II: Simplified Acute Physiology Score version II; SP: *Streptococcus pneumoniae*; SP-P: pneumonia due to *Streptococcus pneumoniae*.

Authors' contributions

EA is the guarantor for the content of the manuscript, including the data and analysis. SV, LB, VL, and EA contributed substantially to the study design, data analysis and interpretation, and the writing of the manuscript. SV, VL, LA, FP, LP, FB, AS, AK, JO, DS, NB, KR, OL, FB, BM, NB, NB, ASM, AL, OP, PP, JM, and EA contributed substantially to patients recruitment, collecting data, and manuscript revision. All authors read and approved the final manuscript.

Author details

[1] AP-HP, Medical ICU, Hôpital Saint-Louis, 1 Avenue Claude Vellefaux, 75010 Paris, France. [2] UFR de Médecine, University Paris-7 Paris-Diderot, Paris, France. [3] AP-HP, DBIM, Hôpital Saint-Louis, Paris, France. [4] Hôpital Edouard Herriot, Service de Réanimation Médicale, Hospices Civils de Lyon, Lyon, France. [5] AP-HP, Réanimation médicale, Hôpital Cochin, Paris, France. [6] Réanimation des Détresses Respiratoires et Infections Sévères, Assistance Publique-Hôpitaux de Marseille, Hôpital Nord, Marseille, France. [7] Service de Réanimation, Centre Hospitalier de Versailles, Le Chesnay, France. [8] Department of Medical Intensive Care, CHU de Caen, Caen, France. [9] Service de Réanimation Médicale et Médecine Hyperbare, Hôpital Angers, Angers, France. [10] AP-HP, Medical-Surgical Intensive Care Unit, Avicenne University Hospital, Bobigny, France. [11] Service de Réanimation polyvalente, Angoulême, France. [12] Intensive Care Unit, Draguignan Hospital, Draguignan, France. [13] AP-HP, Groupe Henri Mondor-Albert Chenevier, Service de Réanimation Médicale, Hôpital Henri Mondor, Créteil, France. [14] Service de Réanimation, CH Saint-Louis, La Rochelle, France. [15] AP-HP, Réanimation médicale, Hôpital Européen Georges Pompidou, Paris, France. [16] AP-HP, Department of Medical and Toxicological Critical Care, Lariboisière Hospital, Paris, France. [17] AP-HP, Medical Intensive Care Unit, Hôpital Saint-Antoine, Paris, France. [18] Medical Intensive Care Unit, Centre Hospitalier Universitaire de Nantes, Nantes, France. [19] Centre de réanimation, Hôpital Salengro, CHU-Lille, Lille, France. [20] Service de Réanimation Médicale Polyvalente, CHU Gabriel Montpied, Clermont-Ferrand, France. [21] AP-HP, Service des urgences, Hôpital Saint-Louis, Paris, France. [22] Service de Réanimation médicale, Hôpital Brabois, Nancy, France. [23] AP-HP, Pneumology and Critical Care Medicine Department, Universitary Hospital La Pitié Salpêtrière-Charles Foix, Paris, France.

Acknowledgements
None.

Competing interests
There is no financial or other competing interest in relation to this manuscript.

Funding
No part of the work presented has received financial support from any source.

References

1. Cillóniz C, Torres A, Niederman M, van der Eerden M, Chalmers J, Welte T, et al. Community-acquired pneumonia related to intracellular pathogens. Intensive Care Med. 2016;42(9):1374–86.

2. Ngeow Y-F, Suwanjutha S, Chantarojanasriri T, Wang F, Saniel M, Alejandria M, et al. An Asian study on the prevalence of atypical respiratory pathogens in community-acquired pneumonia. Int J Infect Dis. 2005;9(3):144–53.

3. Saraya T, Kurai D, Nakagaki K, Sasaki Y, Niwa S, Tsukagoshi H, et al. Novel aspects on the pathogenesis of *Mycoplasma pneumoniae* pneumonia and therapeutic implications. Front Microbiol. 2014 Aug 11. Cited 2015 Jun 24; 5. http://www.ncbi.nlm.nih.gov/pmc/articles/PMC4127663/.

4. von Baum H, Welte T, Marre R, Suttorp N, Lück C, Ewig S. *Mycoplasma pneumoniae* pneumonia revisited within the German Competence Network for Community-acquired pneumonia (CAPNETZ). BMC Infect Dis. 2009;9:62.

5. Marrie TJ. *Mycoplasma pneumoniae* pneumonia requiring hospitalization, with emphasis on infection in the elderly. Arch Intern Med. 1993;153(4):488–94.

6. Dumke R, Schnee C, Pletz MW, Rupp J, Jacobs E, Sachse K, et al. *Mycoplasma pneumoniae* and Chlamydia spp. infection in community-acquired pneumonia, Germany, 2011–2012. Emerg Infect Dis. 2015;21(3):426–34.

7. Spoorenberg SM, Bos WJW, Heijligenberg R, Voorn PG, Grutters JC, Rijkers GT, et al. Microbial aetiology, outcomes, and costs of hospitalisation for community-acquired pneumonia; an observational analysis. BMC Infect Dis. 2014;17(14):335.

8. Sohn JW, Park SC, Choi Y-H, Woo HJ, Cho YK, Lee JS, et al. Atypical pathogens as etiologic agents in hospitalized patients with community-acquired pneumonia in Korea: a prospective multi-center study. J Korean Med Sci. 2006;21(4):602–7.

9. Walden AP, Clarke GM, McKechnie S, Hutton P, Gordon AC, Rello J, et al. Patients with community acquired pneumonia admitted to European intensive care units: an epidemiological survey of the GenOSept cohort. Crit Care. 2014;18(2):R58.

10. Gaillat J, Flahault A, deBarbeyrac B, Orfila J, Portier H, Ducroix J-P, et al. Community epidemiology of Chlamydia and *Mycoplasma pneumoniae* in LRTI in France over 29 months. Eur J Epidemiol. 2005;20(7):643–51.

11. Sopena N, Sabrià M, Pedro-Botet ML, Manterola JM, Matas L, Domínguez J, et al. Prospective study of community-acquired pneumonia of bacterial etiology in adults. Eur J Clin Microbiol Infect Dis. 1999;18(12):852–8.

12. Khoury T, Sviri S, Rmeileh AA, Nubani A, Abutbul A, Hoss S, et al. Increased rates of intensive care unit admission in patients with *Mycoplasma pneumoniae*: a retrospective study. Clin Microbiol Infect. 2016;22(8):711–4.

13. Cillóniz C, Ewig S, Ferrer M, Polverino E, Gabarrús A, de la Bellacasa JP, et al. Community-acquired polymicrobial pneumonia in the intensive care unit: aetiology and prognosis. Crit Care. 2011;15(5):R209.

14. Lui G, Ip M, Lee N, Rainer TH, Man SY, Cockram CS, et al. Role of 'atypical pathogens' among adult hospitalized patients with community-acquired pneumonia. Respirol Carlton Vic. 2009;14(8):1098–105.

15. Miyashita N, Obase Y, Ouchi K, Kawasaki K, Kawai Y, Kobashi Y, et al. Clinical features of severe *Mycoplasma pneumoniae* pneumonia in adults admitted to an intensive care unit. J Med Microbiol. 2007;56(Pt 12):1625–9.

16. Chan ED, Welsh CH. Fulminant *Mycoplasma pneumoniae* pneumonia. West J Med. 1995;162(2):133–42.

17. Yin Y-D, Zhao F, Ren L-L, Song S-F, Liu Y-M, Zhang J-Z, et al. Evaluation of the Japanese Respiratory Society guidelines for the identification of *Mycoplasma pneumoniae* pneumonia. Respirol Carlton Vic. 2012;17(7):1131–6.

18. Guo Q, Li H-Y, Zhou Y-P, Li M, Chen X-K, Peng H-L, et al. Associations of radiological features in *Mycoplasma pneumoniae* pneumonia. Arch Med Sci AMS. 2014;10(4):725–32.

19. Daxboeck F, Krause R, Wenisch C. Laboratory diagnosis of *Mycoplasma pneumoniae* infection. Clin Microbiol Infect. 2003;9(4):263–73.

20. Le Gall JR, Lemeshow S, Saulnier F. A new Simplified Acute Physiology Score (SAPS II) based on a European/North American multicenter study. JAMA. 1993;270(24):2957–63.

21. Waites KB, Talkington DF. *Mycoplasma pneumoniae* and its role as a human pathogen. Clin Microbiol Rev. 2004;17(4):697–728.

22. Norisue Y, Tokuda Y, Koizumi M, Kishaba T, Miyagi S. Phasic characteristics of inspiratory crackles of bacterial and atypical pneumonia. Postgrad Med J. 2008;84(994):432–6.

23. Ruiz-González A, Falguera M, Vives M, Nogués A, Porcel JM, Rubio-Caballero M. Community-acquired pneumonia: development of a bedside predictive model and scoring system to identify the aetiology. Respir Med. 2000;94(5):505–10.

24. Menéndez R, Torres A, Reyes S, Zalacain R, Capelastegui A, Aspa J, et al. Initial management of pneumonia and sepsis: factors associated with improved outcome. Eur Respir J. 2012;39(1):156–62.

25. Medjo B, Atanaskovic-Markovic M, Radic S, Nikolic D, Lukac M, Djukic S. *Mycoplasma pneumoniae* as a causative agent of community-acquired pneumonia in children: clinical features and laboratory diagnosis. Ital J Pediatr. 2014;18(40):104.

21

Brief summary of French guidelines for the prevention, diagnosis and treatment of hospital-acquired pneumonia in ICU

Marc Léone[1*], Lila Bouadma[2], Bélaïd Bouhemad[3], Olivier Brissaud[4], Stéphane Dauger[5], Sébastien Gibot[6], Sami Hraiech[7], Boris Jung[8], Eric Kipnis[9], Yoann Launey[10], Charles-Edouard Luyt[11], Dimitri Margetis[12], Fabrice Michel[13], Djamel Mokart[14], Philippe Montravers[15], Antoine Monsel[16], Saad Nseir[17], Jérôme Pugin[18], Antoine Roquilly[19], Lionel Velly[20], Jean-Ralph Zahar[21], Rémi Bruyère[22], Gérald Chanques[23], ADARPEF and GFRUP

Abstract

Background: The French Society of Anaesthesia and Intensive Care Medicine and the French Society of Intensive Care edited guidelines focused on hospital-acquired pneumonia (HAP) in intensive care unit. The goal of 16 French-speaking experts was to produce a framework enabling an easier decision-making process for intensivists.

Results: The guidelines were related to 3 specific areas related to HAP (prevention, diagnosis and treatment) in 4 identified patient populations (COPD, neutropenia, post-operative and paediatric). The literature analysis and the formulation of the guidelines were conducted according to the Grade of Recommendation Assessment, Development and Evaluation methodology. An extensive literature research over the last 10 years was conducted based on publications indexed in PubMed™ and Cochrane™ databases.

Conclusions: HAP should be prevented by a standardised multimodal approach and the use of selective digestive decontamination in units where multidrug-resistant bacteria prevalence was below 20%. Diagnosis relies on clinical assessment and microbiological findings. Monotherapy, in the absence of risk factors for multidrug-resistant bacteria, non-fermenting Gram-negative bacilli and/or increased mortality (septic shock, organ failure), is strongly recommended. After microbiological documentation, it is recommended to reduce the spectrum and to prefer monotherapy for the antibiotic therapy of HAP, including for non-fermenting Gram-negative bacilli.

Introduction

Hospital-acquired pneumonia (HAP) is the most common infection in the intensive care unit (ICU) [1]. In the ICU, HAP is associated with a mortality rate of 20% and with increased duration of mechanical ventilation and ICU and hospital length-of-stay [2, 3]. The criteria to diagnose pneumonia are shown in Table 1 (Fig. 1).

Method

Sixteen French-speaking experts produce guidelines in three specific areas related to HAP: prevention, diagnosis and treatment as well as the specificities pertaining to different identified patient populations (COPD, neutropenia, post-operative and paediatric). The schedule of the group was defined upstream (Table 2) (Fig. 2).

The questions were formulated according to the PICO (Patient, Intervention, Comparison, Outcome) format. The formulation of the guidelines was conducted according to the GRADE methodology (Grade of Recommendation Assessment, Development and Evaluation) [4, 5]. In the absence of supporting literature, a question could be addressed by a recommendation under the form of an expert opinion ("the experts suggest that…") (Fig. 3).

*Correspondence: Marc.LEONE@ap-hm.fr
[1] Service d'Anesthésie et de Réanimation, Aix-Marseille Universite Hopital Nord, chemin des Bourrely, 13015 Marseille, France
Full list of author information is available at the end of the article

Table 1 Criteria for defining pneumonia

Radiological signs

  Two successive chest radiographs showing new or progressive lung infiltrates

  In the absence of medical history of underlying heart or lung disease, a single chest radiograph is enough

And at least one of the following signs

  Body temperature > 38,3 °C without any other cause

  Leucocytes < 4000/mm^3 or ≥ 12,000/mm^3

And at least two of the following signs

  Purulent sputum

  Cough or dyspnoea

  Declining oxygenation or increased oxygen requirement or need for respiratory assistance

Table 2 Guideline timeline

5 December 2016	Start-up meeting
6 March 2017	Vote: first round
13 March 2017	Post-vote deliberation meeting
1 April 2017	Vote: second round
16 April 2017	Amendment of two guidelines
28 April 2017	Vote of the two amended guidelines
10 May 2017	Guideline finalisation meeting

These guidelines with their arguments were published in the journal Anaesthesia Critical Care and Pain Medicine [6] (Fig. 4).

First area, PREVENTION Which HAP prevention approaches decrease morbidity and mortality in ICU patients?

R1.1   We recommend using a standardised multimodal HAP prevention approach in order to decrease ICU patient morbidity (Grade 1+).

R1.1   Paediatrics We suggest using a standardised multimodal approach aiming at preventing HAP in order to decrease paediatric ICU patient morbidity (Grade 2+).

R1.2   In units where multidrug-resistant bacteria prevalence is low (< 20%), we suggest applying routine selective digestive decontamination using a topical antiseptic administered enterally and a maximal 5-day course of systemic prophylactic antibiotic to decrease mortality (Grade 2+).

R1.3   Within a standardised multimodal HAP prevention approach, we suggest combining some of the following methods to decrease ICU patient morbidity:

- Promote the use of non-invasive ventilation to avoid tracheal intubation (mainly in post-operative digestive surgery patients and in patients with COPD),
- Favour orotracheal over nasotracheal intubation when required

---

Protocol 1

1- Favour non-invasive ventilation (NIV) (mainly following digestive surgery and for COPD patients)

When invasive ventilation is required :

2- Apply* a selective digestive decontamination protocol with prophylactic systemic antibiotic treatment <5 days
   *if the prevalence of multiresistant bacteria is low (<20%)

3- Associate some of the following methods (1st line):
-    Favour the use of NIV to prevent intubation
-    Limit dose and duration of sedatives and analgesics associated with mechanical ventilation
-    Initiate early enteral feeding
-    Regularly verify endotracheal tube cuff pressures
-    Perform sub-glottic suction (/6-8 hours) using an appropriate endotracheal tube
-    Favour the orotracheal route for intubation
NB: The association of head of bed elevation <30 ° and/or oro-pharyngeal decontamination with 0.12 or 0.2% chlorhexidine could be proposed in association to these measures, despite low efficiency, because they do not cost much and are well tolerated.

4- Avoid using the following methods:
-    Systematic early tracheotomy (apart from specific indications)
-    Antiulcer prophylaxis (apart from specific indications)
-    Post-pyloric enteral feeding (apart from specific indications)
-    Probiotics
-    Systematic early changing of humidifier filters (apart from a recommendation from the manufacturer)
-    Closed endo-tracheal suction systems
-    The use of intubation tubes lined/coated or incorporating silver or antiseptics, or with an "optimised" cuff shape
-    Oro-pharyngeal decontamination using povidone-iodine
-    Prophylactic nebulised antibiotics
-    Daily skin decontamination using antiseptics

Fig. 1 Multimodal healthcare associated pneumonia prevention protocol (expert opinion)

Protocol 2

Oro-pharyngeal application (x4/ day, until tracheal extubation) of a paste or gel containing
– polymyxin E (2%)
– tobramycin (2%)
– amphotericin B (2%)
    +

Administration (x4/ day, until tracheal extubation) through a nasogastric tube of 10ml of a suspension containing
– 100 mg Polymyxin E
– 80 mg Tobramycin
– 500 mg Amphotericin B
    +

Intravenous administration of a prophylactic antibiotic treatment during 48 to 72 hours for patients who do not require curative antibiotic therapy
– cefazolin 1 g x 3 / d*
– In case of allergy to cephalosporins:
    – ofloxacin 200 mg x 2 / d*
    – ciprofloxacin 400 mg x 2 / d *

*(*dosages in the absence of renal failure, provided for information purposes only)*

Preparation for *selective digestive decontamination*
(provided for information purposes only)

	Oral gel (jar 125 ml)	Suspension (bottles 15 ml)
polymyxin E	4 g	1 g
gentamicin	4 g	0.8 g
amphotericin B	4 g	5 g
sterile water	134 ml	100 ml
methylcarboxycellulose	6 g	
methylparahydroxybenzoate	0.3 g	
propylene glycol	50 ml	
menthol alcohol	6 ml	

Fig. 2 Selective digestive decontamination protocol (expert opinion)

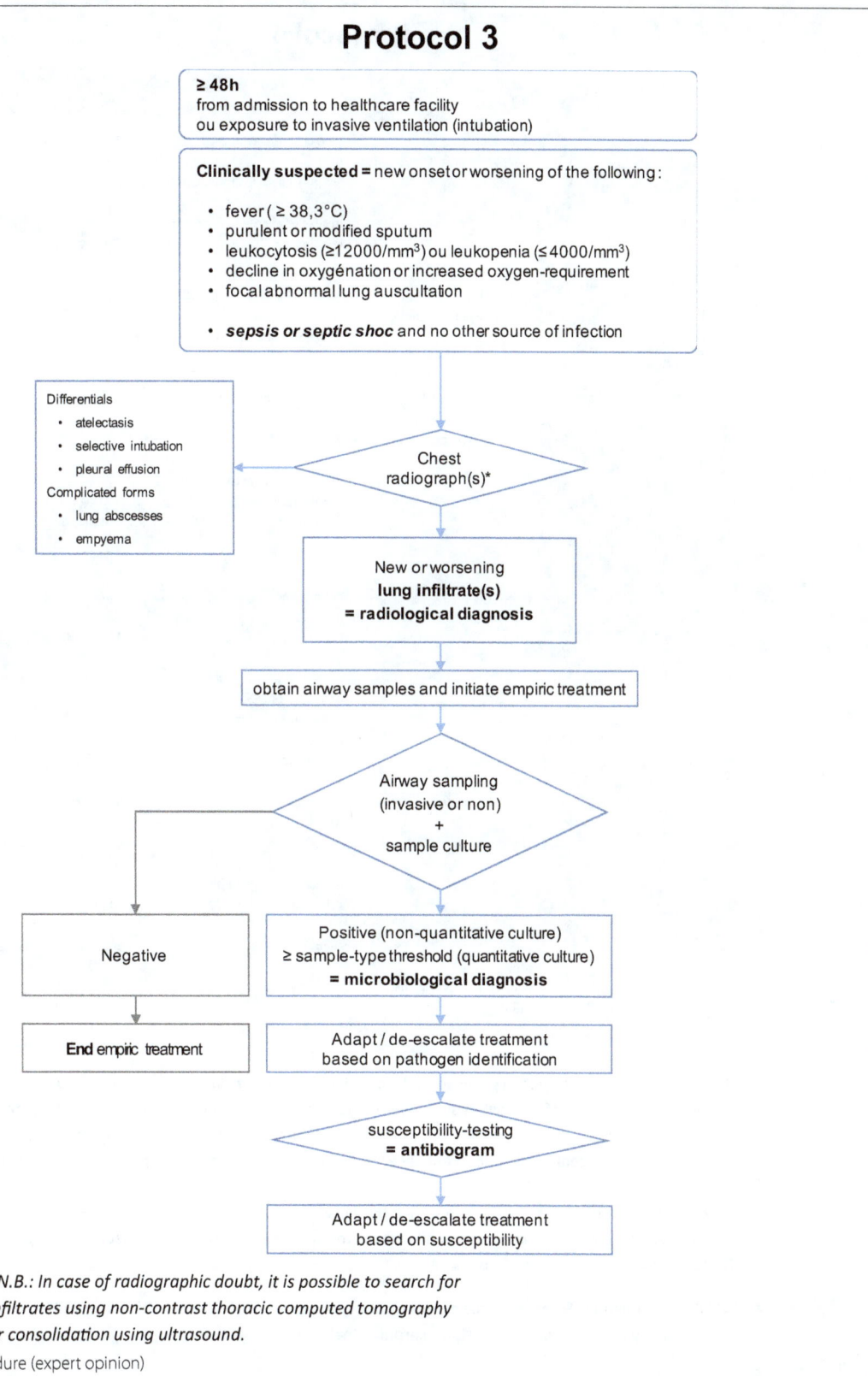

Protocol 3

≥ 48h
from admission to healthcare facility
ou exposure to invasive ventilation (intubation)

Clinically suspected = new onset or worsening of the following :

- fever (≥ 38,3°C)
- purulent or modified sputum
- leukocytosis (≥12000/mm³) ou leukopenia (≤4000/mm³)
- decline in oxygénation or increased oxygen-requirement
- focal abnormal lung auscultation

- ***sepsis or septic shoc*** and no other source of infection

Differentials
- atelectasis
- selective intubation
- pleural effusion
Complicated forms
- lung abscesses
- empyema

Chest
radiograph(s)*

New or worsening
**lung infiltrate(s)
= radiological diagnosis**

obtain airway samples and initiate empiric treatment

Airway sampling
(invasive or non)
+
sample culture

Negative

End empiric treatment

Positive (non-quantitative culture)
≥ sample-type threshold (quantitative culture)
= microbiological diagnosis

Adapt / de-escalate treatment
based on pathogen identification

susceptibility-testing
= antibiogram

Adapt / de-escalate treatment
based on susceptibility

*N.B.: In case of radiographic doubt, it is possible to search for
infiltrates using non-contrast thoracic computed tomography
or consolidation using ultrasound.*

Fig. 3 Diagnostic procedure (expert opinion)

Protocol 4

Nosological framework	Therapeutic class	Antimicrobials	Dosing regimen*
Early pneumonia < 5 days *absence of* septic shock *absence of* MDR bacteria risk factors	β-lactam, inactive against *P. aeruginosa*	amoxicillin/ clavulanic acid or 3rd gen. cephalosporin, cefotaxime	3 to 6 g/d 3 to 6 g/d
		In case of allergy to β-lactam : levofloxacin	500 mg x 2/d
Early pneumonia < 5 days *presence of* septic shock *absence of* MDR bacteria risk factors	β-lactam, inactive against *P. aeruginosa*	amoxicillin/ clavulanic acid or 3rd gen. cephalosporin, cefotaxime	3 to 6 g/d 3 to 6 g/day
	+ Aminoglycoside [b] or + Fluoroquinolone	Example: gentamicin or Example: ofloxacin	8 mg/kg/d 200 mg x 2/d
		In case of allergy to β-lactam : Levofloxacin + Gentamicin	500 mg x 2/d 8 mg/kg/d
Late pneumonia ≥ 5 days or *presence of other* risk factors for nonfermenting Gram-negative bacilli [*]	β-lactam, ACTIVE against *P. aeruginosa*	ceftazidime or cefepime or piperacillin-tazobactam or in case of ESBL [c] Imipenem-cilastatine or meropenem	6 g/d 4 to 6 g/d 16 g/d 3 g/d 3 to 6 g/d
	+ Aminoglycoside [b] or Fluoroquinolone	+ amikacin [d] or ciprofloxacin	30 mg/kg/d 400 mg x 3/d
		In case of allergy to β-lactam aztreonam + clindamycin	3 to 6 g/d 600 mg x 3 to 4/d
Any presentation, *presence of* MRSA risk factors**	add agent active against MRSA	vancomycin or linezolid	15 mg/kg loading followed by 30 to 40 mg/kg/d continuous 600 mg x 2/d

[a] Doses are given for information purposes only in patients with normal renal function and standard weight; [b] Favour the use of aminoglycosides over fluoroquinolones to limit emergence of MDR bacteria; [c] According to the guidelines' criteria « Reduce de use of antibiotics in intensive care unit» ; [d] Favour the use of amikacin over gentamicin due to enhanced efficacy against non-fermenting Gram-negative bacilli.

*Risk factors for non-fermenting Gram-negative bacilli: antibiotic therapy in the previous 90 days, prior hospital stay of more than 5 days, renal replacement therapy requirement during pneumonia, septic shock, acute respiratory distress syndrome.

**Methicillin-resistant *Staphylococcus aureus* (MRSA) risk factors: high local prevalence of MRSA, recent colonisation by MRSA, chronic skin lesions, chronic renal replacement therapy.

Fig. 4 Treatment options (expert opinion)

- Limit dose and duration of sedatives and analgesics (promote their use guided by sedation/pain/agitation scales, and/or daily interruptions),
- Initiate early enteral feeding (within the first 48 h of ICU admission),
- Regularly verify endotracheal tube cuff pressure,
- Perform sub-glottic suction (every 6 to 8 h) using an appropriate endotracheal tube (Grade 2+).

R1.4 Within a standardised multimodal HAP prevention approach, we suggest not using the following methods to decrease ICU patient morbidity:

- Systematic early (< day 7) tracheotomy (except for specific indications),
- Anti-ulcer prophylaxis (except for specific indications),
- Post-pyloric enteral feeding (except for specific indications),
- Administration of probiotics and/or synbiotics,
- Early systematic change of the humidifier filter (except for specific manufacturer recommendations)
- Use of closed suctioning systems for endotracheal secretions,
- Use of antiseptic-coated intubation tubes or with tubes an "optimised" cuff shape,
- Selective oropharyngeal decontamination (SOD) with povidone-iodine,
- Use of prophylactic nebulised antibiotics,
- Daily skin decontamination using antiseptics (Grade 2−).

R1.5 In weaning of COPD patients from ventilation, we suggest using non-invasive ventilation to reduce length of invasive mechanical ventilation, incidence of HAP, morbidity and mortality (Grade 2+).

Second area, DIAGNOSIS What methods to diagnose HAP should be used to decrease ICU patient morbidity and mortality?

R2.1 We suggest not using the clinical scores (CPIS, modified CPIS) for diagnosing HAP (Grade 2−).

R2.2 We suggest collecting microbiological airway samples, regardless of type, before initiation of any change in antibiotic therapy (Grade 2+).

R2.2 Paediatrics   We suggest collecting microbiological airway samples, regardless of type, before initiation of any change in antibiotic therapy (Grade 2+).

R2.3 We suggest not measuring plasma or alveolar levels of procalcitonin or soluble TREM-1 to diagnose HAP (Grade 2−).

Third area, TREATMENT What therapeutic options for HAP should be used to decrease ICU patient morbidity and mortality?

R3.1 We suggest immediately collecting samples and initiating antibiotic treatment taking into consideration risk factors for multidrug-resistant bacteria in patients with suspected HAP and haemodynamic or respiratory compromise (shock or acute respiratory distress syndrome) or frailty such as immunosuppression [95–100] (Grade 2+).

R3.2 We recommend treating HAP in mechanically ventilated immunocompetent patients empirically by a monotherapy, in the absence of risk factors for multidrug-resistant bacteria, non-fermenting Gram-negative bacilli and/or increased mortality (septic shock, organ failure) [101–113] (Grade 1+).

R3.3 The experts suggest not systematically directing empiric antibiotic therapy against methicillin-resistant *Staphylococcus aureus* in the treatment of HAP [114–119] (Experts Opinion).

R3.4 We suggest reducing the spectrum and preferring monotherapy for the antibiotic therapy of HAP after microbiological documentation, including for non-fermenting Gram-negative bacilli [114,115, 120–128] (Grade 2+).

R3.5 We recommend not prolonging for more than 7 days the antibiotic treatment for HAP, including for non-fermenting Gram-negative bacilli, apart from specific situations (immunosuppression, empyema, necrotising or abscessed pneumonia) [129–135] (Grade 1−).

R3.6 We suggest administering nebulised colimycine (sodium colistiméthate) and/or aminoglycosides in documented HAP due multidrug-resistant Gram-negative bacilli documented pneumonia established as sensitive to colimycin and/or aminoglycoside, when no other antibiotics can be used (based on the results of susceptibility testing) [136–152] (Grade 2+).

R3.7 We recommend not administering statins as adjuvant treatment for HAP [153–161] (Grade 1−).

Authors' contributions
Marc Leone and Lila Bouadma proposed the elaboration of this recommendation and manuscript in agreement with the "Société Française d'Anesthésie et de Réanimation" and the "Société de Réanimation de Langue Française";

Gérald Chanques, Rémi Bruyère and Lionel Velly wrote the methodology section and gave the final version with the final presentation. Antoine Roquilly, Charles-Edouard Luyt and Jean-Ralph Zahar contributed to elaborate recommendations and write the rationale of question 1 (prevention). Sébastien Gibot, Bélaïd Bouhemad, Jérome Pugin and Eric Kipnis contributed to elaborate recommendations and to write the rationale of question 2 (diagnosis). Antoine Monsel, Sami Hraiech and Boris Jung contributed to elaborate recommendations and to write the rationale of question 3 (treatment). Djamel Mokart contributed to elaborate recommendations and to write the rationale about neutropenic patients. Saad Nseir contributed to elaborate recommendations and to write the rationale about COPD patients. Olivier Brissaud, Stéphane Dauger and Fabrice Michel contributed to elaborate paediatrics recommendations and to write the rationale of paediatrics issues. Antoine Launey and Dimitri Margetis provide references. Marc Leone and Lila Bouadma drafted the manuscript. All authors read and approved the final manuscript.

Author details
[1] Service d'Anesthésie et de Réanimation, Aix-Marseille Universite Hopital Nord, chemin des Bourrely, 13015 Marseille, France. [2] Service de Réanimation Médicale, Hopital Bichat - Claude-Bernard, AP-HP, Paris, France. [3] Service d'Anesthésie et de Réanimation, Centre Hospitalier Universitaire de Dijon, Paris, France. [4] Unité de Réanimation Pédiatrique, Hôpital Pellegrin, Centre Hospitalier Universitaire de Bordeaux, Bordeaux, France. [5] Service de Réanimation Pédiatrique, Hopital Universitaire Robert-Debre, Paris, France. [6] Service de Réanimation Médicale, CHU de Nancy, Vandoeuvre-les-Nancy, France. [7] Service de Réanimation des Détresses Respiratoires et des Infections Sévères, Aix-Marseille Universite, Hopital Nord, Marseille, France. [8] Service d'Anesthésie et Réanimation, CHU de Montpellier, Montpellier, France. [9] Service d'Anesthésie et Réanimation, CHU de Lille, Lille, France. [10] Service d'Anesthésie et Réanimation, Centre Hospitalier Universitaire de Rennes, Rennes, France. [11] Institut de Cardiologie, Service de Réanimation Médicale, Hopital Universitaire Pitie Salpetriere, AP-HP, Paris, France. [12] Service de Réanimation Médicale - Hôpital Saint-Antoine, Paris, France. [13] Service d'Anesthésie et Réanimation, Hopital La timone, Assistance Publique Hopitaux de Marseille, Marseille, France. [14] Service de Réanimation, Institut Paoli-Calmettes, Marseille, France. [15] Département d'Anesthésie Réanimation, CHU Bichat - Claude-Bernard, AP-HP, Paris, France. [16] Département d'Anesthésie et Réanimation, Université Pierre et Marie Curie, Paris, France. [17] Centre de Soins Intensifs, Service de Réanimation, Centre Hospitalier Regional Universitaire de Lille, Lille, France. [18] Service de Soins Intensifs, Hopitaux Universitaires de Geneve, Geneve, Switzerland. [19] Service d'Anesthésie et Réanimation, CHU de Nantes, Nantes, France. [20] Département d'Anesthésie et Réanimation, Hopital de la Timone, AP-HM, Paris, France. [21] Département de Microbiologie Clinique, Hopital Avicenne, APHP, Paris, France. [22] Service de Réanimation, Centre Hospitalier de Bourg-en-Bresse, Bourg-en-Bresse, France. [23] Département d'Anesthésie Réanimation, Centre Hospitalier Regional Universitaire de Montpellier, Montpellier, France.

Acknowledgements
Guidelines reviewed and endorsed by the SFAR (29/06/2017) and SRLFboards (08/06/2017).

Competing interests
The authors declare the following competing interests: Sébastien Gibot: Inotrem S.A, Eric Kipnis: Astellas; LFB; Pfizer, Marc Leone: MSD; Basilea, Charles-Edouard Luyt: Bayer Healthcare; Thermo Fisher BRAHMS; MSD; Biomerieux, Djamel Mokart: Gilead; Basilea; MSD, Philippe Montravers: Pfizer; MSD; Basilea; AstraZeneca; Bayer; Menari; Parexel; Cubist, Saad Nseir: Medtronic; Cielmedical; Bayer, Jérôme Pugin: Bayer; part of the scientific committee for the Amikacin Inhale study, Jean-Ralph Zahar: MSD; Bard. The remaining authors declare no competing interests.

Funding
This work was financially supported by the Société Française d'Anesthésie et de Réanimation (SFAR) and the Société de Réanimation de Langue Française (SRLF).

References
1. Koulenti D, Tsigou E, Rello J. Nosocomial pneumonia in 27 ICUs in Europe: perspectives from the EU-VAP/CAP study. Eur J Clin Microbiol Infect Dis. 2016;36:1999.
2. Giuliano KK, Baker D, Quinn B. The epidemiology of nonventilator hospital-acquired pneumonia in the United States. Am J Infect Control. 2017;46:322.
3. Melsen WG, Rovers MM, Groenwold RH, Bergmans DC, Camus C, Bauer TT, Hanisch EW, Klarin B, Koeman M, Krueger WA, Lacherade JC, Lorente L, Memish ZA, Morrow LE, Nardi G, van Nieuwenhoven CA, O'Keefe GE, Nakos G, Scannapieco FA, Seguin P, Staudinger T, Topeli A, Ferrer M, Bonten MJ. Attributable mortality of ventilator-associated pneumonia: a meta-analysis of individual patient data from randomised prevention studies. Lancet Infect Dis. 2013;13(8):665–71.
4. Atkins D, Best D, Briss PA, Eccles M, Falck-Ytter Y, Flottorp S, et al. Grading quality of evidence and strength of recommendations. BMJ. 2004;328(7454):1490.
5. Guyatt GH, Oxman AD, Vist GE, Kunz R, Falck-Ytter Y, Alonso-Coello P, et al. GRADE: an emerging consensus on rating quality of evidence and strength of recommendations. BMJ. 2008;336(7650):924–6.
6. Leone M, Bouadma L, Bouhemad B, Brissaud O, Dauger S, Gibot S, Hraiech S, Jung B, Kipnis E, Launey Y, Luyt CE, Margetis D, Michel F, Mokart D, Montravers P, Monsel A, Nseir S, Pugin J, Roquilly A, Velly L, Zahar JR, Bruyère R, Chanques G. Hospital-acquired pneumonia in ICU. Anaesth Crit Care Pain Med. 2018;37(1):83–98.

22

Estimating mean circulatory filling pressure in clinical practice: a systematic review comparing three bedside methods in the critically ill

Marije Wijnberge[1,2,3], Daniko P. Sindhunata[1], Michael R. Pinsky[4*], Alexander P. Vlaar[2,3], Else Ouweneel[1], Jos R. Jansen[5], Denise P. Veelo[1] and Bart F. Geerts[1]

Abstract

The bedside hemodynamic assessment of the critically ill remains challenging since blood volume, arterial–venous interaction and compliance are not measured directly. Mean circulatory filling pressure (P_{mcf}) is the blood pressure throughout the vascular system at zero flow. Animal studies have shown P_{mcf} provides information on vascular compliance, volume responsiveness and enables the calculation of stressed volume. It is now possible to measure P_{mcf} at the bedside. We performed a systematic review of the current P_{mcf} measurement techniques and compared their clinical applicability, precision, accuracy and limitations. A comprehensive search strategy was performed in PubMed, Embase and the Cochrane databases. Studies measuring P_{mcf} in heart-beating patients at the bedside were included. Data were extracted from the articles into predefined forms. Quality assessment was based on the Newcastle–Ottawa Scale for cohort studies. A total of 17 prospective cohort studies were included. Three techniques were described: P_{mcf} hold, based on inspiratory hold-derived venous return curves, P_{mcf} arm, based on arterial and venous pressure equilibration in the arm as a model for the entire circulation, and P_{mcf} analogue, based on a Guytonian mathematical model of the circulation. The included studies show P_{mcf} to accurately follow intravascular fluid administration and vascular compliance following drug-induced hemodynamic changes. Bedside P_{mcf} measures allow for more direct assessment of circulating blood volume, venous return and compliance. However, studies are needed to determine normative P_{mcf} values and their expected changes to therapies if they are to be used to guide clinical practice.

Keywords: Blood pressure, Venous pressure, Blood volume, Intensive care, Critical care, Hemodynamics

Background

It is difficult to determine the cause for hemodynamic instability in patients and to predict the best treatments. Currently, cardiovascular resuscitation options are triggered by arterial pressure and cardiac output (CO) measures, focusing on the oxygen delivery side of the circulation. However, the primary determinants of CO reside on the venous side. Veins are 30–50 times more compliant than arteries and contain approximately 75% of the total blood volume [1–5]. Mean circulatory filling pressure (P_{mcf}) provides vital information on this "forgotten venous side of the circulation" [6].

In 1894, P_{mcf} was defined as the equilibrium pressure throughout the circulation during circulatory arrest [7]. In the 1950s, Guyton and colleagues described a linear relationship between venous return (V_R) and right atrial pressure (P_{ra}), described as: $V_R = (P_{mcf} - P_{ra})/(RVR)$ [8, 9]. RVR is resistance to V_R and defines the slope of the V_R curve. This linearity has been confirmed in intact circulations in animal studies and is not affected by hypo- or hypervolemia [10–15]. V_R curves enable to determine the equilibrium point of the circulation, which

*Correspondence: pinsky@pitt.edu
[4] Department of Critical Care Medicine, University of Pittsburgh Medical Center, 1215.4 Lillian S. Kaufmann Bldg, 3471 Fifth Avenue, Pittsburgh, PA 15213, USA
Full list of author information is available at the end of the article

is the intersection between the CO and V_R curve. Central venous pressure (CVP) is a surrogate of P_{ra} used in clinical practice. CVP at zero flow equals P_{mcf} (Fig. 1).

Vascular volume requires a minimal volume before its distending pressure becomes positive. The amount of blood not causing pressure on the vessels is called unstressed volume (V_u) and reflects intravascular volume present with P_{mcf} of zero. Stressed volume (V_s) is the additional blood causing a distending pressure on the vascular walls and reflects the effective circulating volume. V_u and V_s together define the total blood volume. V_s is approximately 25% of the total blood volume [3–5]. V_s and vascular compliance (Csys) define P_{mcf} [16]. An increase in V_s increases P_{mcf}, and an increase in Csys decreases P_{mcf}. Fluid loading should increase P_{mcf}, but V_R only increases if the pressure gradient for V_R (i.e., P_{mcf} CVP) increases, RVR decreases, or both. Since in the steady state $V_R = CO$, knowing the determinants of V_R is relevant to understanding cardiovascular state.

Recently, methods have emerged to enable clinicians to estimate P_{mcf} at the bedside. Our objectives for this review were to describe the techniques and to highlight their clinical applicability, precision, accuracy and limitations in critically ill patients.

Materials and methods
Publication selection
This review was performed according to PRISMA guidelines [17] (Additional file 1) and methodology outlined in the Cochrane Handbook for systematic reviews [18]. No study protocol was published. A PubMed, Embase and Cochrane Library database search was performed with help of a clinical librarian with no restriction on publication date. The search was performed up to May 18, 2017. The search strategy combined the following concepts: (1) "mean systemic filling pressure" or "mean circulatory filling pressure" or "static filling pressure" and (2) "intensive care" or "critical care" or "perioperative" or "intraoperative" (Additional file 1). Titles, abstracts and full-texts were independently screened by two reviewers (MW and DPS), and discrepancies were resolved by a third reviewer (BFG). The references of the selected articles were examined for additional eligible articles. Studies were included when available in English and full-text, described prospective studies in which P_{mcf} estimation methods were examined in heart-beating ICU patients and contained a description of their clinical applicability, precision and accuracy or limitations.

Data extraction and analysis
Data were extracted into predefined forms. No additional analyses were performed. Critical appraisal was based on the Newcastle–Ottawa Scale for cohort studies [19] to assess the quality of non-randomized studies at study level. A modified version of the scale was used since only five out of nine questions were applicable, resulting in a possible highest score of five stars (Additional file 1).

Results
Study selection and characteristics
The initial search identified 369 articles, of which 300 were excluded after screening title and abstract. A total of 53 articles were excluded based on full-text. Two relevant articles were found by citation tracking. Consequently, 17 prospective cohort studies estimating P_{mcf} in heart-beating ICU patients were included (Additional file 1). Three different bedside measurement techniques were found. Eight studies estimated P_{mcf} applying inspiratory hold maneuvers (P_{mcf} hold), three studies during a circulatory stop-flow in the arm (P_{mcf} arm) and four studies using a mathematical algorithm (P_{mcf} analogue). Two studies compared multiple techniques.

Eleven studies were performed in postoperative cardiac surgery patients (Table 1). All patients were hemodynamically stable without alteration in vasopressor use or fluid therapy during the study protocol. All patients were sedated and mechanically ventilated. In one study, spontaneous breathing efforts were observed [20]. The number of included patients ranged from nine to 80. In all studies, CVP was measured via a catheter in the right internal jugular vein. CO measurement techniques differed between studies (Additional file 1).

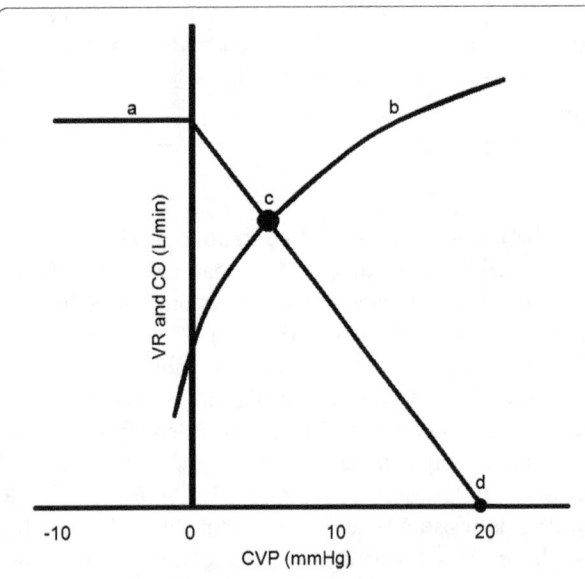

Fig. 1 The venous return curve (*a*) combined with the cardiac output curve (*b*). The intersection of these two curves (*c*) is the working point of the circulation. The central venous pressure when venous return equals zero is the P_{mcf} (*d*). The slope of the V_R is determined by the resistance to venous return

Table 1 Baseline characteristics for included studies

References	Method	N	Patient population (all adult ICU patients)	Age	Male	Timeframe P_{mcf} measurement
Maas et al. [21]	P_{mcf} hold	12	Postoperative cardiac surgery 10 CABG 2 AVR	64 (10)	10 (83%)	Not described
Keller et al. [23]	P_{mcf} hold	9	Postoperative cardiac surgery 3 CABG 6 AVR	Median 61 IQR 55–75	4 (44%)	Not described
Maas et al. [22]	P_{mcf} hold	10	Postoperative cardiac surgery 2 AVR 1 MVP + TVP 7 CABG	64 (11)	9 (90%)	Within 1 h after ICU admission
Persichini et al. [27]	P_{mcf} hold	16	Septic shock	67 (16)	8 (50%)	Not described
Maas et al. [25]	P_{mcf} hold	16	Postoperative cardiac surgery 1 MVP 15 CABG	64 (11)	Not described	Within 1 h after ICU admission
Guerin et al. [28]	P_{mcf} hold	30	Shock	65 (12)	21 (70%)	Not described
De Wit et al. [24]	P_{mcf} hold	17	Postsurgical gastrointestinal 16 esophageal resection 1 pancreaticoduodenectomy	62 (9)	14 (82%)	Not mentioned
Helmerhorst et al. [26]	P_{mcf} hold	22	Postoperative cardiac surgery 22 CABG	63 (59–66)	17 (85%)	1 h after ICU admission
Geerts et al. [43]	P_{mcf} arm	24	Postoperative cardiac surgery 17 CABG 7 CABG plus valve repair	64 (10)	19 (79%)	Within 2 h after ICU admission
Aya et al. [41]	P_{mcf} arm	20	Postoperative cardiac surgery 13 CABG 4 AVR 4 MVR	63 (11)	17 (85%)	Initial period at ICU (not further defined)
Aya et al. [42]	P_{mcf} arm	80	Postoperative cardiac surgery 36 CABG 27 AVR + CABG 12 MVR + CABG 5 Other	70 Range 52–80	62 (78%)	Initial period at ICU (not further defined)
Parkin et al. [49]	P_{mcf} analogue	10	Multi-organ failing patients receiving CVVH for acute renal failure	65 Range 24–77	7 (70%)	Not described
Cecconi et al. [48]	P_{mcf} analogue	39	22 Cardiac surgery 8 Shock 6 Non-cardiac surgery 3 Other	68 (12)	26 (67%)	Not described
Gupta et al. [20]	P_{mcf} analogue	61	Postoperative cardiac surgery 40 CABG 8 CABG + valve replacement 8 Valve replacement 5 Bentall's procedure 7 DDD pacing	63 (11)	46 (75%)	Within 6 h after ICU admission
Aya et al. [51]	P_{mcf} analogue	26	Postoperative fluid challenge 7 Cardiac surgery	68 Range 53–80	16 (62%)	Initial period at ICU (not further defined)

Table 1 (continued)

References	Method	N	Patient population (all adult ICU patients)	Age	Male	Timeframe P_{mcf} measurement
			19 Non-cardiac surgery			
Maas et al. [16]	P_{mcf} hold	11	Postoperative cardiac surgery	64	9 (82%)	Within 2 h after ICU admission
	P_{mcf} arm	11	9 CABG	Range 50–80		
	P_{mcf} analogue	11	2 AVR			
Maas et al. [30]	P_{mcf} arm	15	Postoperative cardiac surgery	64 (11)	Not described	Within 1 h after ICU admission
	P_{mcf} hold	12	9 CABG			
			5 Valve			
			1 CABG + valve			

Age is presented as mean with standard deviation (SD) or median with range or interquartile range (IQR). Number of males per study is presented as counts with percentage

CABG coronary artery bypass, MVR mitral valve replacement, MPV mitral valve prolapse, AVR aortic valve replacement, TVP tricuspid valve prolapse, CVVH continuous veno-venous hemodiafiltration

P_{mcf} hold

Technique description

P_{mcf} hold is based on the linear relation between CVP and V_R ($P_{mcf} = (V_R − CVP)/RVR$). CVP is raised by performing a series of end-inspiratory hold maneuvers. In 2009, the method was first studied in humans [21]. Inspiratory hold maneuvers at 5, 15, 25 and 35 cmH$_2$O incremental ventilatory plateau pressures (P_{vent}) were performed, and CO was measured in the last 3 s of the 12 s inspiratory hold. They validated that after 7–10 s a steady state consists when V_R = CO. By plotting the CVP and CO values, a V_R curve is constructed and the zero-flow pressure (P_{mcf}) extrapolated. Seven studies [16, 21–26] estimated P_{mcf} hold using these four plateau pressures. Two studies [27, 28] used two points (P_{vent} 5 and 30 cmH$_2$O) at 15-s inspiratory and expiratory hold plateau phase. Between the P_{mcf} hold measurements, either 1-min pauses were used to re-establish the initial hemodynamic steady state [16, 21, 22, 24, 28], or the consecutive inspiratory hold was performed when CO had returned to baseline [23, 26, 27].

Clinical applicability

The average baseline P_{mcf} hold values found in the eight included studies range from 19 to 33 mmHg with a wide standard deviation (Tables 2, 3). Five studies [21–23, 26, 28] demonstrated fluid administration caused an increase in P_{mcf} hold, confirming that in humans, as in animals before [14, 15], P_{mcf} hold follows hemodynamic changes (Table 2). One of these studies found passive leg raising (PLR) to significantly increase P_{mcf} hold values [28]. RVR was not significantly affected by different volumetric conditions nor by PLR. V_s was calculated from P_{mcf} as a measure for effective circulating volume [22]. In one study, P_{mcf} was used to assess the

hemodynamic effects of arterial hyperoxia (FiO$_2$ = 90% for 15 min) in ICU patients [26]. During this hyperoxia, left ventricular afterload increased and contractility remained similar; however, CO did not decrease. Both P_{mcf} and RVR increased significantly (Table 3), explaining why V_R (thus CO) remained unaltered.

Studies have used P_{mcf} hold to describe hemodynamic changes caused by propofol [24] and norepinephrine [25, 27] (Table 3). In septic shock patients, decreasing the dose of norepinephrine decreased both P_{mcf} and RVR [27]. Further, after increasing norepinephrine CO decreased in ten patients and CO increased in six patients [25]. In all patients, P_{mcf} and RVR increased, though the "balance" between the two values determined whether CO increased. One study showed an increase in propofol caused a decrease in V_s without a change in CO [24]. These studies show P_{mcf} behaves within the framework of hemodynamic reasoning and lends itself to being used as a less invasive method to assess drug-induced physiology. Since P_{mcf} exists at the intersection of arterial and venous flow, it enables to calculate the true arterial and venous resistance by calculating the critical closing pressure (P_{cc}). P_{cc} is the mean arterial pressure (MAP) to zero CO-intercept. Arterial resistance is calculated as (MAP − P_{cc})/CO [22].

Precision and accuracy

The technique precision has not yet been assessed in humans. However, in an animal study the averaged coefficient of variation for repeated measurements of P_{mcf} hold was 6% [29]. Comparing the techniques' accuracy, no significant differences between P_{mcf} hold and P_{mcf} arm existed, whereas P_{mcf} analogue values were significantly lower [16, 30].

Table 2 Mean circulatory filling pressure during different volumetric state

Study	Method	N	Patient population	Baseline position	Baseline P_{mcf}	Hypervolemia (induced by fluid administration)	p value*	Amount of fluid administered to induce hypervolemia	Hypovolemia (induced by HUT)	p value†
Maas et al. [21]	P_{mcf} hold	12	Cardiac surgery	Supine	18.7 (4.5)	29.1 (5.2)	0.001	500 mL colloid in 15–20 min	14.5 (3.0)	0.005
Keller et al. [23]	P_{mcf} hold	9	Cardiac surgery	Semirecumbent	19.7 IQR 17.0–22.6	26.9 IQR 18.4–31.0	<0.05	500 mL colloid	–	–
Maas et al. [22]	P_{mcf} hold	10	Cardiac surgery	Not described	18.7 (4.0)	26.4 (3.2)	<0.001	500 mL colloid	–	–
Guerin et al. [28]	P_{mcf} hold	30	Shock	Semirecumbent	Responder: 25 (13) Non-responders: 24 (10)	32 (17) 28 (12)	<0.01 <0.01	500 mL saline in 10 min	–	–
Geerts et al. [43]	P_{mcf} arm	24	Cardiac surgery	Supine	Responders: 16.2 (6.3) Non-responders: 24.3 (8.2)	22.0 (7.6) 29.9 (9.1)	<0.001 <0.001	500 mL colloid	–	–
Aya et al. [41]	P_{mcf} arm	20	Cardiac surgery	Supine	22.4 (7.7)	–	–	–	–	–
Aya et al. [42]	P_{mcf} arm	80	Cardiac surgery	Supine	23.0 Range: 17.3–29.8	–	–	–	–	–
Parkin et al. [49]	P_{mcf} analogue	10	CVVH	Not described	Target state=15.9	–	–	CVVHD	–	–
Cecconi et al. [48]	P_{mcf} analogue	39	Heterogenous	Not described	Responders: 17.8 (5.1) Non-responders: 17.9 (5.1)	20.9 (5.1) 21.0 (4.9)	<0.001 <0.001	Mean 252 (8.9) mL 52.5% crystalloid 37.6% colloid 8.8% FFP & RBC	–	–
Gupta et al. [20]	P_{mcf} analogue	61	Cardiac surgery	Supine	Responders: 17 (3.7) Non-responders: 17 (3.6)	19 (4.3) 19 (4.1)	0.02 0.03	Mean 264 (16) mL 50% saline. Other 50%: mix of FFP, platelets, albumin, packed RBC, return of pump blood	–	–
Aya et al. [51]	P_{mcf} analogue	26	Heterogenous	Not described	Responders: 13.7 IQR: 10.9–16.9 Non-responders: 16.7 IQR 10.5–18.9			250 mL crystalloid		
Maas et al. [16]	P_{mcf} hold P_{mcf} arm P_{mcf} analogue	11	Cardiac surgery	Supine	19.7 (3.9) 18.4 (3.7) 14.7 (2.7)	28.3 (3.6) 27.1 (4.0) 19.2 (1.1)	<0.001 <0.001 <0.001	500 mL colloid	16.2 (3.0) 15.4 (3.1) 10.9 (2.0)	0.001 0.001 <0.001
Maas et al. [30]	P_{mcf} arm P_{mcf} hold#	15	Cardiac surgery	Supine	21.0 (6.8)	27.7 (7.4)	<0.001	500 mL colloid (10 steps of 50 mL)	–	–

Data presented as mean with SD or median with interquartile range (IQR). P_{mcf} in mmHg. Hypovolemic state induced by head up tilt (HUT) to 30°. Responders = fluid responsiveness was defined by a 10% increase in CO

* p value, difference between baseline and hypervolemia induced by fluid administration

† p value, difference between baseline and hypovolemic state

Table 3 P_{mcf} and pharmacodynamics

References	Method	n	Situation A	Situation B	p value*	Situation C	p value#
Persichini et al. [27]		16	NE 0.30	NE 0.19			
			Range 0.10–1.40	Range 0.08–1.15			
	P_{mcf} hold (in mmHg)		33 (12)	26 (10)	0.003		
Maas et al. [25]		16	Baseline 1	NE increase of 0.04 (0.02)		Baseline 2	
			NE 0.04 (0.03)			NE 0.04 (0.03)	
	P_{mcf} hold (in mmHg)		21.4 (6.1)	27.6 (7.4)	< 0.001	22.0 (5.3)	
de Wit et al. [24]		17	Propofol low	Propofol medium		Propofol high	
			Cb 3.0 (0.90) µg/mL	Cb 4.5 (1.0) µg/mL		Cb 6.5 (1.2) µg/mL	
	P_{mcf} hold (in mmHg)		27.9 (5.4)	24.6 (4.9)	0.01	21.4 (4.2)	< 0.001
Helmerhorst et al. [26]		22	FiO$_2$ 21–30%	FiO$_2$ 90%			
	P_{mcf} hold (in mmHg)		20.8 (3.5)	23.1 (4.0)	< 0.001		

NE norepinephrine dose in µg/kg/min presented as mean with range or mean with standard deviation. P_{mcf} values are presented as mean with standard deviation. Cb target blood concentration of propofol in µg/mL. P_{mcf} hold values presented in mmHg. FiO$_2$ fractional oxygen concentration

* p value, p value for situation A compared to B

p value, p value for situation A compared to C

Limitations

The use of P_{mcf} hold is restricted to mechanically ventilated and sedated patients with a central venous catheter. The procedure of the inspiratory hold maneuvers is not yet automated and requires a direct link between monitor and ventilator, or advanced monitor analytics to detect the inspiratory holds and to perform the instantaneous CO calculations. Furthermore, it is not suitable during cardiac arrhythmia. This method is not suitable to measure rapid changes in hemodynamic status since it takes a couple of minutes to perform the multiple end-inspiratory (and end-expiratory) holds. Potentially, this technique is operator-dependent because a proper inspiratory plateau pressure is needed. CVP can be altered due to incorrect catheter placement. An absolute CO value is not necessary for P_{mcf} hold as the technique extrapolates to zero CO. If the trend measurements are accurate, the RVR slope might change, but the intersection P_{mcf} point remains constant. The latter holds only true for the P_{mcf} itself, the RVR is dependent of the slope of the curve. In clinical practice, a physician would use P_{mcf} together with RVR; therefore, for clinical use of the P_{mcf} an accurate CO value is needed.

Potentially, the inspiratory hold maneuver overestimates P_{mcf} by the blood translocation from the pulmonary into the systemic circulation [31–33]. However, the potential volume shifts relative to Csys suggest that this effect is minimal [10, 34]. During inspiratory hold maneuvers, arterial pressure decreases. If sustained, baroreflex-induced increased sympathetic tone may cause P_{mcf} to increase [35, 36]. Indeed one study performed in pigs found the P_{mcf} hold overestimating compared to a method using right atrial balloon occlusion

in euvolemic conditions, in bleeding and hypervolemia; however, the values found between the two methods were similar [34]. Two clinical studies [16, 30] have shown P_{mcf} hold and P_{mcf} arm values not being significantly different, debating the former result found in pigs. Future studies in humans are needed. Moreover, all patients undergoing inspiratory holds are on neuro-humoral suppressive agents, probably dampening the baroreflex and other autonomic influences [37–39].

P_{mcf} arm
Technique description

As P_{mcf} is defined as the steady-state blood pressure during no-flow conditions, instantaneously P_{mcf} should mainly be similar for different vascular compartments even though each compartment may have different V_u and V_s [2, 40]. Four studies [16, 41–43] used the arm to estimate P_{mcf}. For arm occlusion, a rapid cuff inflator (inflates in 0.3 s) [16, 43] or a pneumatic tourniquet (inflates in 1.4 s) [41, 42] was inflated around the upper arm to 50 mmHg above systolic blood pressure. Arterial and venous pressures were measured via a radial artery catheter and a peripheral venous cannula in the forearm. When these two pressures equalize, P_{mcf} arm values are achieved. An initial study determined that a 25–30 s stop-flow time was adequate to achieve this equilibration [16]. Following this, in two studies P_{mcf} arm was measured as the average radial arterial pressure at 30 s after stop-flow [16, 43]. One study found the smallest difference between venous and arterial pressure after 60 s of stop-flow [41]. This discrepancy could be explained by different inflation time, i.e., induction of stop-flow.

Clinical applicability

The average baseline P_{mcf} arm values found in the included studies range from 16 to 24 mmHg (Table 2). P_{mcf} arm can be performed in spontaneously breathing subjects and requires only one measure. In two studies, P_{mcf} arm was assessed as a predictor of fluid loading responsiveness (FLR) [16, 43]. One study showed that a low P_{mcf} arm (<22 mmHg) predicts FLR with 71% sensitivity and 88% specificity, where responders were defined when CO increased $>10\%$ after 500 mL colloid administration [43]. Another study showed changes in circulating volume (500 mL colloid) are tracked well by changes in P_{mcf} arm [16]. Finally, one study indicated a minimum of 4 mL/kg fluid challenge was needed to define FLR [42].

Precision and accuracy

Repeated measurements of P_{mcf} arm showed no significant differences [41]. The coefficient of variation for a single measurement was 5%, which reduced to 3% after four measurements. Bland–Altman analysis showed a bias of -0.1 ± 1.68 mmHg for the first two measurements. The least significant change [44] for a single measurement was 14% (i.e., ± 3 mmHg for a P_{mcf} arm of 22 mmHg). One study observed a negligible bias of two P_{mcf} arm determinations at baseline position and after fluid expansion [16]. Two studies [16, 30] found no significant differences in P_{mcf} arm to P_{mcf} hold measures.

Limitations

Theoretically, a limitation of the technique is the influence of an auto regulatory hypoxia-induced response causing arterial vasodilation. The time of measuring P_{mcf} after arm occlusion should be enough for arterial and venous pressures to equilibrate, but before hypoxia-induced vasodilation causes an underestimation of P_{mcf} [45]. One study observed plateau pressures after 20–30 s and saw a further decrement after 35–40 s which indicates hypoxia-induced vasodilation [16]. Potentially, arm occlusion causes a small accumulation of blood volume because the venous outflow stops before the arterial inflow stops [16]. Though, this potential overestimation is negligible since the inflow is small compared to the total distal arm volume as long as cuff inflation is rapid. To note, P_{mcf} arm is only reliable when a stable plateau pressure is achieved [2].

In contrast to P_{mcf} hold, P_{mcf} arm measures can be made in non-sedated patients with cardiac arrhythmias. However, the possible influence of the rapid cuff inflator on reflex mechanisms needs to be studied. In septic patients, central and peripheral vasomotor tone might be altered differently [46]. Shortly after cardiac surgery differences between aortic and radial pressure can occur [47], still, the original validation studies were on postoperative cardiac surgery patients.

P_{mcf} analogue

Technique description

Based on a Guytonian model of the systemic circulation ($CO = V_R = (P_{mcf} - CVP)/RVR$), an analogue of P_{mcf} can be derived using a mathematical model: P_{mcf} analogue $= a \times CVP + b \times MAP + c \times CO$ [5, 20, 48, 49]. In this formula, a and b are dimensionless constants ($a + b = 1$). Assuming a veno-arterial compliance ratio of 24:1, $a = 0.96$ and $b = 0.04$; c resembles arteriovenous resistance and is based on a formula including age, height and weight [5, 48–50].

Clinical applicability

The average baseline P_{mcf} analogue values found in the included studies range from 14 to 18 mmHg (Table 2). One study compared fluid replacement based on target P_{mcf} analogue compared to conventional treatment in continuous veno-venous hemodiafiltration [49]. Fluid replacement based on target P_{mcf} analogue led to significantly less fluid administration with stable cardiovascular variables (CVP, MAP, CO) and no complications. So, P_{mcf} analogue measurement adequately follows intravascular volume status in patients. P_{mcf} analogue measurements are automatic making it an attractive alternative to P_{mcf} hold and P_{mcf} arm.

More recently, the P_{mcf} analogue dynamics, measured with the Navigator™ device (Applied Physiology, Pty Ltd, Australia), were observed [20, 48, 51]. Patients were defined as responders with an increase in stroke volume or CO $>10\%$ after 250 mL fluid administration. P_{mcf} analogue increased after fluid administration; however, baseline P_{mcf} analogue did not differ between responders and non-responders [20, 45, 48] (Table 2). This is contrary to results of another study [43] using P_{mcf} arm, possibly due to different fluid volume (250 vs. 500 mL) [42]. Although the driving pressure for V_R (P_{mcf} CVP) was different between responders and non-responders, it showed low sensitivity (79%) and specificity (56%) to predict FLR [20, 48].

Precision and accuracy

Precision has not been assessed for P_{mcf} analogue (Table 4). Comparing measurement techniques revealed a lower P_{mcf} analogue value compared to P_{mcf} hold [16]. However, a significant regression of P_{mcf} analogue and P_{mcf} hold was observed enabling to adjust the P_{mcf} analogue value using calibration factor [5].

Table 4 Comparison of bedside P_{mcf} measurement techniques

	P_{mcf} hold $CO = (P_{mcf} - CVP)/RVR$	P_{mcf} arm $P_a = P_v$	P_{mcf} analogue $P_{mcf} = a \times CVP + b \times MAP + c \times CO$
Applicability to a broad patient population	−	±	±
	Restricted to fully sedated and mechanically ventilated patients	In theory applicable in all patients (sedated or awake) with an radial artery catheter	In theory applicable in all patients (sedated or awake)
	Restricted to patients without a contraindication for inspiratory holds (such as COPD with bullae)		Continuous and accurate CO, MAP and CVP measurements needed
	Continuous and accurate CO and CVP measurements needed		Not suitable in cardiac arrythmia
	Not suitable in cardiac arrythmia		
Accuracy	+	+	−
	Values interchangeable with P_{mcf} arm	Values interchangeable with P_{mcf} hold	Values significantly lower than derived with P_{mcf} hold
	When sedated baroreflex probably of little influence	Dependent on time of measurement: $> P_a$ and P_v equilibration. < hypoxia-induced vasodilatation	P_{mcf} analogue can be transformed to P_{mcf} hold values (constant error)
	Mechanical ventilation may overestimate P_{mcf} value	Possible influence rapid cuff inflator on reflex mechanism altering P_{mcf} value in non-sedated patients. This is not studied	Mathematical coupling and the equation is based on assumptions that may not be generalizable to all patient populations in ICU
Precision	?	+	?
	Not studied	No significant differences during repeated measurements. LSC for a single measurement is 14%	Not studied
Outcome operator independent	−	±	+
	Inspiratory holds	Timing of measurement	CVP transducer position and CO measurement technique
	CVP transducer position and CO measurement technique		
	Extrapolation of curve		
Responding time	−	+	+
	> 4 min	30–60 s	Fast, no exact times mentioned
Costs	−	+	+
	Theoretically no extra devices needed than standard present in ICU	Rapid Cuff Inflator (Hokanson E20, Bellevue, Washington, USA) = 3000 euro	Navigator™ (Applied Physiology, Pty Ltd, Sydney, Australia)
			Price unknown
Risk of complications	+	±	−
	No complications reported in published studies. In theory:	No complications reported in published studies. In theory:	No complications reported in published studies. In theory:
	Barotrauma from inspiratory holds	In sedated patients attention should be paid deflating the rapid cuff before hypoxemia-induced damage can occur	Complications associated with central venous catheters and CO measurement

Table 4 (continued)

P_{mcf} hold $CO = (P_{mcf} \, CVP)/RVR$	P_{mcf} arm $P_a = P_v$	P_{mcf} analogue $P_{mcf} = axCVP + bxMAP + cxCO$
Severe hemodynamic instability induced by inspiratory holds	In awake patients local pain could be caused by inflating the rapid cuff inflator	
Complications associated with central venous catheters and CO measurement		

CO cardiac output, CVP central venous pressure, RVR resistance to venous return, MAP mean arterial pressure, P_a arterial pressure, P_v venous pressure (the latter two measured in the arm)

Limitations

The mathematical model is based on CVP, MAP and CO measurements. As CVP values vary during ventilation, usually end-expiratory CVP-recordings can be used. Furthermore, CVP values depend on the position of the transducer. Accurate CO values are needed for this method. The limitation of P_{mcf} analogue is that the algorithm is based on a mathematical model with mathematical coupling between CO and P_{mcf} and fixed Csys and resistance parameters [5], therefore presumably not applicable for all patient populations or clinical conditions. We are unable to assess the availability of the Navigator™ for routine care.

Discussion

We found three bedside techniques to measure P_{mcf}: P_{mcf} hold, P_{mcf} arm and P_{mcf} analogue. They were used to follow volumetric state and to study drug-induced hemodynamic changes in patients.

The interpretation of V_R curves and P_{mcf} in clinical practice is subject to debate [52–59]. The values found in heart-beating ICU patients are higher (14–33 mmHg) than in deceased ICU patients (12.8 ± 5.6 mmHg, mean ± sd), probably because of alteration of vasomotor tone after dying [53]. Furthermore, ICU patients often receive vasopressors which increase P_{mcf} and the study populations differed making it not one-to-one comparable. It is also speculated that the pressure described by Guyton is not measurable in heart-beating patients and the extrapolated pressure of the curve represents a different physiological parameter. Nevertheless, in two studies P_{mcf} arm was interchangeable with P_{mcf} hold [16–30]. Furthermore, although P_{mcf} values may differ, the CVP values do as well, which may account for a similar driving pressure for V_R. The reviewed studies illustrate the possible clinical benefits of using the bedside derived P_{mcf} values.

This review is limited since we were unable to pool the data because of the variety in used conditions and interventions. The 16 included studies were performed by only a few research groups with a limited amount of included patients. In most of the studies, each patient served as their own control since it is not clear what would be an appropriate outside control group.

Still, all studies testing the accuracy of P_{mcf} to follow intravascular changes and pharmacodynamics found significant results. Therefore, it is unlikely that a larger number of patients will show different outcomes. It is possible only positive studies were published, indicating publication bias. P_{mcf} values differ between the studies and have a wide range within studies (Table 2). Normal values for different patient populations need to be defined before P_{mcf} can be implemented into standard (ICU)

care. The increase in P_{mcf} values after fluid administration depends on vascular redistribution, vasomotor tone and fluid loss into the interstitial space. Studies focusing on clinical decision-making based on P_{mcf}, driving pressure for V_R, V_s or Csys have not yet been performed. Study designs need to be created to see if using these measures improves outcomes. Also, no precision studies examining P_{mcf} hold or P_{mcf} analogue exist yet.

Conclusions

Presently, three bedside P_{mcf} measurement techniques are available. All require invasive hemodynamic monitoring. Though P_{mcf} measures allow for more direct assessment of circulating blood volume, V_R and Csys, studies are needed to determine cutoff values to allow P_{mcf} to trigger therapeutic interventions and to determine its value in clinical practice.

Abbreviations

CO: cardiac output; Csys: vascular compliance, CVP: central venous pressure; FiO_2: fractional oxygen concentration; FLR: fluid loading responsiveness; ICU: intensive care unit; MAP: mean arterial pressure; RVR: resistance for venous return.

List of symbols

P_{cc}: critical closing pressure; P_{mcf}: mean circulatory filling pressure; P_{ra}: right atrial pressure; V_R: venous return; V_s: stressed volume; V_u: unstressed volume.

Authors' contributions

All authors contributed to the manuscript. MW, DV and BG designed the study. MW performed a systematic search of the literature. MW and DS independently screened articles for relevance and subsequently performed data extraction into predefined forms. Quality assessment of the included articles was also independently performed by MW and DS. MW, DV, BG and MP wrote the manuscript. JJ, EO and AV critically reviewed and revised the manuscript. All authors read and approved the final manuscript.

Author details

[1] Department of Anesthesiology, Academic Medical Center, Amsterdam, The Netherlands. [2] Department of Intensive Care, Academic Medical Center, Amsterdam, The Netherlands. [3] Laboratory of Experimental Intensive Care and Anesthesiology, Academic Medical Center, Amsterdam, The Netherlands. [4] Department of Critical Care Medicine, University of Pittsburgh Medical Center, 1215.4 Lillian S. Kaufmann Bldg, 3471 Fifth Avenue, Pittsburgh, PA 15213, USA. [5] Department of Intensive Care Medicine, Leiden University Medical Center, Leiden, The Netherlands.

Competing interests

None of the authors have relevant conflict of interest present for any aspect of the submitted work. Denise Veelo performed consultancy work for Edwards Lifesciences, Hemologic and Merck outside the submitted work. Bart Geerts performed consultancy work for Edwards Lifesciences and Philips outside the submitted work. Michael Pinsky is a consultant for Cheetah Medical, Edwards Lifesciences, Exotstat Medical, LiDCO Ltd and Cyberonics outside the submitted work.

Funding

None.

References

1. Hainsworth R. The importance of vascular capacitance in cardiovascular control. News Physiol Sci. 1990;5:250–4.
2. Maas JJ. Mean systemic filling pressure: its measurement and meaning. Neth J Crit Care. 2015;19:6–11.
3. Peters J, Mack GW, Lister G. The importance of the peripheral circulation in critical illnesses. Intensive Care Med. 2001;27:1446–58.
4. Gelman S. Venous function and central venous pressure: a physiologic story. Anesthesiology. 2008;108:735–48.
5. Parkin WG. Volume state control: a new approach. Crit Care Resusc. 1999;1:311–21.
6. Jansen JR, Maas JJ, Pinsky MR. Bedside assessment of mean systemic filling pressure. Curr Opin Crit Care. 2010;16:231–6.
7. Bayliss WM, Starling EH. Observations on venous pressures and their relationship to capillary pressures. J Physiol. 1894;16:159–318.
8. Guyton AC, Polizo D, Armstrong GG. Mean circulatory filling pressure measured immediately after cessation of heart pumping. Am J Physiol. 1954;179:261–7.
9. Guyton AC, Lindsey AW, Abernathy B, Richardson T. Venous return at various right atrial pressures and the normal venous return curve. Am J Physiol. 1957;189:609–15.
10. Versprille A, Jansen JR. Mean systemic filling pressure as a characteristic pressure for venous return. Pflugers Arch. 1985;405:226–33.
11. Pinsky MR. Instantaneous venous return curves in an intact canine preparation. J Appl Physiol Respir Environ Exerc Physiol. 1984;56:765–71.
12. Hiesmayr M, Jansen JR, Versprille A. Effects of endotoxin infusion on mean systemic filling pressure and flow resistance to venous return. Pflugers Arch. 1996;431:741–7.
13. den Hartog EA, Versprille A, Jansen JR. Systemic filling pressure in intact circulation determined on basis of aortic vs. central venous pressure relationships. Am J Physiol. 1994;267:H2255–8.
14. Yamamoto J, Trippodo NC, Ishise S, Frohlich ED. Total vascular pressure–volume relationship in the conscious rat. Am J Physiol. 1980;238:H823–8.
15. Samar RE, Coleman TG. Measurement of mean circulatory filling pressure and vascular capacitance in the rat. Am J Physiol. 1978;234:H94–100.
16. Maas JJ, Pinsky MR, Geerts BF, de Wilde RB, Jansen JR. Estimation of mean systemic filling pressure in postoperative cardiac surgery patients with three methods. Intensive Care Med. 2012;38:1452–60.
17. Liberati A, Altman DG, Tetzlaff J, Mulrow C, Gøtzsche PC, Ioannidis JP, et al. The PRISMA statement for reporting systematic reviews and meta-analyses of studies that evaluate health care interventions: explanation and elaboration. PLoS Med. 2009;6:e1000100.
18. Higgins JPT, Green S. Cochrane handbook for systematic reviews of interventions (version 5.1.0). 2011. http://handbook.cochrane.org. Accessed 16 March 2017.
19. Wells G, Shea B, O'Connell J, Peterson J, Welch V, Losos M, et al. The Newcastle–Ottawa Scale (NOS) for assessing the quality of nonrandomised studies in meta-analyses. 2009. http://www.ohri.ca/programs/clinical_epidemiology/oxford.asp. Accessed 20 Feb 2017.
20. Gupta K, Sondergaard S, Parkin G, Leaning M, Aneman A. Applying mean systemic filling pressure to assess the response to fluid boluses in cardiac post-surgical patients. Intensive Care Med. 2015;41:265–72.
21. Maas JJ, Geerts BF, van den Berg PC, Pinsky MR, Jansen JR. Assessment of venous return curve and mean systemic filling pressure in postoperative cardiac surgery patients. Crit Care Med. 2009;37:912–8.
22. Maas JJ, de Wilde RB, Aarts LP, Pinsky MR, Jansen JR. Determination of vascular waterfall phenomenon by bedside measurement of mean systemic filling pressure and critical closing pressure in the intensive care unit. Anesth Analg. 2012;114:803–10.
23. Keller G, Desebbe O, Benard M, Bouchet JB, Lehot JJ. Bedside assessment of passive leg raising effects on venous return. J Clin Monit Comput. 2011;25:257–63.
24. de Wit F, van Vliet AL, de Wilde RB, Jansen JR, Vuyk J, Aarts LP, et al. The effect of propofol on haemodynamics: cardiac output, venous return, mean systemic filling pressure, and vascular resistances. Br J Anaesth. 2016;116:784–9.
25. Maas JJ, Pinsky MR, de Wilde RB, de Jonge E, Jansen JR. Cardiac output response to norepinephrine in postoperative cardiac surgery patients: interpretation with venous return and cardiac function curves. Crit Care Med. 2013;41:143–50.
26. Helmerhorst HJ, de Wilde RB, Lee DH, Palmen M, Jansen JR, van Westerloo DJ, et al. Hemodynamic effects of short-term hyperoxia after coronary artery bypass grafting. Ann Intensive Care. 2017;7:20.
27. Persichini R, Silva S, Teboul JL, Jozwiak M, Chemla D, Richard C, et al. Effects of norepinephrine on mean systemic pressure and venous return in human septic shock. Crit Care Med. 2012;40:3146–53.
28. Guerin L, Teboul JL, Persichini R, Dres M, Richard C, Monet X. Effects of passive leg raising and volume expansion on mean systemic pressure and venous return in shock in humans. Crit Care. 2015;19:411.
29. Maas JJ, Geerts BF, Jansen JR. Evaluation of mean systemic filling pressure from pulse contour cardiac output and central venous pressure. J Clin Monit Comput. 2011;25:193–201.
30. Maas JJ, Pinsky MR, Aarts LP, Jansen JR. Bedside assessment of total systemic vascular compliance, stressed volume, and cardiac function curves in intensive care unit patients. Anesth Analg. 2012;115:880–7.
31. Fessler HE, Brower RG, Wise RA, Permutt S. Effects of positive end-expiratory pressure on the gradient for venous return. Am Rev Respir Dis. 1991;143:19–24.
32. Hedenstierna G. Pulmonary perfusion during anesthesia and mechanical ventilation. Minerva Anestesiol. 2005;71:319–24.
33. Jellinek H, Krenn H, Oczenski W, Veit F, Schwarz S, Fitzgerald RD. Influence of positive airway pressure on the pressure gradient for venous return in humans. J Appl Physiol. 2000;88:926–32.
34. Berger D, Moller PW, Weber A, Bloch A, Bloechlinger S, Haenggi M, et al. Effect of PEEP, blood volume and inspiratory hold maneuvers on venous return. Am J Physiol Heart Circ Physiol. 2016;311:H794–806.
35. Borst C, Karemaker JM. Time delays in the human baroreceptor reflex. J Auton Nerv Syst. 1983;9:399–409.
36. Peters JK, Lister G, Nadel ER, Mack GW. Venous and arterial reflex responses to positive-pressure breathing and lower body negative pressure. J Appl Physiol. 1997;82(6):1889–96.
37. Sato M, Tanaka M, Umehara S, Nishikawa T. Baroreflex control of heart rate during and after propofol infusion in humans. Br J Anaesth. 2005;94:577–81.
38. Ebert TJ. Sympathetic and hemodynamic effects of moderate and deep sedation with propofol in humans. Anesthesiology. 2005;103:20–4.
39. Lennander O, Henriksson BA, Martner J, Biber B. Effects of fentanyl, nitrous oxide, or both, on baroreceptor reflex regulation in the cat. Br J Anaesth. 1996;77:399–403.
40. Anderson RM. Appendix: clinical determination of mean cardiovascular pressure. In: Anderson RM, editor. The gross physiology of the cardiovascular system. 2nd ed. Tucson: Racquet Press; 1993. p. 61–2.
41. Aya HD, Rhodes A, Fletcher N, Grounds RM, Cecconi M. Transient stop-flow arm arterial-venous equilibrium pressure measurement: determination of precision of the technique. J Clin Monit Comput. 2016;30:55–61.
42. Aya HD, Rhodes A, Chis Ster I, Fletcher N, Grounds RM, Cecconi M. Hemodynamic effect of different doses of fluids for a fluid challenge: a quasi-randomized controlled study. Crit Care Med. 2017;45:e161–8.
43. Geerts BF, Maas J, de Wilde RB, Aarts LP, Jansen JR. Arm occlusion pressure is a useful predictor of an increase in cardiac output after fluid loading following cardiac surgery. Eur J Anaesthesiol. 2011;28:802–6.
44. Kawalilak CE, Johnston JD, Olszynski WP, Kontulainen SA. Least significant changes and monitoring time intervals for high-resolution pQCT-derived bone outcomes in postmenopausal women. J Musculoskelet Neuronal Interact. 2015;15:190–6.
45. Betik AC, Luckham VB, Hughson RL. Flow-mediated dilation in human brachial artery after different circulatory occlusion conditions. Am J Physiol Heart Circ Physiol. 2004;286:H4428.
46. Hatib F, Jansen JR, Pinsky MR. Peripheral vascular decoupling in porcine endotoxic shock. J Appl Physiol. 2011;111:853–60.
47. Stern DH, Gerson JI, Allen FB, Parker FB. Can we trust the direct radial artery pressure immediately following cardiopulmonary bypass? Anesthesiology. 1985;62:557–61.
48. Cecconi M, Aya HD, Geisen M, Ebm C, Fletcher N, Grounds RM, et al. Changes in the mean systemic filling pressure during a fluid challenge in postsurgical intensive care patients. Intensive Care Med. 2013;39:1299–305.

49. Parkin G, Wright C, Bellomo R, Boyce N. Use of a mean systemic filling pressure analogue during the closed-loop control of fluid replacement in continuous hemodiafiltration. J Crit Care. 1994;9:124–33.

50. Crozier TM, Wallace EM, Parkin WG. Haemodynamic assessment in pregnancy and pre-eclampsia: a Guytonian approach. Pregnancy Hypertens. 2015;5:177–81.

51. Aya HD, Ster IC, Fletcher N, Grounds RM, Rhodes A, Cecconi M. Pharmacodynamic analysis of a fluid challenge. Crit Care Med. 2016;44:880–91.

52. Brengelmann GL. A critical analysis of the view that right atrial pressure determines venous return. J Appl Physiol. 2003;94:849–59.

53. Repessé X, Charron C, Fink J, Beauchet A, Deleu F, Slama M, et al. Value and determinants of the mean systemic filling pressure in critically ill patients'. Am J Physiol Heart Circ Physiol. 2015;309:H1003–7.

54. Brengelmann GL. Letter to the editor: comments on "Value and determinants of the mean systemic filling pressure in critically ill patients". Am J Physiol Heart Circ Physiol. 2015;309:H1370–1.

55. Repessé X, Vieillard-Baron A. Reply to Letter to the editor: comments on 'Value and determinants of the mean systemic filling pressure in critically ill patients'. Am J Physiol Heart Circ Physiol. 2015;309:H1372–3.

56. Beard DA, Feigl EO. Understanding Guyton's venous return curves. Am J Physiol Heart Circ Physiol. 2011;301:H629–33.

57. Teboul JL. Mean systemic filling pressure: we can now estimate it, but for what? Intensive Care Med. 2013;39:1487–8.

58. Parkin G. Re: mean systemic filling pressure: we can now estimate it but for what? Intensive Care Med. 2014;40:139.

59. Teboul JL. Mean systemic filling pressure: we can now estimate it, but for what? Response to comment by Parkin. Intensive Care Med. 2014;40:140.

Permissions

The contributors of this book come from diverse backgrounds, making this book a truly international effort. This book will bring forth new frontiers with its revolutionizing research information and detailed analysis of the nascent developments around the world.

We would like to thank all the contributing authors for lending their expertise to make the book truly unique. They have played a crucial role in the development of this book. Without their invaluable contributions this book wouldn't have been possible. They have made vital efforts to compile up to date information on the varied aspects of this subject to make this book a valuable addition to the collection of many professionals and students.

This book was conceptualized with the vision of imparting up-to-date information and advanced data in this field. To ensure the same, a matchless editorial board was set up. Every individual on the board went through rigorous rounds of assessment to prove their worth. After which they invested a large part of their time researching and compiling the most relevant data for our readers.

The editorial board has been involved in producing this book since its inception. They have spent rigorous hours researching and exploring the diverse topics which have resulted in the successful publishing of this book. They have passed on their knowledge of decades through this book. To expedite this challenging task, the publisher supported the team at every step. A small team of assistant editors was also appointed to further simplify the editing procedure and attain best results for the readers.

Apart from the editorial board, the designing team has also invested a significant amount of their time in understanding the subject and creating the most relevant covers. They scrutinized every image to scout for the most suitable representation of the subject and create an appropriate cover for the book.

The publishing team has been an ardent support to the editorial, designing and production team. Their endless efforts to recruit the best for this project, has resulted in the accomplishment of this book. They are a veteran in the field of academics and their pool of knowledge is as vast as their experience in printing. Their expertise and guidance has proved useful at every step. Their uncompromising quality standards have made this book an exceptional effort. Their encouragement from time to time has been an inspiration for everyone.

The publisher and the editorial board hope that this book will prove to be a valuable piece of knowledge for researchers, students, practitioners and scholars across the globe.

List of Contributors

David Lagier, Laura Platon, Laurent Chow-Chine, Antoine Sannini, Magali Bisbal, Jean-Paul Brun, Marion Faucher and Djamel Mokart
Intensive Care Unit, Paoli-Calmettes Institute, 232 Boulevard de Sainte-Marguerite,13009 Marseille, France

Jérome Lambert
Biostatistics Department, Saint Louis Teaching Hospital, AP-HP, 1, Avenue Claude Vellefaux, 75010 Paris, France

Karim Asehnoune
Department of Anesthesiology and Critical Care Medicine, Hotel Dieu, University Hospital of Nantes, 1 Place Alexis Ricordeau, 44903 Nantes, France

Marc Leone
Department of Anesthesiology and Critical Care Medicine, Hopital Nord, University Hospital of Marseille, Chemin des Bourrely, 13015 Marseille, France

Izumi Nakayama
Intensive Care Unit, Department of Internal Medicine, Okinawa Chubu Hospital, 281 Miyazato, Uruma, Okinawa 904-2293, Japan

Junichi Izawa
Intensive Care Unit, Department of Anesthesiology, The Jikei University School of Medicine, 3-19-18 Nishi-Shinbashi, Minato-ku, Tokyo 105-8471, Japan
The Center for Critical Care Nephrology, Clinical Research, Investigation, and Systems Modeling of Acute Illness Center, Department of Critical Care Medicine, University of Pittsburgh School of Medicine, Pittsburgh, PA 15213, USA

Hideyuki Mouri and Junji Shiotsuka
Department of Anesthesiology and Critical Care, Jichi Medical University, Saitama Medical Center, 1-847 Amanuma, Oomiya-ku, Saitama, Saitama 330-8503, Japan

Tetsuhisa Kitamura
Division of Environmental Medicine and Population Sciences, Department of Social and Environmental Medicine, Graduate School of Medicine, Osaka University, 1-1 Yamada-oka, Suita, Osaka 565-0871, Japan

David J. Clancy, Timothy Scully, Stephen Huang, Anthony S. McLean and Sam R. Orde
ICU, Nepean Hospital, Kingswood, NSW 2747, Australia

Michel Slama
Medical ICU, Amiens University Hospital, Amiens, France

Joana Gameiro, José Agapito Fonseca, Marta Neves, Sofia Jorge and José António Lopes
Division of Nephrology and Renal Transplantation, Department of Medicine, Centro Hospitalar Lisboa Norte, EPE, Av. Prof. Egas Moniz, 1649-035 Lisbon, Portugal

Ward Eertmans, Cornelia Genbrugge, Dieter Mesotten, Jo Dens, Frank Jans and Cathy De Deyne
Department of Medicine and Life Sciences, Hasselt University, Diepenbeek, Belgium

Ward Eertmans, Cornelia Genbrugge, Margot Vander Laenen, Willem Boer, Dieter Mesotten, Frank Jans and Cathy De Deyne
Department of Anaesthesiology, Intensive Care, Emergency Medicine and Pain Therapy, Ziekenhuis Oost-Limburg, Schiepse Bos 6, 3600 Genk, Belgium

Jo Dens
Department of Cardiology, Ziekenhuis Oost-Limburg, Schiepse Bos 6, 3600 Genk, Belgium

Sebastien Jochmans, Jonathan Chelly and Mehran Monchi
Département de Médecine Intensive et Unité de Recherche Clinique, Groupe Hospitalier Sud Ile-de-France, Hôpital de Melun, 77000 Melun, France

Jean-Emmanuel Alphonsine
Service de Réanimation Médicale, AP-HP, Hôpital Bicêtre, 94270 Le Kremlin-Bicêtre, France

Ly Van Phach Vong, Oumar Sy, Nathalie Rolin and Olivier Ellrodt
Département de Médecine Intensive, Groupe Hospitalier Sud Ile-de-France, Hôpital de Melun, 77000 Melun, France

Christophe Vinsonneau
Service de Réanimation Polyvalente, Hôpital de Bethune, 62408 Bethune, France

Colombe Saillard
Haematology Department, Institut Paoli Calmettes, 232 Boulevard Sainte Marguerite, 13009 Marseille Cedex 09, France

Lara Zafrani and Elie Azoulay
Medical Intensive Care Unit, Saint-Louis University Hospital, AP-HP, Paris, France

Michael Darmon
Medical-Surgical Intensive Care Unit, Hôpital Nord, Université Jean Monnet, Saint Etienne, France

Michael Darmon, Magali Bisbal, Elie Azoulay and Djamel Mokart
GRRR-OH (Groupe de Recherche en Réanimation Respiratoire du patient d'Onco-Hématologie), Paris, France

Magali Bisbal, Laurent Chow-Chine, Antoine Sannini, Jean-Paul Brun, Marion Faucher and Djamel Mokart
Polyvalent Intensive Care Unit, Department of Anesthesiology and Critical Care, Institut Paoli Calmettes, Marseille,France

Jacques Ewald and Olivier Turrini
Surgery Department, Institut Paoli Calmettes, Marseille, France

Elie Azoulay
Faculté de Médecine, Université Paris Diderot, Sorbonne-Paris-Cité, Paris, France

Dana Y. Fuhrman
Children's Hospital of Pittsburgh, 4401 Penn Avenue, Children's Hospital Drive, Faculty Pavilion Suite 2000, Pittsburgh, PA 15224, USA

Sandra Kane-Gill
School of Pharmacy, University of Pittsburgh, 638 Salk Hall, 3501 Terrace Street, Pittsburgh, PA 15261, USA

Stuart L. Goldstein
Center for Acute Care Nephrology, Cincinnati Children's Hospital Medical Center, 3333 Burnet Avenue, Cincinnati, OH 45229, USA

Priyanka Priyanka and John A. Kellum
The Center for Critical Care Nephrology, 3347 Forbes Avenue, Ste 220, Pittsburgh, PA 15213, USA

Ben de Jong and Arthur R. H. van Zanten
Department of Intensive Care Medicine, Gelderse Vallei Hospital, Willy Brandtlaan 10, 6716 RP Ede, The Netherlands

Anne Sophie Schuppers, Arriette Kruisdijk-Gerritsen and Hubertus Laurentius Antonius van den Oever
Department of Intensive Care Medicine, Deventer Hospital, Nico Bolkesteinlaan 75, 7416 SE Deventer, The Netherlands

Maurits Erwin Leo Arbouw
Department of Clinical Pharmacy, Deventer Hospital, Nico Bolkesteinlaan 75, 7416 SE Deventer, The Netherlands

Djillali Annane
Service de Reanimation Medicale, Hopital R. Poincare, 104 Bd Raymond Poincare, 92380 Garches, France

Jean-Paul Mira
Sorbonne Paris Cité, Cochin Hotel-Dieu University Hospital Medical Intensive Care Unit, AP-HP, Université Paris Descartes,75014 Paris, France

Lorraine B. Ware
Departments of Medicine and Pathology, Microbiology and Immunology, Vanderbilt University School of Medicine, 1161 21st Avenue South T1218 MCN, Nashville, TN 37232-2650, USA

Anthony C. Gordon
Section of Anaesthetics, Pain Medicine, and Intensive Care, Charing Cross Hospital, Imperial College London, Fulham Palace Road, London W6 8RF, UK

Charles J. Hinds
Barts and The London School of Medicine, Queen
Mary University of London, London, UK

David C. Christiani
Harvard Medical School and School of Public
Health, 665 Huntington Avenue, Building I Room
1401, Boston, MA 02115, USA

Jonathan Sevransky and Timothy G. Buchman
Emory Center for Critical Care, Woodruff Health
Sciences Center, Emory University, Atlanta, GA,
USA

Kathleen Barnes
Division of Allergy and Clinical Immunology,
Department of Medicine, Johns Hopkins University,
Baltimore, MD, USA

Patrick J. Heagerty
Department of Biostatistics, University of
Washington, F-600, Health Sciences Building,
Office: H-665D HSB, Seattle, WA 98195-7232, USA

**Robert Balshaw, Nadia Lesnikova and Karen de
Nobrega**
Syreon Corporation, Vancouver,BC, Canada

**Hugh F. Wellman, Mauricio Neira and Alexandra
D. J. Mancini**
Formerly with Sirius Genomics Inc, Vancouver, BC,
Canada

Keith R. Walley and James A. Russell
Critical Care Research Laboratories, Centre for Heart
Lung Innovation, St. Paul's Hospital, University of
British Columbia, Burrard Building, Rm 166 - 1081
Burrard St, Vancouver, BC V6Z 1Y6, Canada

**Guillemette Thomas, Sami Hraiech, Samuel
Lehingue, Romain Rambaud, Christophe
Guervilly, Fanny Klasen, Mélanie Adda, Stéphanie
Dizier, Laurent Papazian and Jean-Marie Forel**
Hôpital Nord, Réanimation des Détresses
Respiratoires et des Infections Sévères, Assistance
Publique–Hôpitaux de Marseille, 13015 Marseille,
France

**Sami Hraiech, Nadim Cassir, Samuel Lehingue,
Romain Rambaud, Fanny Klasen, Antoine Roch,
Laurent Papazian and Jean-Marie Forel**
URMITE, UMR CNRS 7278, Faculté de Médecine,
Aix-Marseille Université, 13005 Marseille, France

Sandrine Wiramus
Hôpital de la Conception, Réanimation des brulés
Assistance Publique–Hôpitaux de Marseille, 13005
Marseille, France

Antoine Roch
Hôpital Nord, Service des Urgences, Assistance
Publique–Hôpitaux de Marseille, 13015 Marseille,
France

Xavier Monnet and Jean-Louis Teboul
Hôpital de Bicêtre, Service de Réanimation
Médicale, Hôpitaux Universitaires Paris-Sud, 78,
rue du Général Leclerc, 94270 Le Kremlin-Bicêtre,
France
Université Paris-Sud, Inserm UMR S_999, 94270 Le
Kremlin-Bicêtre, France

**Alette A. Koopman, Robert G. T. Blokpoel and
Martin C. J. Kneyber**
Division of Paediatric Intensive Care, Department of
Paediatrics, Beatrix Children's Hospital, University
Medical Center Groningen, The University of
Groningen, Internal Postal Code CA 62, RB
Groningen, The Netherlands

Leo A. van Eykern
Inbiolab B.V., Groningen, The Netherlands

Frans H. C. de Jongh
Faculty of Science and Technology, University of
Twente, Enschede, The Netherlands

Johannes G. M. Burgerhof
Department of Epidemiology, University Medical
Center Groningen, The University of Groningen,
Groningen, The Netherlands

Martin C. J. Kneyber
Division of Paediatric Intensive Care, Department
of Paediatrics, VU University Medical Center,
Amsterdam, The Netherlands
Critical Care, Anesthesia, Peri-operative Medicine
and Emergency Medicine (CAPE), The University
of Groningen, Groningen, The Netherlands

**Xavier Delabranche, Julie Helms and Ferhat
Meziani**
Université de Strasbourg, Faculté de Médecine &
Hôpitaux Universitaires de Strasbourg, Service de
Réanimation, Nouvel Hôpital Civil, Strasbourg,
France

Xavier Delabranche and Ferhat Meziani
INSERM (French National Institute of Health and Medical Research), UMR 1260, Regenerative Nanomedicine (RNM), FMTS, Université de Strasbourg, Strasbourg, France

Julie Helms
INSERM, EFS Grand Est, BPPS UMR-S 949, Université de Strasbourg, Strasbourg, France

Sophie Emilia Huttmann, Friederike Sophie Magnet, Christian Karagiannidis, Jan Hendrik Storre and Wolfram Windisch
Department of Pneumology, Cologne-Merheim Hospital, Kliniken der Stadt Köln gGmbH, Witten/Herdecke University Hospital, Ostmerheimer Strasse 200, 51109 Cologne, Germany

Jan Hendrik Storre
Department of Pneumology, University Medical Hospital, Freiburg, Germany
Department of Intensive Care, Sleep Medicine and Mechanical Ventilation, Asklepios Fachkliniken Munich-Gauting, Gauting, Germany

Lene Russell, Lars Broksø Holst and Anders Perner
Department of Intensive Care 4131, Copenhagen University Hospital, Rigshospitalet, Blegdamsvej 9, 2100 Copenhagen, Denmark

Lene Russell
Copenhagen Academy for Medical Education and Simulation, University of Copenhagen and The Capital Region of Denmark, Copenhagen, Denmark

Lars Kjeldsen
Department of Haematology, Copenhagen University Hospital, Rigshospitalet, Copenhagen, Denmark

Jakob Stensballe
Section for Transfusion Medicine, Capital Region Blood Bank, Copenhagen University Hospital, Rigshospitalet, Copenhagen, Denmark
Department of Anaesthesia, Centre of Head and Orthopaedics, Copenhagen University Hospital, Rigshospitalet, Copenhagen, Denmark

Yasuhiro Norisue, Jun Kataoka, Yosuke Homma, Shimada Yumiko, Yuiko Hoshina and Eiji Hiraoka
Department of Emergency and Critical Care Medicine, Tokyo Bay Urayasu Ichikawa Medical Center, 3-4-32 Todaijima, Urayasu, Chiba 2790001, Japan

Yasuhiro Norisue, Takaki Naito, Junpei Tsukuda, Kentaro Okamoto, Takeshi Kawaguchi and Shigeki Fujitani
Department of Emergency and Critical Care Medicine, St. Marianna University Hospital, 2-16-1 Sugao, Kawasaki, Kanagawa 2168511, Japan

Lonny Ashworth
Department of Respiratory Care, Boise State University, 1910 W University Drive, Boise, ID 83725, USA

Yasuhiro Norisue
Department of Pulmonary and Critical Care Medicine, Tokyo Bay Urayasu Ichikawa Medical Center, 3-4-32 Todaijima, Urayasu, Chiba 2790001, Japan

F. Sanfilippos
Department of Anesthesia and Intensive Care, IRCCS-ISMETT (Istituto Mediterraneo per i Trapianti e Terapie ad alta specializzazione), Palermo, Italy

S. Scolletta
Unit of Intensive Care Medicine, Department of Medical Biotechnologies, University of Siena, Siena, Italy

A. Morelli
Department of Anaesthesiology and Intensive Care, University of Rome, "La Sapienza", Rome, Italy

A. Vieillard-Baron
Hospital Ambroise Paré, Assistance Publique-Hôpitaux de Paris, Boulogne, France

Moon Seong Baek, Jin Won Huh, Chae-Man Lim, Younsuck Koh and Sang-Bum Hong
Department of Pulmonary and Critical Care Medicine, Asan Medical Centre, University of Ulsan College of Medicine, 88 Olympic-ro 43-gil, Songpa-gu, Seoul 05505, Republic of Korea

MyongJa Han
Medical Emergency Team, Asan Medical Centre, University of Ulsan College of Medicine, Seoul, Republic of Korea

S. Valade, L. Biard and V. Lemiale
AP-HP, Medical ICU, Hôpital Saint-Louis, 1 Avenue Claude Vellefaux, 75010 Paris, France
UFR de Médecine, University Paris-7 Paris-Diderot, Paris, France

L. Biard
AP-HP, DBIM, Hôpital Saint-Louis, Paris, France

L. Argaud
Hôpital Edouard Herriot, Service de Réanimation Médicale, Hospices Civils de Lyon, Lyon, France

F. Pène
AP-HP, Réanimation médicale, Hôpital Cochin, Paris, France

S. Rouleau
Service de Réanimation polyvalente, Angoulême, France

N. Bele
Intensive Care Unit, Draguignan Hospital, Draguignan, France

K. Razazi
AP-HP, Groupe Henri Mondor-Albert Chenevier, Service de Réanimation Médicale, Hôpital Henri Mondor, Créteil, France

O. Peyrony
AP-HP, Service des urgences, Hôpital Saint-Louis, Paris, France

P. Perez
Service de Réanimation médicale, Hôpital Brabois, Nancy, France

J. Mayaux
AP-HP, Pneumology and Critical Care Medicine Department, Universitary Hospital La Pitié Salpêtrière-Charles Foix, Paris, France

Marc Leone
Service d'Anesthésie et de Réanimation, Aix-Marseille Universite Hopital Nord, chemin des Bourrely, 13015 Marseille, France

Lila Bouadma
Service de Réanimation Médicale, Hopital Bichat - Claude-Bernard, AP-HP, Paris, France

Bélaïd Bouhemad
Service d'Anesthésie et Réanimation, Centre Hospitalier Universitaire de Dijon, Paris, France

Olivier Brissaud
Unité de Réanimation Pédiatrique, Hôpital Pellegrin, Centre Hospitalier Universitaire de Bordeaux, Bordeaux, France

Fabrice Michel
Service d'Anesthésie et Réanimation, Hopital La timone, Assistance Publique Hopitaux de Marseille, Marseille, France

Djamel Mokart
Service de Réanimation, Institut Paoli-Calmettes, Marseille, France

Philippe Montravers
Département d'Anesthésie Réanimation, CHU Bichat - Claude-Bernard, AP-HP, Paris, France

Jean-Ralph Zahar
Département de Microbiologie Clinique, Hopital Avicenne, APHP, Paris, France

Rémi Bruyère
Service de Réanimation, Centre Hospitalier de Bourg-en-Bresse, Bourg-en-Bresse, France

Gérald Chanques
Département d'Anesthésie Réanimation, Centre Hospitalier Regional Universitaire de Montpellier, Montpellier, France

Marije Wijnberge, Daniko P. Sindhunata, Else Ouweneel, Denise P. Veelo and Bart F. Geerts
Department of Anesthesiology, Academic Medical Center, Amsterdam, The Netherlands

Marije Wijnberge and Alexander P. Vlaar
Department of Intensive Care, Academic Medical Center, Amsterdam, The Netherlands
Laboratory of Experimental Intensive Care and Anesthesiology, Academic Medical Center, Amsterdam, The Netherlands

Michael R. Pinsky
Department of Critical Care Medicine, University of Pittsburgh Medical Center, 1215.4 Lillian S. Kaufmann Bldg, 3471 Fifth Avenue, Pittsburgh, PA 15213, USA

Jos R. Jansen
Department of Intensive Care Medicine, Leiden University Medical Center, Leiden, The Netherlands

Index